THE VALUE OF PSYCHOLOGICAL TREATMENT

The Collected Papers of
Nicholas A. Cummings
Volume I

THE VALUE OF PSYCHOLOGICAL TREATMENT

The Collected Papers of Nicholas A. Cummings
Volume I

Edited by
J. Lawrence Thomas, Ph.D.
and **Janet L. Cummings, Psy.D.**

Zeig, Tucker & Co., Inc.
Phoenix, Arizona

Published by

ZEIG, TUCKER & CO., INC.
3618 North 24th St.
Phoenix, Arizona 85016

Library of Congress Cataloging-in-Publication Data
Cummings, Nicholas A.
The value of psychological treatment : collected papers of
Nicholas A. Cummings / edited by J. Lawrence Thomas and Janet L.
Cummings.
p. cm.
Includes bibliographical references and index.
ISBN 1-891944-12-6
1. Mental health services—United States.   2. Managed mental
health care—United States.   3. Mental health services—Utilization—
United States.   I. Thomas, J. Lawrence.   II. Cummings, Janet L.
III.   Title.
RA790.6.C85 1999
362.2'0973—dc21 98-50582
CIP

Manufactured in the United States of America

10 9 8 7 6 5 4 3 2 1

C O N T E N T S

S O U R C E S

The following articles are being reprinted by permission of the original publisher and/or the author. The list is in chronological order.

Follette, W. T. & Cummings, N. A. (1967). Psychiatric services and medical utilization in a prepaid health plan setting. *Medical Care, 5*, 25-35.

Cummings, N. A. & Follette, W. T. (1968). Psychiatric services and medical utilization in a prepaid health plan setting: Part II. *Medical Care, 6*, 31-41.

Cummings, N. A. (1975). The health model as entrée to the human services model in psychotherapy. *Clinical Psychologist, 29*, 19-21.

Cummings, N. A. & Follette, W. T. (1976). Brief psychotherapy and medical utilization. In H. Dörken & Associates (Eds.), *The professional psychologist today: New developments in law, health insurance and health practice* (pp. 165-174). San Francisco: Jossey-Bass.

Cummings, N. A. (1977). Prolonged (ideal) versus short-term (realistic) psychotherapy. *Professional Psychology, 8*, 491-501.

Cummings, N. A. (1977). The anatomy of psychotherapy under National Health Insurance. *American Psychologist, 12*,(9), 711-718.

Cummings, N. A. (1979). Turning bread into stones. Our modern antimiracle. *American Psychologist, 34*(12), 1119-1129.

Cummings, N. A. & VandenBos, G. R. (1979). The general practice of psychology. *Professional Psychology, 1*, 430-440.

Cummings, N. A. & VandenBos, G. R. (1981). The twenty year Kaiser-Permanente experience with psychotherapy and medical utilization: Implications for national health policy and National Health Insurance. *Health Policy Quarterly, 1*(2), 159-175.

Cummings, N. A. (1984). The health maintenance organization. In S. Weis, J. Matarazzo, J. A. Herd, N. E. Miller, & S. M. Weiss (Eds.), *Behavioral health: A handbook of health enhancement and prevention* (pp. 1179-1186). New York: Wiley.

Cummings, N. A. (1986). The dismantling of our health system: Strategies for the survival of psychological practice. *American Psychologist, 41*, 426-431.

Cummings, N. A. & Dörken, H. (1986). Corporations, networks, and service plans: Economically sound models for practice. In H. Dörken & Associates (Eds.), *Professional psychology in transition* (pp. 283–312). San Francisco: Jossey-Bass.

Cummings, N. A. (1987). The future of psychotherapy: One psychologist's perspective. *American Journal of Psychotherapy, 61*, 349–360.

Cummings, N. A. & Bragman, J. I. (1988). Triaging the "somaticizer" out of the medical system into a psychological system. *Psychotherapy Patient, 4*(2), 109–112.

Pallak, M. S. & Cummings, N. A. (1989). Review of Kiesler, C. A. & Sibulkin, A. E., Mental hospitalization: Daniel enters the lion's den. *Contemporary Psychology, 34*(8), 736–738.

Cummings, N. A. (1991). Arguments for the financial efficacy of psychological services in health care settings. In J. J. Sweet, R. G. Rozensky, & S. M. Tovian (Eds.), *Handbook of clinical psychology in medical settings* (pp. 113–126). New York: Plenum.

Cummings, N. A. (1991). Inpatient versus outpatient treatment of substance abuse: Recent developments in the controversy. *Contemporary Family Therapy, 13*(5), 507–520.

Cummings, N. A. (1992). Future practice patterns: Independent practice and managed mental health care. Invited Distinguished Centennial Address to the Annual Meeting of the American Psychological Association, Washington, D.C., August 1992.

Cummings, N. A. (1992). The future of psychotherapy: Society's charge to professional psychology. *Independent Practitioner, 12*(3), 126–130.

Cummings, N. A. (1992). Psychologists: An essential component to cost-effective, innovative care. *Psychotherapy in Private Practice, 10*(1/2), 137–143.

Cummings, N. A. (1992). The somatizing patient. In C. S. Austad & W. H. Berman (Eds.), *Psychotherapy in managed care* (pp. 234–247). Washington, DC: American Psychological Association.

Pallak, M. S. & Cummings, N. A. (1992). Inpatient and outpatient psychiatric treatment: The effect of matching patients to appropriate level of treatment on psychiatric and medical-surgical hospital days. *Applied & Preventive Psychology: Current Scientific Perspectives, 1*, 83–87.

Cummings, N. A., Pallak, M. S., Dörken, H., & Henke, C. J. (1993). Medicaid, managed mental healthcare and medical cost offset. *Behavioral Healthcare Tomorrow, 2*(5), 15–20.

Cummings, N. A. (1994). The successful application of medical offset in program planning and in clinical delivery. *Managed Care Quarterly, 2*(2), 1-6.

Pallak, M. S. & Cummings, N. A. (1994). Outcomes research in managed behavioral health care: Issues, strategies, and trends. In W. G. Troy, S. Shueman, S. L. Mayhugh, & B. S. Gould (Eds.), *Managed behavioral health care: A search for precision.* (pp. 205-221). Springfield, IL: Charles C Thomas.

Cummings, N. A. (1995). Impact of managed care on employment and training: A primer for survival. *Professional Psychology: Research and Practice, 26*(1), 10-15.

Cummings, N. A. (1995). Behavioral health after managed care: The next golden opportunity for professional psychology. *Register Report, 20*(3), 1, 30-33.

Cummings, N. A. (1996). Practitioner-driven managed care: The quality solution. In C. E. Stout, G. A. Theis, & J. M. Oher (Eds.), *The complete guide to managed behavioral healthcare* (pp. II.F.2—II.F.11). New York: Wiley.

Cummings, N. A. & Cummings, J. L. (1997). The behavioral health practitioner of the future: The efficacy of psychoeducational programs in integrated primary care. In N. A. Cummings, J. L. Cummings, & J. N. Johnson (Eds.), *Behavioral health in primary care: A guide for clinical integration* (pp. 325-346). Madison, CT: Psychosocial Press.

As Nicholas Cummings and I were walking away from one of his conference presentations, I casually mentioned that someone should collect his papers into several volumes, so that all of his articles and chapters on a given subject could be in one place. Warning: Do not bring up the idea of a project to Nick Cummings unless you plan to stand behind it!

A year passed, and then he said that he wanted me to edit his collected papers. Why should Nick Cummings' papers be brought together into several volumes?

One of the most important phenomena that Dr. Cummings discovered early in his career (from about 1955 to 1979) is that if psychotherapy (or, more accurately, psychological treatment) were included and blended into a healthcare system, the cost of medical care could be reduced by as much as 60 percent. The label or term that has emerged from this work and its replications is "medical cost offset." But before all of you mental health professionals get too excited, this does not mean that doing just any kind of psychotherapy will produce this phenomenon. Of central importance is the fact that one can achieve this offset of costs only with brief and targeted psychotherapy.

In 1958 Cummings was hired by Dr. Sidney Garfield to be Chief Psychologist at Kaiser Permanente, one of the earliest health maintenance organizations (HMOs) in the country, and known as a very efficient system of providing healthcare. Since it is a prepaid healthcare system, all of the medical costs are included, or, in a sense, "free." It had become apparent to Garfield that more than 60 percent of the doctor visits were to people who had no discernible physical cause for their complaints. It seemed reasonable that if these patients could be treated effectively to solve their underlying psychological issues, then their medical problems could be helped a great deal, if not solved completely. Further, those patients who had a chronic disease, such as arthritis, diabetes, or chronic pain, could be taught to manage their condition largely by themselves, thus reducing their utilization of medical services. As a bonus, these people would feel more in control of their lives.

Dr. Garfield was clear that he wanted to hire a psychologist to develop programs and to do the careful research necessary to flesh out this curious phenomenon: He did not want there to be a tendency to slip into the medical model of treating the psychological issues. Much of the rest of this story is told in the collected articles in this book, since this has been a central focus of Dr. Cummings' career.

The implication of understanding and utilizing these ideas is nothing short of monumental. Can you imagine all health costs being cut in half? And people feeling more in control of their destinies to boot? Even if there were only a 10 percent reduction in costs, billions of dollars would be saved! Thus, the importance of these papers and chapters is self-evident.

Another reason for collecting these papers into one volume is that many are hard to find, even in the best of libraries. Some of these articles were published in journals that no longer exist; likewise, some of the chapters Cummings wrote are in books now out of print. In fact, even Cummings does not have copies of all of the articles he has written! To bring these pioneering articles together would be reason enough to justify the publication of this book.

But there is an added contribution I thought would make such volumes particularly important. Cummings has been uncannily accurate in his predictions about where healthcare is going—particularly mental healthcare. Although he has been warning psychologists about what the future trends would be, few have heeded his advice. Luckily, even as a septuagenarian, Cummings is still incredibly active in the profession. I thought it would be interesting to have him comment on these articles, to see if the ideas he generated over three decades ago are still valid. What is still relevant today, and what would need to be readjusted to fit the current and future climate of behavioral healthcare?

To say that currently the mental health professions are in turmoil is an understatement. Every mental health professional is aware of the problems involved in dealing with managed care, and the struggles we go through justifying our very existence. For the past few decades, psychotherapists had been getting reimbursed for their fees at a good rate, and no one seemed to be able to stop the upward spirals of mental health costs. More and more young people wanted to become therapists and open $100-per-hour private practices. The universities and professional schools obliged, and have been making their own profits producing psychotherapists. As a result, the field of psychotherapy is flooded with licensed professionals. Yet the trend is to reduce the number of sessions to a single digit! What a mess!

Interestingly, Nick Cummings predicted the current period of chaos over a decade ago (Cummings, 1985). In fact, many of his publications have predicted how and why the mental health terrain would change, but from an optimistic point of view—how psychologists could prepare for the coming changes and control. And that is the underlying theme of this book: the value of psychological treatment not only for mental healthcare, but for the entire arena of healthcare. If the psychological issues seen in healthcare are treated effectively and efficiently by those best trained for this work—mental health professionals, the overall cost of healthcare not only can be reduced by a tremendous amount, but patients will be more in control of their own destinies and human suffering will be lessened by an untold amount.

The next volume of Cummings' collected papers will include a detailed explanation in concrete terms of how this clinical work is done. What does the therapist do so that good results can be produced? And efficiently, no less! How exactly is psychotherapy conceptualized so that people who are *not* psychologically minded nonetheless can benefit from talking to and working with a mental health professional?

A third volume will offer a collection of papers and commentaries about the organizations and institutions that Cummings created in order to address certain critical issues at specific historic points in the profession of psychology. These include founding, or being instrumental in creating, the California Schools of Professional Psychology, the National Academies of Practice, American Biodyne, the American Psychological Association Task Force on Insurance, and CAPPS. Some of the stories are amusing, and have never been told before. There will also be a commentary by Cummings as to the lessons that can be gleaned from these developments.

As I learned what Nicholas Cummings has given to the profession of psychology, I realized that many of his contributions have been monumental. For example, when the profession of clinical psychology was dying in the mid-1960s, Cummings took it upon himself to create a professional psychology school in California, which, in turn, provided a model for other training programs in the field. In a sense, he has given us our profession. He was also on the first Congressional and American Psychological Association committees to advocate for psychologists to be reimbursed by insurance companies for their professional work. So he helped get us paid for our work. He created a brain trust of health professionals who could advise our Congressional leaders as to the proper direction to take healthcare issues, without bloody turf wars. So he has asked that we become honorable. And the list goes on. He gave us our profession, got us paid, and now wants us to be honorable as well as efficient. Not bad for a lifetime of work. And it has all been aimed at reducing human suffering and enhancing control over one's own destiny.

These are some of the values that Cummings has stood for, and the meaning behind the creation of these volumes of his collected papers. I am proud to be involved with this project and grateful for the faith that Nicholas Cummings has had in my small part in bringing them to the professional healthcare community. It is a fine legacy and one worthy of our best efforts to continue this work.

—J. Lawrence Thomas, Ph.D.

ABOUT
NICHOLAS
CUMMINGS

NICHOLAS CUMMINGS, THE 87th president of the American Psychological Association (APA) (1979–1980), is a professional psychologist who has always discerned what the profession needs in order to advance, and has developed effective and innovative ways to meet those challenges. As a result, he has had a number of careers, as he puts himself directly into the solutions he fosters. Throughout his 45 years in the profession, however, there was one activity that was consistent and the most enjoyable for him: he did 40 to 50 psychotherapy sessions per week, from 3:00 a.m. every Monday morning until 2:00 a.m., Wednesday morning. He was able to do this because he has always been able to survive with only three hours of sleep a night.

Beginning private practice as a master's-level psychologist in the late 1940s, and realizing how scary this was with no licensure for psychologists, he became instrumental, with a handful of others, in California's becoming one of the first states to provide statutory recognition. Grandfathered on an M.A. level, he saw the importance of the doctorate and he traveled to Adelphi University in New York to obtain his Ph.D. degree and analytic training.

In the 1950s, no insurance company reimbursed for psychotherapy, believing that it was not economically viable to do so. Dr. Cummings was able to persuade Kaiser Permanente, the first health maintenance organization (HMO) in northern California, to make psychotherapy a covered benefit. He and his colleagues conducted extensive research that determined that psychotherapeutic interventions, especially with the somatizers who were high utilizers, save medical and surgical dollars far beyond the money necessary to provide the psychological services. What has become known as the "medical cost offset phenomenon" is now in its third generation of research, and Dr. Cummings remains its seminal investigator.

Medical cost offset persuaded insurers to pay for psychotherapy, but only psychiatrists were eligible for reimbursement. As the first chair of the APA's Committee on Health Insurance (COHI), Dr. Cummings developed the freedom-of-choice legislation that amended the insurance codes of every state so that if an insurer reimbursed psychiatrists, it must also reimburse psychologists. It was with this legislation passed in all 50 states that the private practice of psychology began to flourish, a course later followed by social work and other professions.

Dr. Cummings spent years attempting to influence the APA's Education and Training Board to change its rules so that practitioners could serve on faculties with the same prestige as academicians. Failing to do so, he founded the four campuses of the California School of Professional Psychology, the nation's first such professional school, which resulted in the Vail Conference and the changes in graduate education whereby psychotherapy and other subjects are taught by practitioners.

In 1985 Dr. Cummings foresaw the impending industrialization of healthcare and warned the profession in his historic article in the *American Psychologist*, "The Dismantling of Our Health System." He published a blueprint on how psychologists could own what came to be known as managed care and keep business interests out. He formed American Biodyne, a practitioner-driven national company, as a model he intended to limit to 500,000 enrollees. When his colleagues ignored the plan as grandiose, he took his foot off the brake and American Biodyne grew to 14.5 million enrollees in 39 states. He then sold the company to MedCo/Merck in 1992 and once again set about flunking retirement.

This practitioner-driven national behavioral healthcare delivery system still stands as the model to be emulated. It earned Dr. Cummings the appellation of "Father of Behavioral Healthcare Delivery," conferred upon him at the opening session of the 1997 Behavioral Healthcare Tomorrow Conference in Washington, D.C.

In 1981 Dr. Cummings formed the Foundation for Behavioral Health, which conducted the seven-year longitudinal study on behavioral-care services known as the Hawaii Project. It remains *the* definitive research that the government uses to this date in planning.

Dr. Cummings then served as the executive director of the Mental Research Institute (MRI) in Palo Alto, where he continued his work in brief therapy with that group. Previously, while still at Kaiser Permanente, he had developed a type of focused psychotherapy known as Brief Intermittent Psychotherapy Throughout the Life Cycle.

In advancing psychology, Dr. Cummings has served on two Presidential Mental Health Commissions: those of Presidents Kennedy and Carter. He was advisor to the U.S. Senate Subcommittee on Health (Senator Edward Kennedy, chair) for three years, the U.S. Senate Finance Committee for four years, and the Health Economics Branch of what is now the Department of Health and Human Services for six years. He has testified before the U.S. Congress 18 times on behalf of psychology and mental health, and his research has been entered into the *Congressional Record* eight times. He has also found the time to publish 11 books and over 400 refereed journal articles and book chapters.

He found time as well to found the National Academies of Practice in Washington, D.C., the nation's interdisciplinary national health forum composed of 100 of the most prestigious practitioners in each of nine academies: dentistry, medicine, nursing, optometry, osteopathic medicine, podiatric medicine, psychology, social work, and veterinary medicine. He also founded the National Council of Schools of Professional Psychology, the American Managed Behavioral Healthcare Association, and several other national organizations. At the present time, he is the president of the Foundation for Behavioral Health and chair of the Nicholas and Dorothy Cummings Foundation.

Nicholas Cummings has received every honor and award the profession has to bestow, and is the recipient of three honorary doctorates for his work in education, practice, and the Greek classics. His greatest joy is that he has been married for over 50 years to Dorothy Mills, a psychiatric social worker. His favorite colleague is his psychologist daughter (more recently, his co-author), and he boasts that his son is one of the five honest lawyers in the nation. Practicing and ranching for 45 years in his birth state of California, he is now a resident of the nation's fastest growing state, Nevada, where he holds the position of Distinguished Professor at the University of Nevada, Reno.

—Janet L. Cummings, Psy.D.

THE VALUE OF PSYCHOLOGICAL TREATMENT

The Collected Papers of
Nicholas A. Cummings
Volume I

1955–1975
The Era of Discovery

A Commentary by Nick Cummings

T HE ARTICLES IN this section will be more meaningful if certain historical facts are recalled. First, when Kaiser Permanente, the prototype of the modern health maintenance organization (HMO), discovered that 60 percent of physician visits were by patients who had no demonstrable physical disease, the relationship of stress to physical symptoms was not understood as it is today. The physicians, when confronted with a patient for whom exhaustive tests and repeated visits had revealed no physical disease, would invoke the diagnosis of "hypochondriac," and such an entry would be made on the patient's medical chart. When I was asked to help implement a program to address the "hypochondriacs" who were inundating the medical system, the first thing I sought to do was to replace the term itself. It seemed pejorative, as if the physicians were holding these patients responsible for wasting valuable medical time and expertise. A series of alternative terms put forth over several months were resoundingly rejected until in a late-night brainstorming session on other issues, I suggested that these patients were "somaticizing," defined as translating emotional problems into physical symptoms, and could thus be referred to as "somatizers." Dr. Sidney Garfield, the founder of Kaiser Permanente, responded enthusiastically to my proposal, stating that it sounded acceptably medical. Thus, a new diagnosis was coined, and it has remained an important term in medical parlance.

Second, in the middle to late 1950s, no health plan, including that of Kaiser Permanente, listed psychotherapy as a covered benefit. The conventional wisdom was that psychotherapy was too vague and ethereal to be taken seriously by the insurance world. My suggestion that it should be an integral part of the health benefit was met with staunch resistance by my superiors. Yet somatizers were flooding the system, and the Kaiser Permanente physicians, who were on capitation, would not profit one iota from these patients as would a practitioner on fee-for-service reimbursement. All it meant for the former was a much longer working day, one that often continued into the night. Out of desperation, a noncovered "benefit" was approved: for a $5 co-payment, a patient could be seen in psychotherapy, but by physician referral only. When one considers the value of the dollar in the 1950s, and that a private practitioner would charge $15 to $20 per session for psychoanalysis, this co-payment was substantial. This was the population upon which the first pilot studies on psychotherapy were conducted, with the consequent reduction in medical utilization. It was these findings that persuaded Kaiser Permanente to make psychotherapy an integral part of its health system. Years later, after funding over two dozen replications of the Cummings and Follette findings, the National Institute of Mental Health (NIMH) referred to the phenomenon as "medical cost offset," thus coining the second enduring term in this area. Medical cost offset was the fact that persuaded Kaiser Permanente to implement the nation's first comprehensive psychotherapy benefit, and even today the continued research finding that behavioral interventions reduce medical costs remains the most important argument for the inclusion of mental health services as part of healthcare.

A third historical consideration is: Who were our patients when all psychotherapy was paid out of pocket? They were undoubtedly from the more affluent and better educated segments of our society. One might even say that we were specializing in the diseases of the rich. Once Kaiser Permanente opened the prepayment gates, who were the patients who made up the membership of the health plan? They were essentially blue-collar workers, tradespeople, and laborers, for it was the labor unions of the time that strongly supported the concept of healthcare implemented by Kaiser Permanente. These patients simply did not behave or respond as did those I saw in my psychoanalytic training in New York. A series of mishaps occurred, some comical and some tragic, which eventually forced us to question many of our preconceived notions, and even to abandon our psychoanalytic couches.

I recall one man who had been suffering low back pain for over a year. Finally, his exasperated orthopedic surgeon sent him to us. Once in my office, I motioned for him to lie on the couch, and he promptly complied, but face down. Indicating that he didn't understand, I asked him to turn over. Again he complied, but while doing so, he asked in bewilderment, "Sure, Doc, but how are you going to examine my back if I am lying on it?" I explained that I was not going to examine his back; rather, we were going to talk. "Oh," he exclaimed as he arose from the couch. He grabbed a chair, and placing it opposite me, he sat down and looked at me expectantly. For the very first time, it occurred to me that everyone in the world except psychoanalysts knew that the best way to converse is face-to-face. After a number of even more amusing mishaps, I complained to Dr. Garfield that this was not going to work because his patients were not "psychologically minded." He shot back that this was the only kind of patient Kaiser Permanente had, and asked what I was going to do about it. What we did was to get rid of our couches and to begin listening to our working-class patients. We quickly learned a great deal about the real world, and to this day, I marvel when I still hear a colleague refer to a patient as not being "psychologically minded," as if this were some kind of mandated responsibility for the distressed person seeking our help.

What was our therapy like? As we became more active, our patients became more able to solve their own problems. We experimented with various techniques that were once a part of our psychotherapeutic folklore: the paradoxes of Harry Stack Sullivan, the strategic interventions of Milton Erickson, the developmental models of Erik Erikson, longer or shorter sessions with alterations in spacing as necessitated by our patients and as modeled by our medical colleagues, house calls for those too distressed to leave the safety of the home, the mobilization of rage in the service of health exquisitely utilized by Frieda Fromm-Reichman, briefer approaches pioneered by Thomas and French. We also employed a host of other techniques, such as skills training, desensitization, and relaxation, that were being perfected by the behavioral psychologists. But in everything we did, we had the good sense to subject each intervention to empirical research using medical cost offset as the outcome measure. Then we discovered homework, along with highly therapeutic ways of enforcing it. From then on, things moved rapidly as we developed targeted, focused interventions. We abandoned the notion of keeping the patient in therapy until the ultimate "cure," or some elusive plane of "self-actualization," and began to practice brief, intermittent psychotherapy throughout the life cycle.

During this time, the importance of psychotherapy in the health system began to be accepted by employers and other purchasers of health insurance. In response to consumer demand, health plans began to include a psychotherapy benefit, but reimbursed the cost only when the patient was in treatment with a psychiatrist. Medical cost offset research had been persuasive, but psychologists were cut out of the process. At that point, I became very active in the American Psychological Association (APA), which was extremely reluctant to tangle with the American Psychiatric Association (ApA) in support of the increasing number of psychologists who had gone into independent practice and were struggling to make a living with only out-of-pocket patients. I became the first chair of a brand-new APA committee, the Committee on Health Insurance (COHI), and during my first year, devised the strategy of amending the state insurance codes so that if an insurer paid psychiatrists, it also had to reimburse psychologists. We were able to get the law enacted in six states before the APA adopted the strategy as policy. Named the "freedom-of-choice" legislation by my successor and the second chair of COHI, Jack Wiggins, it required only a few word changes in each state insurance code to accomplish that which the ApA steadfastly, and the APA initially, opposed: the independent practice of psychotherapy by psychologists.

By the end of this era (1955–1975), and thanks to the early discoveries and the subsequent work at Kaiser Permanente, society had accepted the value of psychotherapy sufficiently so that many states had freedom-of-choice legislation and insurers were persuaded to include psychologists in independent practice as reimbursable practitioners. This, as well as licensure in every state (the last state, Missouri, enacted licensure for psychology in 1977), launched the golden era of the private practice of psychology. Those were wonderful, exciting years for the psychologist in private practice. Indeed, they were so wonderful that our colleagues were reluctant to acknowledge the winds of impending change.

{ 1 }

PSYCHIATRIC SERVICES AND MEDICAL UTILIZATION IN A PREPAID HEALTH PLAN SETTING*

IN TWO PREVIOUS STUDIES (Cummings, Kahn, & Sparkman, 1964; Follette & Cummings, 1962), the psychiatric practitioner's contention that emotionally disturbed patients do not seek organic treatment for their complaints following the intervention of psychotherapy has been investigated. Although it has long been recognized that a large number of the physical complaints seen by the physician are emotionally, rather than organically, determined, the more precise relationship between problems in living and their possible expression through apparent physical symptomatology has been difficult to test experimentally. As noted in the previous study, the GHI Project demonstrated that users of psy-

* With William T. Follette, M.D.

Presented at one of the Contributed Papers Sessions sponsored by the Medical Care Section at the 94th Annual meeting of the American Public Health Association, San Francisco, Calif., October 31–November 4, 1966.

This study was primarily financed by Grant PH 108-64-100 (P), U.S. Public Health Service. The authors gratefully acknowledge the assistance and cooperation of Mr. Royal Crystal, Deputy Chief, Health Economics Branch. Secondary financial support for this study was through Grant No. 131-7241, Kaiser Foundation Research Institute.

This paper is a report of the first of two investigations seeking to develop and test methods of assessing the effect of psychiatric services on medical utilization in a comprehensive medical program.

chiatric services were also significantly frequent users of medical services, but the Project was not able to answer the question of whether there is a reduction in the use of medical services following psychotherapy.

Because the facilities and structure of the Kaiser Foundation Health Plan accord an experimental milieu not available to Avnet, the original pilot project in San Francisco was able to demonstrate a significant reduction in medical utilization between the year prior to psychotherapy, and the two years following its intervention. Certain methodologic problems inherent to the pilot study indicated caution and the need for refinement and replication to avoid arriving at premature conclusions. The lack of a control group of what might be termed psychologically disturbed high utilizers who did not receive psychotherapy was a serious omission in the first experiment.[†] Furthermore, an error in the tabulation of inpatient utilization was discovered after the experiment had been concluded.[††] In addition, the question was raised whether the patients studied might, subsequent to the two years following psychotherapy, revert to previous patterns of somatization or, as a new pattern, merely substitute protracted and costly psychotherapy for previous medical treatment.

THE PROBLEM

This study investigated the question of whether there is a change in patients' utilization of outpatient and inpatient medical facilities after psychotherapy, comparing the patients studied to a matched group who did not receive psychotherapy.

Psychotherapy was defined as any contact with the Department of Psychiatry, even if the patient was seen for an initial interview only. The year prior to the initial contact was compared with the five subsequent years in both groups.

The problem can be stated simply: Is the provision of psychiatric

[†]The authors acknowledge their debt to Dr. M. F. Collen for this and other suggestions, and to Arthur Weissman, Medical Economist, Kaiser Foundation Medical care entities, for his expert consultation.

[††]At that time days of hospitalization per patient and by year were tabulated from each patient's outpatient medical records. Subsequent investigation has revealed that only about a third of the outpatient charts reviewed contained summaries of hospital admissions, and that tabulation of inpatient utilization must be made directly through the separately kept inpatient records.

services associated with a reduction of medical services utilization (defined as visits to other medical clinics, outpatient laboratory and x-ray procedures, and days of hospitalization)?

METHODOLOGY

The setting: The Kaiser Foundation Health Plan in the Northern California Region is a group-practice prepayment plan offering comprehensive hospital and professional services on a direct service basis. Professional services are provided by the Permanente Medical Group—a partnership of physicians. The Medical Group has a contract to provide comprehensive medical care to the subscribers, of whom there were more than a half million at the time of this study. The composition of the Health Plan subscribers is diverse, encompassing most socioeconomic groups. The Permanente Medical Group comprises all major medical specialties; referral from one specialty clinic to another is facilitated by the organizational features of group practice, geographical proximity and use of common medical records. During the years of this study (1959–1964), psychiatry was essentially not covered by the Northern California Health Plan on a prepaid basis, but in some areas of the Northern California region psychiatric services were available to Health Plan Subscribers at reduced rates. During the six years of the study, the psychiatric clinic staff in San Francisco consisted of psychiatrists, clinical psychologists, psychiatric social workers, resident psychiatrists at the third- or fourth-year level, and psychology interns, all full-time. The clinic operates primarily as an outpatient service for adults (age eighteen or older), for the evaluation and treatment of emotional disorders, but it also provides consultation for non-psychiatric physicians and consultation in the general hospital and the emergency room. There is no formal "intake" procedure, the first visit with any staff member being considered potentially therapeutic as well as evaluative and dispositional. Regardless of professional discipline, the person who sees the patient initially becomes that patient's therapist unless there is a reason for transfer to some other staff member, and he continues to see the patient for the duration of the therapy. An attempt is made to schedule the first interview as soon as possible after the patient calls for an appointment. There is also a "drop-in" or non-appointment service for emergencies so that patients in urgent need of psychiatric help usually can be seen immediately or at least within an hour or two of arrival at the clinic.

One of the unique aspects of this kind of associated health plan and medical group is that it tends to put a premium on health rather than on illness, i.e., it makes preventive medicine economically rewarding, thereby stimulating a constant search for the most effective and specific methods of treatment. The question of how psychiatry fits into comprehensive prepaid medical care is largely unexplored; there are not many settings in which it can be answered. Another feature of group practice in this setting is that all medical records for each patient are retained within the organization.

Subjects: The experimental subjects for this investigation were selected systematically by including every fifth psychiatric patient whose initial interview took place between January 1 and December 31, 1960. Of the 152 patients thus selected, 80 were seen for one interview only, 41 were seen for two to eight interviews (mean of 6.2) and were defined as "brief therapy," and 31 were seen for nine or more interviews (mean of 33.9) and were defined as "long-term therapy."

To provide a control group, the medical records of high medical utilizers who had never presented themselves to the Department of Psychiatry were reviewed until a group was selected which matched the psychotherapy sample in age, sex, socioeconomic status, medical utilization in the year 1959, Health Plan membership including at least the years 1959 through 1962, and criteria of psychological distress. Thus, each experimental patient was matched with a control patient in the criteria above, but without reference to any other variable. Both samples ranged in age from 24 to 62, with a mean of 38.1. Of these, 52 percent were women and 63 percent were blue-collar workers or their dependents. The satisfaction of so many criteria in choosing a matched control group proved to be a tedious and time-consuming procedure.

Review of the medical records of the psychiatric sample disclosed consistent and conceptually useful notations in the year prior to the patients' coming to psychotherapy, which could be considered as *criteria of psychological distress*. These consisted of recordings, made by the physicians on the dates of the patients' visits, which were indicative of those patients' emotional distress, whether or not the physicians recognized this when they made the notations. These (38) criteria were assigned weights from one to three in accordance with the frequency of their appearance in medical records and in accordance with clinical experience about the significance of the criteria when encountered in psychotherapeutic practice. The criteria, with

Table 1. *Criteria of Psychological Distress with Assigned Weights*

One point	Two points	Three points
1. Tranquilizer or sedative requested.	23. Fear of cancer, brain tumor, venereal disease, heart disease, leukemia, diabetes, etc.	34. Unsubstantiated complaint there is something wrong with genitals.
2. Doctor's statement pt. is tense, chronically tired, was reassured, etc.	*24. Health Questionnaire: yes on 3 or more psych. questions.	35. Psychiatric referral made or requested.
3. Patient's statement as in no. 2.	25. Two or more accidents (bone fractures, etc.) within 1 yr. Pt. may be alcoholic.	36. Suicidal attempt, threat, or preoccupation.
4. Lump in throat.		37. Fear of homosexuals or of homosexuality.
*5. Health Questionnaire: yes on 1 or 2 psych. questions.	26. Alcoholism or its complications: delirium tremens, peripheral neuropathy, cirrhosis.	38. Non-organic delusions and/or hallucinations; paranoid ideation; psychotic thinking or psychotic behavior.
6. Alopecia areata.		
7. Vague, unsubstantiated pain.	27. Spouse is angry at doctor and demands different treatment for patient.	
8. Tranquilizer or sedative given.		
9. Vitamin B_{12} shots (except for pernicious anemia).	28. Seen by hypnotist or seeks referral to hypnotist.	
10. Negative EEG.	29. Requests surgery which is refused.	
11. Migraine or psychogenic headache.	30. Vasectomy: requested or performed.	
12. More than 4 upper respiratory infections per year.	31. Hyperventilation syndrome.	
13. Menstrual or premenstrual tension; menopausal sx.	32. Repetitive movements noted by doctor: tics, grimaces, mannerisms, torticollis, hysterical seizures.	
14. Consults doctor about difficulty in child rearing.		
15. Chronic allergic state.	33. Weight-lifting and/or health faddism.	
16. Compulsive eating (or overeating).		
17. Chronic gastrointestinal upset; aereophagia.		
18. Chronic skin disease.		
19. Anal pruritus.		
20. Excessive scratching.		
21. Use of emergency room: 2 or more per year.		
22. Brings written list of symptoms or complaints to doctor.		

* Refers to the last 4 questions (relating to emotional distress) on a Modified Cornell Medical Index—a general medical questionnaire given to patients undergoing the Multiphasic Health Check in the years concerned (1959–62).

weights assigned, are presented in Table 1. In comparing the charts of the psychiatric patients with those of Health Plan patients randomly drawn, it was determined that although some criteria were occasionally present in the medical records of the latter, a weighted score of three within one year clearly differentiated the psychiatric from the non-psychiatric groups. Accordingly, therefore, in matching the control (non-psychotherapy) group to the experimental (psychotherapy) group, the patients selected had records which indicated scores of three or more points for the year 1959. The mean weights of the three experimental groups and the control group in terms of the 38 criteria of psychological distress are presented in Table 2: note that there was no significant difference between this dimension of the two groups in 1959.

In order to facilitate comparison of the experimental (psychotherapy) and control (non-psychotherapy) groups, one last criterion for inclusion in the matched group was employed. Each subject in the control group had to be a Health Plan member for the first three consecutive years under investigation inasmuch as the experimental group, though demonstrating attrition in continued membership after that time, remained intact for those years.

Dependent variable: Each psychiatric patient's utilization of health facilities was investigated first for the full year preceding the day of his initial interview, then for each of the succeeding five years beginning with the day after his initial interview.

The corresponding years were investigated for the control group which, of course, was not seen in the Department of Psychiatry. This investigation consisted of a straightforward tabulation of each contact

Table 2. *Scores for Criteria of Psychological Distress, for the Experimental Groups and the Control Group During the Year Prior to Psychotherapy (1959)*

Group	Total Score	No. of Patients	Average Score
One session only	264	80	3.30
Brief therapy	134	41	3.27
Long-term therapy	246	31	7.94
All experimental (psychotherapy) groups	644	152	4.24
Control (nonpsychotherapy) group	629	152	4.13

*These procedures were counted as one even if there were more than one laboratory or x-ray procedure per report in the chart

with any outpatient facility, each laboratory report and x-ray report.* In addition a tabulation of number of days of hospitalization was made without regard to the type or quantity of service provided. Each patient's utilization scores consisted of the total number of separate outpatient and inpatient tabulations.

RESULTS

The results of this study are summarized in Table 3, which shows the differences by group in utilization of outpatient medical facilities in the year before and the five years after the initial interview for the psychiatric sample, and the utilization of outpatient medical services for the corresponding six years for the non-psychotherapy sample.

The data of Table 3 are summarized as percentages in Table 4, which indicates a decline in outpatient medical (not including psychiatric) utilization for all three psychotherapy groups for the years following the initial interview, while there is a tendency for the non-psychotherapy patients to increase medical utilization during the corresponding years. Applying t-tests of the significance of the stan-

Table 3. *Utilization of Outpatient Medical Services (Excluding Psychiatry) by Psychotherapy Groups for the Year Before (1-B) and the Five Years After (1-A, 2-A, 3-A, 4-A, 5-A) the Initial Interview, and the Corresponding Years for the Nonpsychiatric Group*

Group	1-B	1-A	2-A	3-A	4-A	5-A
One session only, unit score	911	815	612	372	321	217
No. of pts.	80	80	80	57	53	49
Average	11.4	10.2	7.7	6.5	6.1	4.4
Brief therapy, unit score	778	471	354	202	215	155
No. of pts.	41	41	41	32	30	27
Average	19.0	11.5	8.6	6.3	7.2	5.7
Long-term therapy, unit score	359	323	279	236	151	108
No. of pts.	31	31	31	27	24	19
Average	11.6	10.4	9.0	8.7	6.5	5.7
All experimental (psychotherapy) groups, unit score	2048	1609	1245	810	687	480
No. of pts.	152	152	152	116	107	95
Average	13.5	10.6	8.2	6.4	6.4	5.1
Control (nonpsychotherapy) group, unit score	1726	1743	1718	1577	1611	1264
No. of pts.	152	152	152	127	111	98
Average	11.4	11.5	11.3	12.4	14.5	12.9

dard error of the difference between the means of the "year before" and the means of each of the five "years after" (as compared with the year before), the following results obtain. The declines in outpatients (non-psychiatric) utilization for the "one session only" and the "long-term therapy" groups are not significant for the first year following the initial interview while the declines are significant at either the .05 or .01 level for the remaining four years. In the "brief therapy" group, there are statistically significant declines in all five of the years following the initial interview. As further indicated in Table 4, there is a tendency for the control group to *increase* its utilization of medical services, but this proved significant for the "fourth year after" only.

The question was raised as to whether the patients demonstrating declines in medical utilization have done so because they have merely substituted protracted psychotherapy visits for their previous medical visits.

Table 4. *Comparison of the Year Prior to the Initial Interview with each Succeeding Year, Indicating Per Cent Decline or Per Cent Increase (Latter Shown in Parentheses) in Outpatient Medical (Nonpsychiatric) Utilization by Psychotherapy Grouping, and Corresponding Comparisons for the Control Group, with Levels of Significance*

	1-A		2-A		3-A		4-A		5-A	
	%		%		%		%		%	
Group	Change	*Signif.*	Change	*Signif.*	Change	*Signif.*	Change	*Signif.*	Change	*Signif.*
One session only	10.5	NS	32.8	.05	44.75	.05	46.5	.05	61.4	.01
Brief therapy	39.5	.05	53.2	.05	66.8	.01	62.1	.01	70.0	.01
Long-term therapy	10.0	NS	22.3	.05	25.0	.05	43.0	.05	50.9	.05
All experimental (psychotherapy) groups	21.4	.05	39.2	.01	48.2	.01	52.3	.01	62.5	.01
Control (nonpsychotherapy) group	None	—	None	—	(8.8)	NS	(27.2)	.05	(13.2)	NS

Table 5. *Average Number of Psychotherapy Sessions per Year for Five Years by Experimental Group*

Group	1-A	2-A	3-A	4-A	5-A
One session only	1.00	0.00	0.00	0.02	0.06
Brief therapy	6.22	0.00	0.09	0.57	0.52
Long-term therapy	12.33	5.08	5.56	5.88	5.05

As shown in Table 5, the number of patients in the one-session-only group who return in the third to fifth years for additional visits is negligible. Comparable results are seen in the brief-therapy group. In contrast, the long-term-therapy group reduces its psychiatric utilization by more than half in the "second year after," but maintains this level in the succeeding three years. By adding the outpatient medical visits to the psychiatric visits, it becomes clear that whereas the first two psychotherapy groups have not substituted psychotherapy for medical visits, this does seem to be the case in the long-term psychotherapy group. These results are shown in Table 6, and indicate that the *combined* outpatient utilization remains about the same from the "year before" to the "fifth year after" for the third psychotherapy group, while declines are evident for the first two psychotherapy groups. As regards the combined (medical plus psychiatric) utilization, the long-term psychotherapy group is not appreciably different from the control (non-psychiatric) group.

Investigation of inpatient utilization reveals a steady decline in utilization in the three psychotherapy groups from the "year before" to the "second year after," with the three remaining "years after" maintaining the level of utilization attained in the "second year after." In contrast, the control sample demonstrated a constant level in number of hospital days throughout the six years studied. These results are shown in Table 7, which indicates that the approximately 60 percent decline in number of days of hospitalization between the "year before" and the "second year after" for the first two psychotherapy groups is maintained to the "fifth year after"; this decline is significant at the .01 level. The inpatient utilization for the "long-term therapy" group in the "year before" was over twice that of the non-psychiatric sample, and about three times that of the first two

Table 6. *Combined Averages (Outpatient Medical plus Psychotherapy Visits) of Utilization by Years Before and After Psychotherapy for the Experimental Groups, and Total Outpatient Utilization by Corresponding Years for the Control (Nonpsychiatric) Group*

Group	1-B	1-A	2-A	3-A	4-A	5-A
One session only	11.4	11.2	7.7	6.5	6.1	4.5
Brief therapy	19.0	17.7	8.6	6.4	7.7	6.2
Long-term therapy	11.6	22.7	14.1	14.3	12.4	10.8
All experimental (psychotherapy) groups	13.5	15.3	9.2	8.3	7.9	6.2
Control group	11.4	11.5	11.3	12.4	14.5	12.9

Table 7. *Number of Days of Hospitalization and Averages by Psychotherapy Group for the Year Before and the Five Years After Psychotherapy, and the Corresponding Period for the Nonpsychotherapy Group* (Note: Health Plan average is .8 per year for patients 20 years old or older.)

Group	1-B	1-A	2-A	3-A	4-A	5-A
One session only, days/year	117	78	52	32	33	31
No. of pts.	80	80	80	57	53	49
Average	1.46	0.98	0.65	0.56	0.62	0.63
Brief therapy, days/years	66	44	31	24	23	23
No. of pts.	41	41	41	32	30	27
Average	1.61	1.07	0.76	0.75	0.77	0.85
Long-term therapy, days/year	153	37	19	18	16	13
No. of pts.	31	31	31	27	24	19
Average	4.94	1.09	0.61	0.67	0.67	0.68
All experimental (psychotherapy) groups, days/year	336	159	102	74	72	67
No. of pts.	152	152	152	116	107	95
Average	2.21	1.05	0.68	0.64	0.67	0.71
Significance		*.05*	*.02*	*.05*	*.05*	*.05*
Control (nonpsychotherapy) group, days/year	324	307	477	255	208	197
No. of pts.	152	152	152	127	111	98
Average	2.13	2.02	3.07	2.02	1.87	2.01
Significance		*NS*	*.05*	*NS*	*NS*	*NS*

psychotherapy groups. The significant (.01 level) decline of 88 percent from the "year before" to the "second year after" is maintained through the "fifth year after," rendering the inpatient utilization of the third psychotherapy group comparable to that of the first two psychotherapy groups.

In terms of decline in use of inpatient services (days of hospitalization), however, the long-term psychotherapy group and the control group are different, in that the former patients significantly reduce their inpatient utilization from the "year before" to the "fifth year after." However, the small size of the samples limits the conclusions that can be drawn.

DISCUSSION

The original pilot study of which this project is an outgrowth was proposed by the senior author as an aid in planning for psychiatric care as part of comprehensive prepaid health-plan coverage. It had long been observed that some of this psychiatric clinic's patients, as well as many patients in the hospital for whom a psychiatric consultation was requested, had very thick medical charts. It was also repeatedly noted that when these patients were treated from a psychiatric point of reference, i.e., as a person who might have primarily emotional distress which was expressed in physical symptoms, they often abandoned their physical complaints. It seemed reasonable to expect that for many of these people, psychiatrically oriented help was a more specific and relevant kind of treatment than the usual medical treatments.

This would be especially true if the effects of psychiatric help were relatively long-lasting, or if a change in the patient affected others in his immediate environment. In the long run, the interruption of the transmission of sick ways of living to succeeding generations would be the most fundamental and efficient kind of preventive medicine. It therefore seemed imperative to test the intuitive impressions that this kind of patient could be treated more effectively by an unstructured psychiatric interview technique than by the more traditional medical routine with its directed history.

The Balints (1957, 1961) have published many valuable case reports which describe the change in quantity and quality in patients' appeals to the general practitioner after the latter learns to listen and understand his patients as people in distress because of current and past life experiences. It would be difficult, however, to design a statistical study of those patients and of a matched control group treated for similar complaints in a more conventional manner.

Psychiatry has been in an ambivalent position in relation to the rest of medicine: welcomed by some, resented by others, often, however, with considerable politeness which serves to cover up deep-seated fears of and prejudices against "something different." In a medical group associated with a prepaid health plan, conditions are favorable for integrating psychiatry into the medical fraternity as a welcomed and familiar (therefore nonthreatening) member specialty. The inherent ease of referral and communication within such a setting would be much further enhanced by the factor of prepayment, which eliminates the financial barrier for all those who can afford health insurance. For many reasons, then, this setting provides both the impetus and the opportunity to attempt an integration of psychiatry into general medical practice and to observe the outcome. In the past two decades, medicine has been changing in many significant ways, among which are prepaid health insurance, group practice, increasing specialization, automation, and a focus on the "whole person" rather than on the "pathology."

Forsham (1959) and others have suggested that at some not-too-distant date the patient will go through a highly automated process of history, laboratory procedures and physical tests, with the doctor at the end of the line doing a physical examination but occupying mainly the position of a medical psychologist. He will have all the results of the previously completed examinations which he will interpret for the patient, and he will have time for listening to the patient, if he wishes to do so. The "Multiphasic Health Check," which has been used for many years in the Northern California Region in the Kaiser Foundation Medical Clinics and which is constantly being expanded, is just such an automated health survey, and Medical Group doctors are in the process of becoming continually better psychologists. Eventually many more of the patients who are now seen in the psychiatric clinic will be expertly treated in the general medical clinics by more "compleat physicians."

A study such as this raises more questions than it provides answers. One question alluded to above is whether, with an ongoing training program such as Balint has conducted for general practitioners at Tavistock Clinic, internists might not be just as effective as psychiatric personnel in helping a greater percentage of their patients. A training seminar such as this has been conducted by Dr. Edna Fitch in the Department of Pediatrics of Permanente Medical Group in San Francisco for many years and has been effective in helping pediatricians to treat, with more insight and comfort, emotional problems of children and their families and physical disorders which are an expression of emotional distress.

Using a broader perspective than the focus on the clinical pathology, one can wonder what social, economic or cultural factors are related to choice of symptoms, attitudes toward being "sick" (mentally or physically), attitudes toward and expectations of the doctor, traditions of family illness, superstitions relating to bodily damage, child raising practices, etc. How often is the understanding of such factors of crucial importance for effective and efficient treatment for the patient? Of special interest in general medical practice and overlooked almost routinely by physicians (and by many in the psychological field) are the "anniversary reactions" in which symptoms appear at an age at which a relative had similar symptoms and/or died.

Health Plan statistics indicate an increase in medical utilization with increasing age in adults. This is consistent with the relatively flat curve seen in the "medical utilization" of the control sample over the six year period and is in marked contrast to that of the experimental sample.

There is the implication in this that some of the increasing symptoms and disability of advancing years are psychogenic and that psychotherapeutic intervention may in some cases function as preventive medical care for the problems associated with aging as well as preventive medicine in children.

A certain percentage of the long-term psychotherapy group seems to continue without diminution of number of visits to the psychiatric clinic; these patients appear from the data to be interminable or lifelong psychiatric utilizers just as they had been consistently high utilizers of non-psychiatric medical care before. They seem merely to substitute psychiatric visits for some of their medical clinic visits. A further breakdown of the long-term group into three parts, e.g., less than 50, 50 to 150, and more than 150 visits, would probably help to sort this population's utilization into several patterns. More precise data on these groups would suggest modifications in classifications and methods of therapy or might suggest alternatives to either traditional medical or traditional psychiatric treatment in favor of some attempt to promote beneficial social changes in the environments of these chronically disturbed people.

Sources of Criticism

1. One problem in providing a control group comparable to an experimental group in this kind of study is that, although undoubtedly having emotional distress, and in a similar "quantity" according to our yardstick, the control group did *not* get to the psychiatric clinic by either self- or physician referral. The fact that the control patients had not sought psychiatric help may reflect a more profound difference between this group and the experimental group than is superficially apparent. One cannot assume that the medical utilization of this control group would change if they were seen in the Psychiatry Clinic. Although the average inpatient utilization for the three combined psychotherapy groups is the same as that of the control group in the year before (1959), the inpatient utilization of the long-term psychotherapy group is two and a half times that of the control group. If the study were extended to several years before, rather than just one year, it would become evident whether this was just a year of crisis for the long-term group or whether this had been a longer pattern of high inpatient utilization.

2. Patients who visit the psychiatric clinic may, for one reason or

another, seek medical help from a physician not associated with the Medical Group so that his medical utilization is not recorded in the clinic record, the source of information about utilization. In the long-term-therapy group the therapist is usually aware if his patient is visiting an outside physician, and although it is an almost negligible factor in that group, there can be no information in this regard for the one-session-only and brief-therapy groups without follow-up investigation.

3. There is no justification in assuming that decreased utilization means better medical care, necessarily. Criteria of improvement would have to be developed and applied to a significantly large sample to try to answer this important question.

4. Patients may substitute for physical or emotional symptoms behavioral disturbances which do not bring them to a doctor but may be just as distressing to them or to other people.

5. The "unit" of utilization cannot be used as a guide in estimating costs, standing as it does for such diverse items. In itself the units are not an exact indicator of severity of illness nor of costs. A person with a minor problem may visit the clinic many times, while a much more severely ill person may visit the clinic infrequently. Even more striking is the variation in the cost of a unit, varying from about a dollar for certain laboratory procedures to well over a hundred dollars for certain hospital days (with admissions procedures, laboratory tests, x-rays, consultations, etc.) each worth one "unit." To arrive at an approximation of costs, the units have to be retabulated in cost-weighted form.

Suggested Further Studies

1. The question of treatment of patients by nonmedical professional clinicians has been argued for more than a half century. It is generally recognized that there are not enough psychiatrists now and that there will not be enough in the foreseeable future to treat all those persons who have disabling emotional disorders. In the late President Kennedy's program for Mental Health this lack was recognized; the recommendation for professional staff for community Mental Health Centers included clinical psychologists, psychiatric social workers and other trained personnel. Having little distinction in our psychiatric clinic between the various disciplines as far as their functions are concerned, it would be feasible and interesting to compare therapeutic results of the disciplines as well as individuals with various

types of patients and various types of psychotherapy.

2. Is length of treatment correlated with diagnostic category, original prognosis by therapist, socioeconomic level of patient, discipline and orientation of therapist, or "severity of pathology"?

3. What happens to the spouse, parents, and children of the patients who are seen in psychiatry?

4. Are there distinguishing patterns of complaints in the three psychotherapy groups?

5. How do blue-collar patients differ from white-collar or professional patients in number of interviews, diagnostic label, use of medication, recommendation of hospitalization, and type of complaints?

6. What is the nature of the illness that resulted in hospitalization before the patient came to psychiatry—and after? How often was this a diagnostic work-up because the internist could not find "anything wrong" in the clinic?

SUMMARY

The outpatient and inpatient medical utilization for the year prior to the initial interview in the Department of Psychiatry as well as for the five years following were studied for three groups of psychotherapy patients (one interview only, brief therapy with a mean of 6.2 interviews, and long-term therapy with a mean of 33.9 interviews) and a control group of matched patients demonstrating similar criteria of distress but not, in the six years under study, seen in psychotherapy. The three psychotherapy groups as well as the control (non-psychotherapy) group were high utilizers of medical facilities, with an average utilization significantly higher than that of the Health Plan average. Results of the study indicated significant declines in medical utilization in the psychotherapy groups when compared with the control group, whose inpatient and outpatient utilization remained relatively constant throughout the six years. The most significant declines occurred in the second year after the initial interview, and the one-interview-only and brief-therapy groups did not require additional psychotherapy to maintain the lower utilization level for five years. On the other hand, after two years the long-term-psychotherapy group attained a level of psychiatric utilization which remained constant through the remaining three years of study.

The combined psychiatric and medical utilization of the long-term-therapy group indicated that for this small group there was no overall decline in outpatient utilization inasmuch as psychotherapy visits seemed to supplant medical visits. On the other hand, there was a significant decline in inpatient utilization, especially in the long-term-therapy group from an initial utilization of several times that of the Health Plan average, to a level comparable to that of the general adult Health Plan population. This decline in hospitalization rate tended to occur within the first year after the initial interview and remained generally comparable to the Health Plan average for the five years.

Weighing the Charts as an Index of
Psychological Distress

After working at Kaiser for a few years in the late 1950s, we saw that psychotherapy could reduce medical costs, and we kicked around all sorts of ways to measure this phenomenon. Today, of course, there are a number of scales and various measures for assessing outcome, but these weren't around in the late 1950s and early 1960s. As can be seen in our 1967 and 1968 articles, we developed the method of weighting the signs of emotional distress. This involved using the notes the doctors made on their charts. We also found that weighing the charts was a good way to find out who the somatizers were. It wasn't the intensity of services (i.e., surgery versus an ordinary office visit) but the frequency of the visits that mattered. When the frequent users of medical services came in, a new sheet was found, and the new note was entered. Somatizers came in so often that the charts had not made it back to the medical records storage, so extra sheets were added to the record, and the charts became very thick. With other patients, there were several notations on one page, and the charts were thinner. Weighing the charts became an excellent way to tell if the patient was a somatizer.

There is another aspect to this idea of "what one should measure" when trying to judge the effectiveness of psychological work with medical patients. We did not want to ask the doctors to fill out special forms, or have them rate their patients in special ways. We used what was already there—their own notations. Although this method of doing things was almost forced on us, I can look back now and say that it was fortuitous. The research was integral to the system, and I think we were lucky to have developed this way of studying these issues.

{ 2 }

PSYCHIATRIC SERVICES AND MEDICAL UTILIZATION IN A PREPAID HEALTH PLAN SETTING: PART II*

DOES PSYCHOTHERAPY ALTER the pattern of medical care? Can emotionally distressed patients who might benefit from psychotherapy be identified by screening a group of patients taking a health checkup? Will an automated psychological test be useful in such a screening process? These are the questions we set out to answer in this study.

The first question has been studied and the results reported by the authors (Follette & Cummings, 1967) It was found that psychotherapy patients initially were high "utilizers," but that after psychotherapy their utilization declined significantly. On the other hand, the utilization of the matched "control" group (not receiving psychotherapy) did not decline. The brief therapy and one-session-only psychotherapy groups had the largest decline in outpatient utilization, which theoretically helped to offset the cost of providing the psychotherapy. The decline in outpatient utilization of the long-term psychotherapy group was not enough to offset the cost of psychiatric and non-psychiatric treatment, being greater than the cost of prior medical utilization alone. However, this group showed considerable decline in days of

* With William T. Follette, M.D.

hospitalization, which helped to make their psychiatric care financially less costly in this setting.

A major criticism of Part I (Follette & Cummings, 1967) was that, although the psychotherapy and "control" groups were matched socioeconomically and demographically, in medical utilization and in degree of emotional distress, the groups remained different in one crucial respect: the psychotherapy sample, whether self- or physician-referred, voluntarily presented themselves to the psychiatric clinic. In contrast, the matched group did not come to the psychiatric clinic even if referred by their physicians. The nature of the difference between the two groups made conclusions tentative. The question is crucial, because it may be that the group which did not come to the psychiatric clinic is *unable* to make use of psychiatric services in a meaningful manner, and that psychotherapy would not decrease the medical utilization of this group. The most obvious way to provide a valid control group would be to choose a large sample by uniform criteria and randomly divide it into two parts, then treat the two parts differently and observe the results. The present paper is a report on such a prospective study.

METHOD

The setting: The Kaiser Foundation Health Plan of Northern California is a group-practice prepayment plan offering comprehensive hospital and professional services on a direct-service basis. Professional services are provided by the Permanente Medical Group—a partnership of physicians. The Medical Group has a contract to provide comprehensive medical care to the members of the Plan, of whom there were three-quarters of a million at the time of this study. The composition of the Health Plan membership is diverse, encompassing most socioeconomic groups. The Permanente Medical Group comprises all major medical specialties; referral from one specialty clinic to another is facilitated by the organizational features of group practice, geographical proximity and the use of common medical records. During the years of this study (1965–1966), only 17 percent of Health Plan members were eligible for psychiatric benefits on a prepaid basis, but in most areas of the Northern California region psychiatric services were available to Health Plan subscribers at reduced rates. The psychiatric staff in the San Francisco Clinic, where the present study took place, consists of psychiatrists, clinical psychologists, psychiatric social workers, and psychology and social work interns. The clinic operates primarily as an outpatient service for adults and children for the evaluation and treatment of emotional disorders, but it also provides consultation for non-psychiatric physicians and consultation in the general hospital and the emergency room. There is no formal "intake" procedure, the first visit with any staff member being considered potentially therapeutic as well as evaluative and dispositional. Regardless of professional discipline, the person who see the patients initially becomes the patient's therapist unless there is reason for transfer to some other staff member, and he continues to see the patient's therapist unless there is reason for transfer to some other staff member, and he continues to see the patient for the duration of the therapy. An attempt is made to schedule the first interview as soon as possible after the patient calls for an appointment. There is also a "drop-in" or non-appointment service for emergencies so that patients in urgent need of psychiatric help usually can be seen immediately or at least within an hour or two after arrival at the clinic.

One of the unique aspects of this kind of associated health plan and medical group is that it tends to put a premium on health rather than on illness, i.e., it makes preventive medicine economically rewarding, thereby stimulating a constant search for the most effective and specific methods of treatment. Another feature of group practice in this setting is that all medical records for each patient are maintained within the organization.

The subjects: The source of the population for this study was 10,667 patients who voluntarily presented themselves in a six-month period to the San Francisco Kaiser Permanente Automated Multiphasic Clinic for a health check, part of which includes 19 computerized procedures, ranging from simple body measurements to complex laboratory tests (Collen, 1966). A routine part of the three-hour series of examinations is the administration of a psychological test known as the Neuro-Mental Questionnaire, or NMQ (Cummings, Siegelaub, Follette, & Collen, 1968). This consists of 155 dichotomous questions which (eventually, when the test is fully developed) will identify approximately 60 psychological categories. Each question is printed on a separate prepunched card, which the patient must deposit in either the "true" or the "false" section of a divided box. For this study only the six major psychological categories were used: depression, hysteria, obsessional, panic and anxiety attacks, passive-aggressive, and schizophrenia. (This probably would identify most of the patients who could be identified by the full test, because 87 percent of the patients seen in the Department of Psychiatry fall into one or more of these six categories.)

The NMQ was computer-scored, and results were sent to the investigators within 24 hours of the time the patient had the questionnaire. The medical charts of the patients identified by the test were reviewed for evidences of psychological distress in the 12-month period prior to the Multiphasic examination.

"*Criteria of psychological distress*" (developed in Part I [see previous article] and presented in Table 1) refer to physicians' notes in the patients' medical charts which indicated emotional distress, whether or not the physicians recognized them as such. These 38 criteria have assigned weights from one to three, a weighted score of three within one year being accepted as an indication that a patient is in psychological distress. Accordingly, patients for the present study had 1) a "positive NMQ," and 2) a score of three or more points in "Criteria of Psychological Distress," for the 12 months prior to taking the Multiphasic examination.

Of the 10,667 patients who took the NMQ, 3,682, or 36.4 percent, yielded a positive score in one or more of the six NMQ categories (depression, hysteria, obsessional, panic-anxiety, passive-aggressive, schizophrenic). Of this group, 822 (7.7 percent) also scored three points or more on "Criteria of Distress." Of the 6,985 patients who did not score positively on the NMQ, only 56 (0.8 percent) scored three or more points on the "Criteria of Distress." Thus the use of scales in only six categories of the NMQ proved to be a useful method of eliminating two-thirds of the Multiphasic population in our search for a group of experimental subjects.

The psychological, socioeconomic and demographic characteristics of the 822-patient sample are given in Table 2. It will be noted that the mean age of 45.1 years is higher than the mean age of 38.1 years for patients generally seen in the Department of Psychiatry. Because the NMQ was administered to only the first 100 patients taking the Multiphasic examination each day, rather than the full 130, appreciably more women were tested than men, because the men tend to make evening appointments. Consequently, 71.0 percent of the sample is composed of women. It will be noted further that in the 822-patient sample 43 percent were categorized as neurotic, 32 percent as having

Table 1. *Criteria of Psychological Distress with Assigned Weights*

One point	Two points	Three points
1. Tranquilizer or sedative requested.	23. Fear of cancer, brain tumor, venereal disease, heart disease, leukemia, diabetes, etc.	34. Unsubstantiated complaint there is something wrong with genitals.
2. Doctor's statement pt. is tense, chronically tired, was reassured, etc.	*24. Health Questionnaire: yes on 3 or more psych. questions.	35. Psychiatric referral made or requested.
3. Patient's statement as in no. 2.	25. Two or more accidents (bone fractures, etc.) within 1 yr. Pt. may be alcoholic.	36. Suicidal attempt, threat, or preoccupation.
4. Lump in throat.		37. Fear of homosexuals or of homosexuality.
*5. Health Questionnaire: yes on 1 or 2 psych. questions.	26. Alcoholism or its complications: delirium tremens, peripheral neuropathy, cirrhosis.	38. Non-organic delusions and/or hallucinations; paranoid ideation; psychotic thinking or psychotic behavior.
6. Alopecia areata.		
7. Vague, unsubstantiated pain.	27. Spouse is angry at doctor and demands different treatment for patient.	
8. Tranquilizer or sedative given.		
9. Vitamin B$_{12}$ shots (except for pernicious anemia).	28. Seen by hypnotist or seeks referral to hypnotist.	
10. Negative EEG.		
11. Migraine or psychogenic headache.	29. Requests surgery which is refused.	
12. More than 4 upper respiratory infections per year.	30. Vasectomy: requested or performed.	
13. Menstrual or premenstrual tension; menopausal sx.	31. Hyperventilation syndrome.	
14. Consults doctor about difficulty in child rearing.	32. Repetitive movements noted by doctor: tics, grimaces, mannerisms, torticollis, hysterical seizures.	
15. Chronic allergic state.		
16. Compulsive eating (or overeating).		
17. Chronic gastrointestinal upset; aereophagia.	33. Weight-lifting and/or health faddism.	
18. Chronic skin disease.		
19. Anal pruritus.		
20. Excessive scratching.		
21. Use of emergency room: 2 or more per year.		
22. Brings written list of symptoms or complaints to doctor.		

* Refers to the last 4 questions (relating to emotional distress) on a Modified Cornell Medical Index—a general medical questionnaire given to patients undergoing the Multiphasic Health Check in the years concerned (1959–62).

Table 2. Psychological, Socioeconomic, and Demographic Characteristics of 822-Patient Sample with Positive NMQ and Plus-3 or More on Criteria of Distress

NMQ categories (with category number)		Blue collar			White collar			Totals
		Urban	Suburban	Rural	Urban	Suburban	Rural	
Neurotic								352 (42.8 per cent)
Depressive	30	37	11	2	43	2	1	96
Hysteric	16	12	5	1	2	4	2	26
Obsessional	25	23	6		35	6		70
Obs. hysteric	16, 25	10	3	2	12	3		30
Panic/anxiety	22	25	11		13	7	1	57
Phobic	24	28	9	2	19	15		73
Character disorders								261 (31.8 per cent)
Anal char.	13, 25	4	2		3	2		11
Depressive	25, 30 (13)	26	7	2	18	3		56
Hysterical	13, 16	15	8	1	14	2	1	41
Phobic	16, 24	21	12	1	20	7	1	62
Passive/aggr.	13	27	5	1	25	13		71
Sado-masoch.	13, 16, 30	6	3	1	8	2		20
Psychotic								209 (25.4 per cent)
Schizophrenic	37	55	19	3	44	20	1	142
Pseudo-neur.	37, 25, 30	21	8	2	24	11	1	67
Schiz..	(plus 1 more)							
TOTALS		310	109	18	280	97	8	

Totals:

Mean age:	45.1 yrs.
No. women:	70.1 %
Blue collar:	53.2 %
Urban:	71.8 %
Suburban:	25.0 %
Rural:	3.2 %
Neurotic:	42.8 %
Char. dis.:	31.8 %
Psychotic:	25.4 %

character disorders and 25 percent as psychotic. There was no difference between the percentages of blue-collar patients and white-collar patients diagnosed "psychotic."

Experimental condition: All patients with both positive NMQ's and three or more "distress" points were alternately assigned to either the referred or non-referred ("control") groups. For the referred patients the computer printed out the following "consider-rule": *Consider referral to psychiatry for emotional problems*. The 411 patients assigned to the control group did not, of course, have such a consider-rule on their print-outs.

The physician participants: A few weeks after the Multiphasic screening, every patient has a routine follow-up office visit with one of 32 internists. At this time the physician interviews the patient, completes the physical examination, reviews the clinical information from all sources, and provides appropriate treatment or referral. Prior to conducting the present experiment, the physician co-author of this paper met with the internists, explained the nature of the study and solicited their individual cooperation. They were informed that they would be seeing patients whose Multiphasic print-outs would contain the consider-rule suggesting referral to psychiatry. This was to be regarded as one more item of information to the physician, who would weigh it along with his total knowledge of the patient and make the ultimate decision whether to make such a referral. The internists also were advised that other patients would comprise the control group of the study, would not have the consider-rule in their print-outs, and would be undistinguishable from the other Multiphasic patients they would see routinely on follow-up visits.

Thus, "referred" patients (consider-rule) might or might not be referred to psychiatry, and, if referred, might or might not choose to come; or, if not referred by the internist, they might come to the psychiatric clinic through other channels. On the other hand, control patients (no consider-rule) might be referred to psychiatry as the result of the routine practice of medicine in this setting and without regard to the experiment, and, again, might choose to come or not to come to the psychiatric clinic. The various possibilities are shown in Figure 1.

RESULTS

No Experimental Generation of a Psychiatric Population

Six months after the last experimental subject consulted with his internist on his Multiphasic follow-up visit, only five of the 411 patients given the consider-rule had made and kept appointments in the psychiatric clinic! This figure is exactly the same as the number of patients from the control group who made and kept appointments in the psychiatric clinic. Thus, the experimental conditions failed to generate a psychiatric population, and were in no way superior in obtaining early referral to psychiatry than the usual, routine medical practice in this setting. (See Fig. 1.)

Figure 1

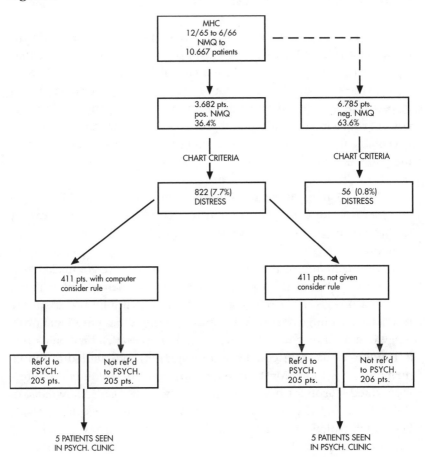

Within the referred group there were found to be 40 patients who had previously been seen in the psychiatric clinic, and in the control group there were 42. None of the 82 patients previously seen in psychotherapy returned during the course of the experiment.

Usefulness of Automated Screening

The NMQ, as part of an automated Multiphasic screening, proved to be a useful instrument in identifying a population within which the patients in emotional distress would be found. As seen in Figure 1, 36.4 percent of the patients with positive NMQ's also were in emotional distress, while less than 1 percent of the patients who did not have positive NMQ's were found to be in emotional distress.

Degree of Internists' Participation

At the conclusion of the primary phase of this study, and after the last patient had undergone his follow-up visit, 30 of the 32 participating internists were interviewed individually to determine their reactions to the computerized procedure and why they did or did not refer to psychiatry. As noted in Figure 1, about half the patients given the consider-rule in their computer print-outs actually were referred to psychiatry by their internists according to notations to that effect in the patients' charts.

a. Ten (33 percent) of the internists did not even recall seeing a consider-rule for referral to psychiatry; 20 (67 percent) stated they saw instances of such a consider-rule, but the number seen varied from one to 15.

b. Of the 20 internists who saw the consider-rule, eight made no referrals, four referred all such patients, and eight referred half or more.

c. Reasons given for reluctance to refer centered mostly about the physician's feelings regarding having to deal with an emotional problem when his time with the patient was limited. He felt he would open a "Pandora's box" that could not appropriately be handled in the fifteen minutes allotted for the initial return visit. The second most often-mentioned reason for not referring was the physician's knowledge of the patient and his circumstances. Typical of this was the reply: "I know this patient well. I referred him before and he wouldn't go. I had no reason to believe he would go this time." Or, "I know this patient has emotional problems, but we have been handling them here because she is reluctant to see a psychiatrist." A third type of response by the physician was one of antagonism to the procedure. A few internists complained that it was "cold" or "impersonal."

d. Internists who made referrals remarked that it made their job somewhat easier. They were startled by the accuracy of the consider-rule, for after opening up the issue of emotional problems, they found their patients eager to discuss them. One physician stated he felt more comfortable referring a patient to psychiatry when the patient could blame the computer and not the doctor.

e. Ultimately, the internist's individual procedure regarding referral to psychiatry seemed little affected by the consider-rule. Physicians who routinely and easily refer to psychiatry continued to do so in the experiment, while physicians who usually do not refer to psychiatry essentially ignored the consider-rule. For the most part, it was the individual physician's mode of practice that mattered.

Degree of Outpatient and Inpatient Medical Utilization

Each referred and control patient's utilization of health facilities was investigated for the full year prior to the patient's having taken the Multiphasic screening. This investigation consisted of a straightforward tabulation of each contact with any outpatient facility, each laboratory report and x-ray report. In addition, a tabulation of number of days of hospitalization was made without regard to the type or quantity of service provided. Each patient's utilization scores consisted of the total number of separate outpatient tabulations. These results are summarized in Table 3 (outpatient) and Table 4 (inpatient). The rural patients were excluded, inasmuch as their number was too small to contribute significantly to the results. As expected, no significant differences were found between the experimental and control groups, and both groups are combined (with rural patients excluded) in Tables 3 and 4.

All 796 patients (26 rural patients excluded) were significantly high utilizers of both outpatient and inpatient medical services.

A $2 \times 3 \times 4$ analysis of variance of the 796 patients indicated no significant difference in terms of blue versus white collar, or urban versus suburban conditions, as regards the utilization of both outpatient and inpatient medical services.

There was a significant difference in the degree of utilization of both

Table 3. *Average Utilization of Outpatient Medical Services for the Year Prior to the Multiphasic Screening for Both Referred and Control Groups by Diagnosis, Socioeconomic Status, and Residence (Excluding Rural)*

	Blue collar		White collar		
	Urban	Suburban	Urban	Suburban	Totals
Neurotic					
No. patients	135	45	124	37	341
Score	2538	886	2505	673	6602
Mean	18.8	19.6	20.2	18.4	19.4
Character disorder					
No. patients	99	37	88	29	253
Score	1168	396	994	336	2894
Mean	11.8	10.7	11.3	11.6	11.4
Psychotic					
No. patients	55	19	44	20	138
Score	677	217	480	234	1608
Mean	12.3	11.4	10.9	11.7	11.6
Pseudo-neurotic					
No. patients	21	8	24	11	64
Score	452	158	571	289	1470
Mean	21.5	19.7	23.8	26.3	22.9

Table 4. *Average Utilization of Inpatient Medical Services (Days of Hospitalization) for the Year Prior to the Multiphasic Screening for Both Referred and Control Groups by Diagnosis, Socioeconomic Status, and Residence, Excluding Rural**

	Blue collar		White collar		
	Urban	suburban	Urban	Suburban	Totals
Neurotic					
No. patients	135	45	124	37	341
Score	170	60	165	48	443
Mean	1.26	1.34	1.33	1.29	1.30
Character disorder					
No. patients	99	37	88	29	253
Score	285	93	239	84	701
Mean	2.88	2.51	2.72	2.91	2.77
Psychotic					
No. patients	55	19	44	20	138
Score	235	94	200	79	608
Mean	4.27	4.95	4.54	3.95	4.41
Pseudo-neurotic					
No. patients	21	8	24	11	64
Score	105	39	122	58	324
Mean	5.00	4.88	5.08	5.27	5.03

*(Note: Health Plan Average is 0.8 per year for patients 20 years old or older.)

outpatient and inpatient medical services in terms of diagnostic category. The neurotic patients had the highest outpatient utilization, whereas the psychotic patients had the highest inpatient utilization.

The outpatient utilization of the pseudoneurotic schizophrenic resembled that of the neurotic, while the inpatient utilization of the pseudoneurotic schizophrenic is not significantly different than that of the psychotic.

Patients with character disorders utilize outpatient services at the same rate as psychotics, but their inpatient rate is approximately halfway between neurotic and psychotic inpatient rates.

DISCUSSION

Research in human behavior is easy to do, but difficult to do well. A research design may look fine on paper, but may not be feasible in fact. Such was the case with the present experiment: no experimental population was generated. This result can be instructive, however, and we will proceed to search for serendipitous results. Human subjects cannot be manipulated for experimental or therapeutic purposes in the same way that animals or machines can. This applies to the doctors in this experiment as well as the patients.

This observation may be timely and relevant now when vast sums of money are being spent in developing mental health programs, many of which are designed on paper from an armchair and have never been proven to be clinically effective.

A recent paper from the University of California at Los Angeles Alcoholism Research Clinic found the results to be the same in a group of alcoholics randomly assigned by court probation to one of three treatment conditions: (1) a psychiatrically oriented outpatient alcoholic clinic, (2) Alcoholics Anonymous, (3) no treatment. One might conclude that the answer to the problem of alcoholism *may not* be the provision of a multitude of "alcoholic clinics" across the country. Similarly, it has never been demonstrated that a "suicide prevention center" has lowered the incidence of suicide in any community. We might, on the other hand, expect that such a center would be likely to increase (1) preoccupation with suicide in the community, (2) the number of suicidal threats, and (3) the number of suicidal gestures. In other words, if people volunteer to play dramatic life-saver, we can confidently expect others to volunteer to threaten self-destruction.

Nevertheless, we have suicide prevention centers popping up all over the land.

The question is to what extent psychiatric patients can be "found" in the community and then successfully treated. Is it possible and worthwhile to induce an ever-greater percentage of the population to get some treatment to improve mental health? Are the patients who come to a psychiatric clinic via the common traditional channels (referral by self, relative, friend, family doctor) more or less treatable than those produced by newer "case finding" methods in the community?

The setting in which this study was done is unusual in having had a psychiatric clinic as part of comprehensive health services for about 15 years. For this reason there was no large reservoir of patients needing and wanting psychiatric services which they could not afford. Note that 10 percent of the patients identified as emotionally disturbed and in acute distress already had been seen in the psychiatric clinic. Many of the others in this group undoubtedly have been referred but will never be seen in psychiatry for a number of reasons, among which may be the following: (1) they have too much invested in their roles of being (physically) sick; (2) they have major physical illnesses which they and their doctors use to ignore the emotional illness; (3) they are terrified by the idea of mental illness ("craziness"); (4) there is often a payoff for "real," i.e. physical, illness, but not for emotional disturbance from family, friends, doctors, insurance companies. The fact that 90 percent of these patients have never gotten to the psychiatric clinic demonstrates that non-psychiatric physicians have been treating and will continue to treat the bulk of the emotionally disturbed people in the population.

While we have demonstrated that emotionally disturbed patients who are seen in psychiatry reduce their use of other medical services, we are still unable to determine whether this would hold true for all those patients identified by our double-screening technique as likely candidates for psychotherapy.

One should be cautious in using statistics from mental health clinics when they deviate from the averages reported by most other clinics. It has often been reported that about one percent of a population will seek psychiatric services per year. The Group Health Insurance study (Avnet, 1962) showed the pattern of response that is usually seen when a population is offered low-cost psychiatric services for the first time: increased utilization for the first few months due to an accumulation of need for such services. After that, the demand stabilizes. Active "promotion" of psychiatric benefits did not increase the utilization of psychiatric services in their population.

It is possible to report a much higher rate of utilization, e.g., 5 percent/year, if one organizes his psychiatric clinic in the following manner: (1) "crisis" orientation; (2) very brief therapy and counselling; (3) representing the psychiatric staff member as "your friendly family counselor"; (4) fostering dependency relationship by encouraging patients to return frequently—whenever they have to make decisions, feel anxious or depressed, etc.; (5) counting each family member as a separate patient when a family is seen together; (6) most of all—by counting each return to the clinic a "new patient." Unfortunately, the higher the percentage, the more effective the service.

Antes muerto que mudado (death rather than change), a Spanish proverb quoted by Lichtenstein (1961) in his classic monograph on identity, dramatizes the tremendous dynamic force behind the human being's need to maintain his identity—a force that has priority over all forces motivating a person's behavior and lifestyle. Many otherwise baffling aspects of the behavior of individuals, groups and nations become clear if this force is recognized. Patients do not want to change, in fact resist change, even though their lives are full of misery and pain. A psychotherapist, then, is relatively helpless unless the patient is highly motivated, i.e., in a great deal of "pain." Getting a patient to the office of a psychotherapist is likely to be a waste of everybody's time unless the patient is "ready" or motivated for some kind of change. It is, of course, the psychotherapist's job to foster and capitalize on every shred of motivation he can find. Many emotionally disturbed people in the community may seem to "need help" but are not at all interested in change. This is certainly true of a high percentage of alcoholics, "hippies," addicts, "psychopaths," criminals and many other types whom the community at large thinks "need help."

The assessment of the effectiveness of psychotherapy has always presented great difficulties, conclusions varying from "psychotherapy is worthless" to the behavior therapists' claim of as high as 86–95 percent effectiveness in 30 interviews or fewer. By far the best investigation of brief psychotherapy was done by the Tavistock group, reported by Malan (1963). We need much more high-quality research of this kind in assessing the value of mental health programs.

It is interesting to note the few differences between blue-collar and white-collar workers (Table 2). The blue-collar patients are more apt to be in only three (of 14) categories: hysteric; panic and anxiety attacks;

and depressive character; and less likely to be obsessional. Otherwise, the two groups are comparable in percentages in the other neurotic and character-disorder categories and in all the psychotic categories. The "pseudoneurotic schizophrenic" category defines a group of patients who have a wealth of symptoms of many kinds. These patients are the ones that seek professional help constantly, who "never get well" and may make up a large percentage of those long-term patients in the office of every physician, psychotherapist and psychoanalyst.

The similar percentages of incidence of psychoses in blue-collar and white-collar groups may reflect the greater impartiality of the computer than the clinician, if we accept the contention of Hollingshead (1958) that middle-class psychotherapists tend to over-diagnose psychosis in patients of lower socioeconomic classes as compared with those of middle or upper classes.

SUMMARY

During a six-month period, 10,667 patients taking the Automated Multiphasic Screening Examination (Kaiser Permanente Medical Center, San Francisco) were given a computerized psychological test as a routine part of that screening. The tests revealed that 3,682 patients, or one third, had evidence of neurosis, personality disorder, or psychosis. Of these, 822 (or 7.7 percent of the total Multiphasic patients tested) also had high degrees of "emotional distress." The 32 internists conducting the Multiphasic follow-up examinations received computer-printed "consider-rules" suggesting referral to psychiatry for half (411) of these patients, while the other half served as a control group and did not have such a "consider-rule."

It was found that attempts at early detection of emotional problems did not generate more psychiatric clinic patients than those generated through routine medical practice in this setting. There was considerable resistance on the part of physicians to the "artificiality" of referral by automated procedures, and there was a comparable rejection by patients of a referral made as a result of such procedures.

The population selected by this automated psychological screening method were high utilizers of medical services. Where neurotics tend to use outpatient medical services, psychotic patients tend to use inpatient medical services. Patients with personality disorders seem to use both. No differences in utilization rates were found in terms of blue collar versus white collar, or urban versus suburban.

The implications of these findings are: (1) attempts at early detection of psychiatric problems will not create as great a demand for psychiatric services as might be expected; (2) whereas many patients seeking outpatient medical treatment may be reflecting neurotic problems, psychotic patients often manifest symptoms which so simulate a variety of baffling problems that they are hospitalized for medical diagnostic workups. Patients with personality disorders seem to require both outpatient and inpatient attention in above-average amounts.

The Early Days at Kaiser

In 1955 I was in private practice in San Francisco and having some significant doubts concerning my treatment of private patients in psychotherapy. As a trained psychoanalyst, I was treating people with that method—they would lie on the couch and free-associate. I saw many of them several times per week. Erik Erikson had been my analyst, so I had one of the best training experiences possible.

I learned that I could extend the therapy for an extra six months by simply saying a certain phrase, essentially manipulating them into doing many more sessions of analysis. This method, which had been part of my training, was justified as preventing a patient from terminating before analysis was completed and becoming what was known as a "psychoanalytic dropout." It meant that my income would remain steady, but I began to wonder, "Is this serving the patient or is it serving me?" This bothered me a great deal. Somewhere inside me I knew that psychotherapy and the variations of psychological treatment I had learned—especially my experience in helping paratroopers survive their fourth, fifth, and sixth jumps—did not need to take so many sessions.

One day I saw an ad in a San Francisco newspaper for chief psychologist at Kaiser, and I applied for the position. Of the 38 applicants, I survived the first interview, and was invited to a second interview to meet with Sidney Garfield, the physician who founded Kaiser. In some ways, Garfield was a very advanced thinker for that time, and he can be credited as one of the first people to clearly recognize that many patients—in fact, a slight majority—who visited doctors had a very strong psychological component to their presenting problem. That is one reason he insisted on hiring a psychologist as Chief of the Mental Health Service at Kaiser Permanente: He wanted to make sure that patients came to realize that their problems were not only medical. Garfield definitely did not want a psychiatrist in that role for just this reason. He also wanted to have the research training that a psychologist would offer in order to study scientifically the issue of medical/psychological overlap. So, in a way, this was a very special mandate for me, although I did not clearly understand that at the time. It was a challenge to spot the psychological problems embedded within the medical problems. And, of course, many presenting problems were purely psychological.

Over the years while working at Kaiser, my creative juices started flowing, but only after making some funny mistakes and learning lessons that have stayed in my mind over four decades. Looking back, I have to smile at my naiveté. But this was pioneering work, and I was creating a new way of being a psychologist. To a large extent, the lessons that I and others learned are still valid. Unfortunately, the field of professional psychology still has not grasped this way of working. The first studies that Bill Follette and I put out, in 1967 and 1968, were preceded by a great deal of research carried out in the late 1950s and early 1960s. I have not been able to find the very early papers of those years, which were published in-house at Kaiser.

I suppose that one of the reasons that this model is hard to grasp is that it cuts across the usual categories in our profession: The boundary between what is psychological and what is medical is blurred, and the mental health therapist must work within that blurred area, sometimes not letting the patient know that psychological treatment is being provided. Plus, the traditional schools of psychotherapy are also blurred, and the therapist utilizes parts of different schools at different times—all in the service of helping patients improve their health and their lives. This requires a very flexible way of conceptualizing psychological treatment, and the contexts within which the therapist works. As we developed this method of working, I found that many professionals were not able to operate in this way, and this led to many disappointments. I think that in today's climate of justifying psychological work, this kind of conceptual flexibility is even more important, if the professional psychotherapist is to survive.

1975–1984:
Change Is on the Horizon

A Commentary by Nick Cummings

W HILE PROFESSIONAL PSYCHOLOGISTS were experiencing the golden age of the private practice of psychotherapy, the health system in the United States was already in economic trouble. There were national voices that were actively attempting to signal these impending changes to psychology's leadership, but a profession that was at the pinnacle of its success was not in the mood for predictions of trouble ahead. Some of these efforts to alert the profession, like the book by Kiesler, Cummings, and VandenBos (1979), *Psychology and National Health Insurance*, received little attention even though it had the blessing of the board of directors of the American Psychological Association (APA) and two of the coauthors were the APA's then-current executive officer (Kiesler) and president (Cummings). The sampling of articles chosen by the coeditors of this section of the *Collected Papers* reflects the broad range of issues confronting professional psychology during this period. To make these writings more understandable to the reader, it would be worthwhile to recall the successes and difficulties of this era that not only contributed to the changes that would occur in the succeeding years (1985-1997), but also sowed the seeds for psychology's eventual state of denial in the face of the overwhelming changes that were to come.

The inflationary spiral of healthcare was gaining momentum because the federal government had fueled a noncompetitive health economy. Beginning with the Hill–Burton legislation that spurred the proliferation of hospitals from a shortage in rural areas to beyond the point of real need anywhere, to Medicare, and finally to Medicaid, the federal government set the stage for the spending of unpredictable billions of dollars without putting into place sound economic controls. It was courting the medical profession, which had been successful in blocking previous Congressional efforts at health reform. The result was best described by Professor Eli Ginsberg, the Columbia University health economist, who parodied, "The government gave the keys to the U.S. Treasury to the hospitals and the medical profession, and invited them to help themselves" (Personal communication, March 1986). The government was relying on the predictable glut of healthcare practitioners to introduce competition and reduce costs. For years, it had been subsidizing medical and allied medical training, beginning with the shortages immediately following World War II, not only because of a benevolent interest in eliminating such shortages, but also in the erroneous belief that an oversupply of doctors would result in competition and the subsequent lowering of costs. Again, Professor Ginsberg had attempted to persuade the government economists that this was faulty thinking because healthcare does not follow the laws of supply and demand. Quite the contrary, since doctors control both supply (the patients) *and* demand (what and how many procedures each patient should receive), the greater the number of doctors, the greater are the resulting costs. Hospitals grew fat on a "cost plus 15 percent reimbursement," and physicians cynically stated at their practice-building seminars that income is predicated not on how many patients are seen, but on how many costly procedures are performed. In large measure, taxpayers and employers were footing the bill. This is the backdrop against which psychotherapy practice was enjoying its golden era.

By this time, U.S. society had espoused psychotherapy, as witnessed by both the many articles in the popular press and the ever-increasing numbers of psychotherapy patients. The American Psychiatric Association (ApA) was beginning its "remedicalization," which resulted in its eventually virtually abandoning psychotherapy to psychologists and social workers. Psychology became the preeminent psychotherapy profession in the land. The so-called human potential movement was at its height, and many psychologists were achieving guru status in fringe endeavors. The APA swelled to a membership of over 100,000 while psychology became the most popular undergraduate major. Everyone wanted to be a psychologist, and the demand for training was so great that professional schools of psychology, both excellent and disgraceful, proliferated beyond any expectation. Psychologists were entering private practice in large numbers, and almost everyone thought it would never end.

During this exuberance, there were signs pointing to trouble on the horizon. The government was intent on bringing costs down, and hoped to do so by enacting a program of National Health Insurance. This would extend coverage to all Americans, but would entail strict federal control over doctors' fees and hospital charges. It would also regulate what services were provided. The ominous picture for psychology was that either psychological services would not be covered, or they would be covered only as ancillary to psychiatry. The American Medical Association, and the ApA, clearly had the attention of the government policy makers. Psychology was on the defensive, and it was an uphill fight to demonstrate our effectiveness. On one of the several occasions I testified to the Congress, I was fortunate to catch the attention of Senator Edward Kennedy, who was chairing the U.S. Senate Subcommittee on Health. He asked that I consult with his committee, and I did so for several years, until Senator Russell Long, as chair of the U.S. Senate Finance Committee, replaced Senator Kennedy with a far less progressively minded chair, Senator Herman Talmadge. What had interested Senator Kennedy was our medical cost offset research, and the emerging innovative therapies that would make psychologists more effective, and consequently more attractive to National Health Insurance (NHI). These were our entrées to an otherwise closed door. Many of my writings during this era addressed NHI, the need for more controlled studies in medical cost offset, and the reluctance of the profession to move beyond traditional psychotherapy.

During the same period, I was fortunate in being named to Walter Reuther's Committee of 100. Reuther was the charismatic head of the United Auto Workers (UAW) who was later assassinated by a shotgun blast through his living room window. His Committee of 100 advocated NHI, and he had the ear of Senator Kennedy and other influential members of the Congress. The UAW's Vice President for Health and Welfare at the time was a social worker, Mel Glasser, who despised and distrusted psychologists. The rumor was that he had been flunked out of a doctoral program in clinical psychology, and although this was never confirmed, his rage at psychology (and toward me) was commensurate with that kind of experience. I was never able, therefore, to convince Reuther of the need for psychological services and, consequently, I failed to obtain Ted Kennedy's full support.

Senator Long's chief clerk was a lawyer named Jay Constantine. In the course of my testimonies before the U.S. Senate Finance Committee, during which I sought to demonstrate the cost-effectiveness of psychological services, Mr. Constantine and I became very good friends. He distributed our medical cost offset literature throughout the Congress, and was keenly and genuinely interested in the more time- and cost-effective psychotherapies. He was blunt in telling me that psychologists would never be included in NHI as long as they were viewed as "junior psychiatrists." They would have to demonstrate their unique contributions. Whereas in my discussions with Senator Kennedy, I had the backing of the APA, many of our colleagues were uncomfortable with time/cost-effective psychotherapies. I was aware of their opposition to my negotiations with Jay Constantine, but it became clear when Clarence Martin, the APA lobbyist, leaked a statement critical of Constantine, and even accused him of conspiracy. This is a word that has a specific and serious meaning in Washington, and although Martin later stated that he meant it only in its broadest sense, Constantine was infuriated and was essentially unavailable to me thereafter. He did, however, keep his word and backed the funding of the Hawaii Medicaid Project, along with Senator Daniel Inouye, who later made such a project by the Health Care Financing Administration (HCFA) part of the budget resolution bill in 1982.

Another warning cloud was forming during this same period. The Nixon administration decided that health reform would be better accomplished through health maintenance organizations (HMOs) than through NHI. Following the White House lead, the Congress passed the HMO bill, which provided three years of start-up funding for new HMOs. Suddenly, where there had been only a handful of HMOs, there were now scores of companies, with more and more psychologists joining them as congenial, rewarding places in which to practice. Some psychologists, such as Rogers Wright, were vehement in their opposition to HMOs, but most took little note of them because they were not yet a threat to independent practice. In the golden age of psychotherapy, there was enough clientele for all. My own role in the three years following the enactment of the HMO legislation was to consult, encourage, and help implement the fledgling health plans. Edgar Kaiser, son of the late Henry Kaiser, decided on behalf of Kaiser Permanente that we would give away the HMO technology. In spite of

our help, five out of every eight new HMOs went bankrupt or were acquired once the federal subsidy expired. I was fortunate to have
worked in those early days with the Group Health Cooperative of
Puget Sound (Seattle) and the Harvard Community Health Plan
(Boston), both of which are highly successful to this day.

{ 3 }

THE HEALTH MODEL AS ENTREE TO THE HUMAN SERVICES MODEL IN PSYCHOTHERAPY

BEFORE ONE CAN appreciate where psychology's role in the delivery of psychotherapy may be going, one must first understand where modern psychotherapy has been these past three decades. Psychology entered the field of psychotherapy essentially in the post-World War II era of the late 1940's, a period which can now be designated as the "golden age of psychotherapy." The art of dynamic healing through verbal understanding became an essential service in the military whose casualties in the war just having ended were one-third mental and emotional. The two decades immediately following World War II saw the popularization of psychoanalysis and the seemingly overnight public acceptance of the private psychotherapists. Psychoanalysis was inordinately successful, creating throughout the United States an enormous demand for its services. Psychologists aped the medical model and rode the crest of this "golden age of psychotherapy" as they flourished in private practice. There seemed to be no end to the number of patients seeking psychotherapy, giving rise to the myth there could never be enough professionals trained. This grand illusion helped spawn the paraprofessional model as a response to the belief in the perennial shortage of professionals, and gave impetus to the mental health movement, which sought to prevent the eruption of three new patients by the problems of society for every one that was cured on the couch. The community mental health centers were launched with the golden promise that given enough dollars and trained workers the ills of a sick society could be alleviated if not eradicated. This application of psychotherapeutic techniques to social structures was heralded as infinitely more efficient than the tedious one-to-one, fifty-minute hour.

In its golden age psychotherapy tragically oversold itself to the American public in three specific areas. First, it promised a level of freedom from anxiety that is neither realistic nor possible in reacting, pulsating, functioning human beings. Americans accepted the notion that relief from tension and a permanent sense of well-being were within the grasp of our society, and it can never be adequately determined to what extent this iatrogenic "delusion" paved the way for the subsequent espousing by the public of alcohol and drugs as natural agents in the right to feel good, and the concomitant, almost universal push of the tranquilizer by physicians. Secondly, psychotherapy promised a freedom from guilt that was equally unrealistic. Guilt is a necessary condition of human life. It is the basis of moral, ethical and empathic behavior; it is neurotic guilt that is the legitimate target of psychotherapy. Thirdly, psychotherapy promised a cure for mental and emotional illnesses and, even worse, it promised the cure for society's illnesses. It became apparent by the late 1950's and early 1960's that psychotherapy had oversold itself, and the mental health movement looked nervously to community psychiatry and psychology to deliver the golden promise that psychotherapy admittedly could not deliver. The realization was not long in coming that this, too, had been oversold. The power structure in Washington began to ask embarrassing questions: How long could the government be expected to finance social revolution, alias community psychology?

As the mental health professions themselves began to realize they could not make good their promise to the American public, the oversell approach collapsed and a profound despair, characterized by two self-destructive phenomena, appeared. The first of these was a pervasive, overly critical re-evaluation of psychotherapy which soon took on all of the overtones of self-flagellation. What should have been a healthy re-examination emulated in its despair the excesses of the oversell. The medical model needed to be criticized, but taken full-blown, the position of Thomas Szasz is an absurdity. Eysenck found no good in psychotherapy whatsoever, and Schofield labelled it "paid friendship."

Behavior modification proponents attacked the dynamic therapies unmercifully, and everyone joined in to make orthodox psychoanalysis the scapegoat for all of psychotherapy's tarnished promises. And now, in a plethora of popularized articles negative to psychotherapy, the public is being invited to join the pitiful flagellation.

The second symptom of despair, equally destructive by its intensity and excesses, was an almost instantaneous espousal of every new kind of treatment that a seemingly endless array of proponents presented. This, too, had its healthy and necessary elements, for many of these new techniques, once the initial huckstering was removed from them, expanded our ability to treat heretofore stubborn, resistive conditions. The despair was reflected in the irresponsibility of grasping at any straw in the slim hope that the golden promise would yet be fulfilled. Psychotherapy owes much to these fresh approaches even though they may have been born out of despair. The less efficacious techniques will be taken care of by the legions of malpractice suits that will follow the attorneys' discovery of fertile new ground.

Given the unbridled continuation of the excesses of this despair, psychotherapy could be a dirty word in our society within ten years. We have seen this happen to the field of education, and we are watching it happen to medicine. In response essentially two outcomes could be undertaken by this profession. One of these could be a retreat into therapy for therapy's sake. This is no longer acceptable, as this will no longer be financed or tolerated by society. Therapy for the ethereal, unattainable goal of a total personality revamping is a luxury and a myth that has had its day. On the other hand, the future of psychotherapy can be bright and productive if we follow a model that is responsive to the needs of individuals and society within a modified health model. We are literally at the threshold of national health care for all the American people. No comprehensive health system can be delivered on a cost-effective basis without a psychotherapy component. A decade-and-a-half of research in prepaid psychotherapy has demonstrated this, and it is to this health model, as an entree to the eventual human services model, to which this paper addresses itself. At the present time the Congress is interested in paying for health, not human services. It will eventually include a mental health component because it must, otherwise medical services per se will become bogged down in overutilization by persons having no discoverable "medical" cause. To the extent that professional psychology can demonstrate its responsiveness to this need, to that extent it will be included as a health service provider under whatever national health care system is finally adopted.

The Kaiser Permanente Health Plan on the West Coast flourished in the post–World War II era because it provided comprehensive treatment at low subscriber rates for all a person's ills without the exclusions, limitations, co-insurance and other troublesome features common to health plans at that time. Kaiser Permanente, as the forerunner of the modern Health Maintenance Organization (HMO), soon found to its dismay that once a health system makes it simple and free for the patient to see a physician, an alarming inundation of medical clinics by seemingly physically healthy persons occurred. This has always been relatively true in private practice where the doctor's fee was somewhat of a deterrent to overutilization of services. Furthermore, since the financial base at Kaiser Permanente is one of per capitation (subscription) and neither the physician nor the Health Plan derives an additional fee for seeing the patient, rather than becoming wealthy from imagined physical ills, the system could be bankrupted by what was regarded as abuse by the hypochondriac. Early in its history Kaiser Permanente added psychotherapy to its list of services, first on a courtesy reduced fee of five dollars per visit and eventually as a prepaid benefit. Initially this was motivated not so much by a conviction in the efficacy of psychotherapy, but in the urgent need to get the so-called hypochondriac out of the doctor's office. From this initial perception as a dumping ground began sixteen years of expensive research which has led to the conclusion that no comprehensive prepaid health system can survive without providing a psychotherapy benefit.

The author and his colleagues (Follette & Cummings, 1967) initially found that the term "hypochondriac" did not adequately describe the overutilizer of medical services. It was immediately determined that patients eventually seen in psychotherapy were high utilizers of medical services. From the review of hundreds of medical charts of persons seen in psychotherapy, they developed a series of thirty-eight criteria of emotional distress, weighted from one to three points each, application of which permitted psychologically untrained physicians to validly and reliably differentiate between health plan members who subsequent to their overutilization were seen in psychotherapy and those health plan members who were not. These criteria were based on notations in the medical charts by physicians who were making medical judgments, the psychological significance of which they were unaware. In later studies the same authors discovered that patients with emotional distress can be identified rather consistently by weighing their medical records. The conclusion from these studies is that in an HMO-type of health plan patients in emotional distress, finding an unsympathetic or uncomprehending ear when they attempt to discuss their distress with their physician, quickly begin to translate their emotional distress into physical symptoms for which they receive a great deal of attention in the form of X-rays, laboratory tests, prescriptions and return visits to this doctor. The question then remained that, given psychotherapy as the treatment of choice for their emotional ills, would these patients demonstrate a subsequently different utilization of health plan services.

In the first of a series of investigations into the relationship between psychological services and medical utilization in a prepaid health plan setting, the author and his colleagues (Follette & Cummings, 1967) compared the number and type of medical services sought before and after the intervention of psychotherapy in a large group of randomly selected patients. The outpatient and inpatient medical utilization for the year prior to the initial interview in the Department of Psychotherapy as well as for the five years following were studied for three groups of psychotherapy patients (one interview only, brief therapy with a mean of 6.2 interviews, and long-term therapy with a mean of 33.9 interviews) and a control group of matched patients demonstrating similar criteria of distress but not, in the six years under study, seen in psychotherapy. Their findings indicated that: (1) persons in emotional distress were significantly higher users of both inpatient and outpatient medical facilities as compared to the Health Plan average; (2) there were significant declines in medical utilization in those emotionally distressed individuals who received psychotherapy as compared to a control group of matched emotionally distressed Health Plan members who were not accorded psychotherapy; (3) these declines remained constant during the five years following the termination of psychotherapy; (4) the most significant declines occurred in the second year after the initial interview, and those patients receiving one session only or brief psychotherapy (two to eight sessions) did not require additional psychotherapy to maintain the lower level of utilization for five years; (5) patients seen two years or more in regular psychotherapy demonstrated no overall decline in total outpatient utilization inasmuch as psychotherapy visits tended to supplant medical visits. However, there was significant decline in inpatient utilization in this long-term therapy group from an initial hospitalization rate several times that of the Health Plan average, to a level comparable to that of the general adult Health Plan population. In a subsequent study the same authors (Cummings & Follette, 1968) found that intensive efforts to increase the number of referrals to psychotherapy by computerized psychological screening with early detection and alerting of the attending physicians did not increase significantly the number of patients seeking psychotherapy. The authors concluded that in a prepaid health plan setting already maximally employing educative techniques to both patients and physicians, and already providing a range of prepaid psychological services, the number of Health Plan subscribers seeking psychotherapy reached an optimal level and remained fairly constant thereafter.

In summarizing sixteen years of prepayment experience these same authors (Cummings & Follette, 1975) demonstrate that there is no basis for the fear that an increased demand for psychotherapy will financially endanger the system, for it is not the number of referrals received that will drive costs up, but the manner in which psychotherapy services are delivered that determines optimal cost-therapeutic effectiveness. The finding that one session only, with no repeat psychological visits, could reduce medical utilization by 60% over the following five years, was surprising and totally unexpected. Equally surprising was the 75% reduction in medical utilization over a five-year period in those patients initially receiving two to eight psychotherapy sessions (brief therapy). The data offered no conclusive reason as to how and why this early, brief psychotherapeutic intervention resulted in a persistent reduction in medical utilization throughout the following half decade. The authors speculated that the results obtained demonstrated a psychotherapeutic effect, inasmuch as the clinic procedure was to offer early and incisive intervention into the patient's crisis problem, get beneath the manifest symptoms to his/her real concerns and offer understanding and therapy within the very first session itself. Such a hypothesis would suggest that a patient's understanding or appreciation of the problem and its relationship to his/her symptoms would result in a diminution of the somaticizing of emotions, and a consequent reduction in medical visits. This is in keeping with the experiences of providing psychotherapy under national health care in Great Britain (Balint, 1957). Perhaps a less satisfactory, but an equally plausible hypothesis would hold that the patient attained no mastery over his/her problems and that subsequent to the psychological visit s/he found ways other than visiting the doctor to express emotional distress.

In a further present study the authors sought to answer in an eighth-year telephone follow-up whether the results described previously were a therapeutic effect, or the consequence of extraneous factors, or a deleterious effect. It was hypothesized that if better understanding of the problem had occurred in the psychotherapeutic sessions, the patient would recall the actual problem rather than the presenting symptom, and would have both lost the presenting symptom and coped more effectively with the real problem.

The results suggest that the reduction in medical utilization was the consequence of resolving the emotional distress that was being reflected in symptoms and doctors' visits. The modal patient in this eighth-year follow-up may be described as follows: "s/he denies ever having consulted a physician for the symptoms for which s/he had been originally referred. Rather, the actual problem discussed with the psychotherapist is recalled as the reason for the 'psychiatric' visit, and although the problem is resolved, this resolution is attributed to the patient's own efforts and no credit is given the psychotherapist." This reaffirms the contention that the reduction in medical utilization reflected the diminution in the emotional distress which had been expressed in symptoms which were presented to the doctor.

The findings suggest that the expectations of the therapist influence the outcome of psychotherapy, for if the first interview is merely "evaluation" or "intake," not much of therapeutic value is likely to occur in the first interview. If the therapist's attitude is that no real help is forthcoming from less than prolonged "intensive" psychotherapy, s/he may be right (for his/her own patients). Malan (1963), in his classic study of brief psychotherapy, was able to honestly examine the prejudices of his group of psychiatrists about brief therapy: the kinds of benefit possible, the kinds of patients who could utilize it, the permanency of the results, and so forth. He concluded that traditional attitudes about very brief therapy were mostly in the nature of unjustified prejudices. It would appear that therapeutic effects of brief therapy, which can be labelled "transference cure," "flight into health," "intellectualization," and other derogatory terms, can often be long-lasting and result in a major change in the person's symptoms, relationships and even lifestyle. Many of the patients in this study would undoubtedly be called "poorly motivated for treatment" or "dropouts from therapy" in many psychotherapy clinics.

The Kaiser Permanente studies have been replicated in a variety of prepaid settings with similar findings. Recently Karon and VandenBos (1975) reported in a study of hospitalized schizophrenic patients that despite the expense of psychotherapy, there were savings of 22% to 36% in total treatment costs because of the shorter hospitalization of patients receiving psychotherapy as compared to patients who received medication and no psychotherapy. This growing body of evidence reflects the rightful place of psychotherapy in any health delivery system, and suggests that the health model is the present entree for the psychologist into the health delivery system. Inclusion of psychologists as health service providers in national healthcare within a relatively short time after its enactment will conclude a difficult decade-and-a-half struggle for recognition on the part of the dedicated professional leadership of psychology. But this will occur not only because there is a need for psychotherapy within any comprehensive health delivery system, but also because psychologists are beginning to recognize the contribution of psychotherapy in such a setting. Once within the health system, psychologists will then commence a second struggle, predictably of eight to ten years' duration, before the government is persuaded that the human services model is more efficacious than the health services model for the delivery of psychotherapy. But while the second battle is being waged, professional psychologists will have a viable economic base within the health system from which to practice. The professional school movement essentially has gambled that the much larger numbers of practitioners that can be trained by such schools will be absorbed by the national healthcare system. If psychology were not to be included in national healthcare as a provider, this would not only spell the end of professional schools, but essentially the end of the entire field of professional psychology as well. Given the health model as the entrée, the future offers to professional psychology a bright challenge.

The Balints: Pioneers in Integrated
Behavioral Healthcare

*In 1957 Michael Balint, an English physician, published his land-
mark book,* The Doctor, His Patient and the Illness. *When you try to
trace brief psychotherapy to its roots, the path always leads back to
this very important book. In fact, it is also one of the first books on
integrated behavioral healthcare, although he did not call it that.
The book is now long out of print, but it showed the first efforts to
help the ordinary patient, who goes to a general practice doctor
with a medical complaint, to understand many of the underlying
psychological issues. Balint and the small group of physicians with
which he worked reported their beginning attempts to deal with
these issues. It was a very influential book at the time. Of course, at
Kaiser, we were developing our own way of working, and we were
enjoying some success. I later learned that, in some ways, we were
ahead of Balint.*

*I think it was 1960 or 1961 when we brought Michael and Alice
Balint to the Kaiser San Francisco Medical Center. We then brought
in about 1,000 physicians to interact with them. Imagine, in 1960,
we were talking about integration! Nobody else was thinking about
integrated behavioral healthcare. But England had had socialized
medicine since 1946, and very early on realized the inefficiencies of
medical treatment for those in emotional distress. It wreaked havoc
with the system, and there were not enough psychotherapists in England to deal with it. That is one reason why the English developed
group therapy models to such a sophisticated level.*

*Initially, Balint utilized five sessions of assessment to determine
whether or not a person was a good candidate for brief therapy. I remember looking at Michael with my jaw somewhere around my
belly button—I was shocked! The average number of sessions we
were doing at Kaiser was only 6.2! If we used five of them to determine who was going to get sessions, then we would have 11.2 sessions. I suggested to Balint that, instead of determining who was a
good candidate for brief therapy, we would put everybody in brief
therapy, and if they benefited and resolved their distress, we could
say, "It worked!" If it didn't work, we could go on to long-term ther-*

apy. Why screen out people for brief therapy in long-term therapy? He looked at me and said, with his lovely British accent, "Well, that's brilliant."

Balint at first had adopted David Malan's techniques. Malan had developed a way of working in a brief-therapy model, but it was still very tied to classic psychoanalytic theory, and it was still a relatively time-consuming method of therapy—at that time, probably 50 or more sessions. Balint went along with Malan's method, but found out that it didn't do the trick. Remember, Balint was a physician in general practice, and he couldn't take the time to assess someone for five sessions to see if the person would be a good candidate for brief psychotherapy. But he was very squeamish about standing up and declaring that he didn't use Malan's methods. Alice Balint saw the point, and said to Michael and me, after one of his San Francisco talks, "Yes, Michael, that's the right answer to David." She knew that five sessions of assessment was not going to work for the general physician, but her husband did not know how to tell this to David Malan. Now he knew. I sometimes wonder how it turned out, and if he told Malan about this new approach.

The Balints influenced me tremendously. After their visit, a lot of things gelled in my mind. I began to appreciate that we knew more than they knew in England. And we had the courage to say, "Damn the torpedoes! Full speed ahead!" And we knew what we were doing, because it was working. They were a wonderful couple, the Balints, and I am very grateful for having known them.

{ 4 }

BRIEF PSYCHOTHERAPY
AND MEDICAL UTILIZATION*

IT HAS BEEN suggested that hospital overutilization is caused partly by the very nature of hospital insurance benefits—services are reimbursable if done in the hospital, but not in the practitioner's office. Pacific Mutual's five years of experience with a health maintenance plan in Southern California (Gamblin, 1975), administered through the Orange Country Medical Foundation, clearly supports this view by demonstrating that when the traditional benefits are reversed, there is an actual decrease in dollars paid out. Contrary to common practice, the foundation placed a $100 deductible on hospital stays while offering first-dollar coverage for outpatient physicians' services. Claims increased 30 percent but dollars paid out decreased. This refutation of traditional fears has been demonstrated by the Kaiser Health Plan for years as illustrated in the eight-year follow-up study reported in this chapter.

In the first of a series of investigations into the relationship between psychological services and medical utilization in a prepaid health plan setting, the authors (Follette & Cummings, 1967) found that (1) persons in emotional distress were significantly higher users of both inpatient and outpatient medical facilities as compared to the health plan

*With William T. Follette, M.D.

average; (2) medical utilization declined significantly in those emotionally distressed individuals who received psychotherapy as compared with a control group of matched emotionally distressed health plan members who were not accorded psychotherapy; (3) these declines remained constant during the five years following the termination of psychotherapy; (4) the most significant declines occurred in the second year after the initial interview, and those patients receiving one session only or brief psychotherapy (two to eight sessions) did not require additional psychotherapy to maintain the lower level of utilization for five years; and (5) patients seen for two years or more in regular psychotherapy demonstrated no overall decline in total outpatient utilization, since psychotherapy visits tended to supplant medical visits. However, there was significant decline in inpatient utilization in this long-term therapy group from an initial hospitalization rate several times that of the health plan average, to a level comparable to that of the general adult health plan population. In a subsequent study the same authors (Cummings & Follette, 1968) found that intensive efforts to increase the number of referrals to psychotherapy by computerized psychological screening with early detection and alerting of the attending physicians did not increase significantly the number of patients seeking psychotherapy. The authors concluded that in a prepaid health plan setting already maximally employing educational techniques for both patients and physicians, and already providing a range of prepaid psychological services, the number of health plan subscribers seeking psychotherapy reached an optimal level and remained fairly constant. During the entire period of the study, as well as in the insured years before and after the eight years of this study, the utilization of mental health services was consistently 0.5 per 1,000 insureds for inpatient (hospitalization), and 9 per 1,000 insureds for outpatient services. The average length of hospitalization remained under eight days, and the average outpatient psychotherapy series remained at 6.6 visits.

Sixteen years of prepayment experience demonstrates that there is no basis for the fear that an increased demand for psychotherapy will financially endanger the system. It is not the number of referrals received, but the manner in which psychotherapy services are delivered, that determines optimal cost-therapeutic effectiveness. The finding that one session only, with no repeat psychological visits, could reduce medical utilization by 60 percent over the following five years, was surprising and totally unexpected. Equally surprising was the 75 percent reduction in medical utilization over a five-year period in those patients initially receiving two to eight psychotherapy sessions (brief therapy). The data offered no conclusive reason as to how and why this early, brief psychotherapeutic intervention resulted in a persistent reduction in medical utilization throughout the following half decade. The authors speculated that the results obtained demonstrated a psychotherapeutic effect, inasmuch as the clinic procedure was to offer early and incisive intervention into the patient's crisis problem, to get beneath the manifest symptoms to his or her real concerns, and to offer understanding and therapy in the very first session. Such a hypothesis would suggest that a patient's understanding or appreciation of his or her problem and its relationship to symptoms would diminish the somaticizing of emotions, and consequently reduce medical visits. This speculation is in keeping with the experiences of providing psychotherapy under national health care in Great Britain (Balint, 1957). Perhaps a less satisfactory but an equally plausible hypothesis might be that the patient attained no mastery over his problems and that after the psychological visit he found ways other than visiting the doctor to express emotional distress. The present eight-year follow-up tried to clarify the effect of brief psychotherapy previously reported.

It is important to describe the setting in which the past and present studies were conducted. The Kaiser Foundation Health Plan of Northern California is a group-practice prepayment plan offering comprehensive hospital and professional services on a direct-service basis to 1,250,000 subscribers in the greater San Francisco Bay Area. Professional services are provided by the Permanente Medical Group, a partnership of physicians that uniquely and effectively utilizes an impressive number of non-medical doctors (such as clinical psychologists and optometrists) as primary health service providers. The San Francisco Kaiser Permanente Medical Center, where the studies were conducted, is one of ten centers in the San Francisco Bay Area offering direct and indirect mental health services. Its staff of six clinical psychologists, four psychiatrists, and two psychiatric social workers reflects the fact that throughout the Northern California facilities it is typically the nonmedical and particularly the psychological personnel that provide the bulk of the psychotherapy and consultation. Working on an equal patient-responsibility level with their psychiatric colleagues, clinical psychologists and psychiatric social workers assume full responsibility for their patients; admit and discharge from the hospital; provide consultation for nonpsychiatric physicians and consultation in the general hospital; participate in twenty-four-hour "on call" duty; and make determinations of mental health emergencies (such as suicidal attempts and acute psychotic episodes) appearing at night in the emergency room of the general hospital. The ability of a psychologist or social worker to function effectively as a primary health service provider with full patient responsibility is a condition of employment at Kaiser Permanente, San Francisco.

As the original health maintenance organization (HMO), one of the heretofore unique aspects of this setting is that it tends to put a premium on health rather than on illness, by making preventative medicine economically rewarding. The same principle holds true for the delivery of mental health services where there is a constant search for the most effective and specific methods of treatment. Consequently, effective cost-therapeutic techniques have been developed for the treatment of alcoholism, suicidal activity, drug abuse, heroin addiction, and a variety of other conditions often excluded from insurance coverage. To deny psychotherapeutic intervention in these problems merely results in having to medically and surgically treat their expensive physical consequences. On the other hand, traditional intake procedures, waiting lists, and protracted therapies have been eliminated in favor of rapid, immediate intervention with individual and group psychotherapy, which is most often relatively brief, but which occurs in programs specifically designed to promote maximum patient recovery to his effective state. All therapists perform long-term psychotherapy when indicated, but other dynamic modalities are most often the treatment of choice.

The present study investigated the question of whether the reduction in outpatient and inpatient medical utilization following brief psychotherapeutic intervention reflects a positive, or therapeutically defined change in the patient's behavior. The hypothesis can be stated simply: if the reduction in medical utilization is the result of the patient's having coped more effectively with emotional distress, then the presenting symptom (called the "manifest problem") should disappear, and the patient should have an awareness of the real or underlying concern that produced his or her symptom.

The psychotherapy charts of the eighty patients seen for one session only and the forty-one patients seen for brief therapy (a total of 121 patients seen eight years previously) were drawn and reviewed for the following information obtained from the psychotherapists' notes:

1. What is presenting symptom, problem, or "manifest" reason why patient was referred or is here?

2. What is the underlying psychological reason for patient's symptom, problem, or complaint?

3. Did the therapist suggest that patient return, or did he or she ask patient to return? Did patient express an interest in returning? Did patient make return appointment?

4. From the therapist's notes, did you get the feeling that anything was dealt with by the patient that would be of value? Was patient unduly resistive, angry; or was patient friendly, impressed?

This information was necessary as background orientation for a telephone questionnaire conducted by a master's-level psychology assistant. Whenever possible each patient, when located, was individually interviewed. It was not possible to locate all patients after eight years, as over 50 percent of each group were no longer members of the health plan, a typical situation in the highly mobile California labor force. Meticulous tracing, often out of state and sometimes as far away as the East Coast, resulted in telephone contact with fifty-six of the eighty one-session-only group, and thirty-one of the forty-one brief-psychotherapy group. The telephone interviewers employed the following questionnaire as a guide:

Telephone Call to Patient
(Try to record extensively patient's exact words.)
I am _____, a psychologist at Kaiser Permanente. We are following up on some of the people we saw sometime back, and would like to know how you are getting along.

1. Do you remember your appointment or visit with a psychotherapist? How long ago was it?

2. Do you remember whom you saw?

3. How did you know of our service? Did a doctor refer you, or did you ask for a referral?

4. What was the reason you consulted a psychotherapist? (If patient says something to the effect that "my doctor wanted me to go," try to elicit the reason [such as symptom, complaint, problem] why the doctor thought the referral a good idea. We are interested here in what the patient remembers, whether he focuses on the manifest problem or the psychological problem.)

5. What do you recall was discussed with your psychotherapist (if this has not been spelled out in No. 4 above)?

6. Do you feel the visit with a psychotherapist was of any benefit to you? If so, how? If not, why not?

7. How have you been getting along? (Here if the patient has not recalled the manifest symptom or complaint, remind him and ask about it. If he has not recalled the psychological problem that was discussed, remind him and ask about it.)

In the telephone interviews the researchers were interested in whether the patient recalled the presenting symptom (manifest problem) as the reason for having consulted a psychotherapist, or whether, instead, he or she remembered the actual focus and direction taken by the therapist in bringing to awareness the patient's real concern as the reason for the consultation. Of importance, also, was the patient's own perception of the degree of help derived from the single consultation or brief series of sessions. Of the eighty-seven patients located and interviewed, only two refused to cooperate. A third who initially refused cooperation changed her mind after verifying the legitimate nature of the research project.

All 85 patients contacted and who were diagnosed in terms of anxieties, phobias, somaticization, depression, and psychosis in their presenting problems could readily be categorized in terms of the actual problem that was creating the symptom, and on the basis of even one interview. They could be classified as marital difficulties, problems with children or pregnancy, alcohol or drugs, job problems, and so forth, and all cut across psychodiagnostic categories. The therapist was quick in eliciting the patient's immediate life problem, but it must be emphasized that often he was also able to formulate for the patient the immediate crisis in terms of his dominant psychological dynamics and life-style. This formulation was made without fostering long-term dependency or plans for a complete personality overhaul, and within the context of immediate, brief, incisive therapeutic intervention.

The telephone interviews found that although all but one of the eighty-five persons responding remembered seeing a psychotherapist, only two could recall the therapist's name. There was a tendency to underestimate the eight years elapsed since the last session, with "two or three years ago" being the response in almost 60 percent of the cases. The patients were nearly equally divided between those who recalled being referred by a physician (forty-four) and those who were self-referred, or by the spouse, a relative or a friend (forty-one).

The crucial question was whether the patient remembered the manifest or the actual problem in recalling the interview. The results are unequivocal, for seventy-eight patients, or 92 percent, recalled the problem discussed (marital, familial, job, and so forth) rather than the presenting symptom as the reason for the referral. In fact, when these seventy-eight patients were asked directly about the presenting symptom (such as, "Did you ever have severe headaches?"), all but five denied ever having consulted a doctor for such a complaint. Thus the patient seems to have understood that the problem was more "real" than the symptom.

In view of the latter finding, it is somewhat surprising that the patients generally felt their psychotherapeutic contact had not been helpful. This trend existed in spite of the response that they were getting along well and had either resolved the psychological conflict or were coping with the problem. The responses elicited were as follows:

	Yes	No
1. Do you feel the visit with the "psychiatrist" was of any benefit to you?	9	76

	Well	Not well
2. How have you been getting along (in regard to the psychological problem)?	83	2

The patients tended to attribute their coping with the problem to their own, rather than the therapist's solution, with "I just worked it out" being the frequent answer. On further consideration, this finding need not be surprising, as real insight becomes part of the patient's own belief system.

In several instances the patient reported being very angry with the psychotherapist, but in each case the patient added, "He made me so mad I realized I had to solve this myself." Two illustrative cases might be helpful.

CASE 1

Mrs. W., age thirty-nine, married sixteen years, with three children, was referred by her internist for severe headaches that had become less and less responsive to medication for the past ten months. She was seen by a psychologist three times, during which time her anger at her husband (whom she reluctantly said was seeing his secretary) was discussed, along with her feelings of being old at thirty-nine and unattractive. Between the second and third sessions she blew up at her husband, put her foot down regarding his staying out at night, and was surprised to find he was remorseful and eager to make amends. On telephone interview eight years later she denied ever having suffered from severe headaches, and recalled clearly that she consulted a psychotherapist for a marital problem. She did not find the sessions helpful, and stated flatly that she and husband worked it all out and they have been happier than ever.

CASE 2

Mrs. S., age fifty-four, office worker, divorced after one year of marriage at age forty-seven, has no children, and lives alone. She was diagnosed as an involutional psychotic after being referred by her internist for delusions in which her neighbor was wiring her house to kill her with electricity. She saw the psychiatrist only once and left in a rage when, after discussing her lifelong loneliness, isolation and feelings of uselessness, he suggested she was envious of a neighbor woman's happy marriage, her four older children, and her new baby. On telephone interview eight years later she expressed frank hostility toward her psychiatrist and was outspoken in stating he made her worse. On the other hand, she recalled discussing her loneliness, denied ever having had her delusion, and insisted the neighbor had always been her best friend. In fact, the patient was the neighbor's frequent and only babysitter and had become "like a member of the family." At the conclusion of the interview she could not resist adding heatedly that "psychiatry is bunk; they try to make lonely people think they're crazy."

The results suggest that the reduction in medical utilization was the consequence of resolving the emotional distress being reflected in symptoms and doctors' visits. The modal patient in this eighth-year follow-up may be described as follows: "He denies ever having consulted a physician for the symptoms for which he had been originally referred. Rather, he recalls the actual problem discussed as the reason for the "psychiatric" visit, and although he reports the problem is resolved, he attributes this to his own efforts and does not give credit to his psychotherapist." This description reaffirms the contention that the reduced medical utilization reflected the diminished emotional distress expressed in symptoms presented to the doctor.

The findings suggest that the expectations of the therapist influence the outcome of psychotherapy, for if the first interview is merely "eval-uation" or "intake," not much of therapeutic value is likely to occur in the first interview. If the therapist's attitude is that no real help is forth-coming from less than prolonged "intensive" psychotherapy, he may be right (for his own patients). Malan (1963), in his classic study of brief psychotherapy, was able to examine honestly the prejudices of his group of psychiatrists about brief therapy and the kinds of benefit possible, the kinds of patients who could utilize it, the permanency of the results, and so forth. He concluded that traditional attitudes about very brief therapy were mostly in the nature of unjustified prejudices. It would appear that therapeutic effects of brief therapy that can be labeled "transference cure," "flight into health," "intellectualization," and other derogatory terms can often be long-lasting and result in a major change in the person's symptoms, relationships, and even life-style. Many of the patients in this study would undoubtedly be called "poorly motivated for treatment" or "dropouts from therapy" in many psy-chotherapy clinics.

Immediacy of availability and treatment is probably a very important aspect of this study. The results tend to support the crisis-clinic thesis that a great deal more can be done in less time during a time of emo-tional disturbance than during a period when a patient is relatively comfortable (such as often occurs after being on a waiting list for sev-eral months). The lack of "intake procedure" and the beginning of psy-chotherapeutic intervention in the first interview—sometimes even in the waiting room before the first interview—are probably crucial in obtaining psychotherapeutic results in a minimum amount of time and maintaining cost-effectiveness as well.

Should Healthcare Keep the Psychological and the Medical Separate?

Although I was hired to help with the problem of somatizers at Kaiser, at times I was even going against my boss, Sidney Garfield, who had brought me to Kaiser. He wanted two different systems— the psychological and the medical. He wanted to use the automated multiphasic screening system to identify whether a patient had a psychological problem or a medical one. If it was a psychological problem, the patient would go to that area, and not to the medical treatment system.

My point of view was that healthcare should always be integrated, and that having two separate systems was not going to work. We now know that there is a 60 percent overlap of medical and psychological issues in healthcare, and that by treating the psychological problems properly, the medical problems can be ameliorated, and a great deal of money and time saved. We have proved this with our research, and others have replicated this finding.

David Mechanic, an academic psychologist, wrote about this overlap of medical and psychological issues shortly after our early research at Kaiser. He said he believed that the overlap was 90 percent, and it may be as much as that.

L. T.: If I were a psychologist working in such a setting at that time, would I be working with six doctors and have a few specialties?

N. C.: Essentially, yes. In the Back Pain Clinic, for example, there would not be an orthopedic surgeon because, of course, orthopedic surgeons like to operate. Also, the six people you would be working with would not necessarily be M.D.'s. There might be two nurses, and some other health professionals.

{ 5 }

PROLONGED (IDEAL) VERSUS SHORT-TERM (REALISTIC) PSYCHOTHERAPY

It is argued that not only can psychotherapy be included economically in a prepaid insurance plan such as national health insurance, but also that the failure to include psychotherapy in prepaid insurance schemes would deprive a substantial proportion of patients (with emotional as opposed to organic etiology) of the benefits they might enjoy under such plans. A series of studies examining the outcomes of therapy of varying durations showed that the cost of the psychotherapy was more than offset by the savings in medical visits. A cost–therapeutic-effectiveness index shows that it is not the provision of a mental health component that determines optimal cost–therapeutic effectiveness but the manner in which psychotherapeutic services are delivered. It is shown also that for the vast majority of patients studied, innovative short-term psychotherapy is more effective than long-term psychotherapy.

AS WE APPROACH the inevitable enactment of national health care in the United States, there is occurring within the larger context of the pros and cons of national health insurance itself a heated debate as to whether any national health scheme can feasibly include a mental health component. The dubious experiences of Medicaid, Medicare, and the Civilian Health and Medical Program of the Uniformed Services (CHAMPUS) have left some members of the Congress with the conclusion that the inclusion of mental health would disproportionately overinflate what is already expected to become a staggering price tag for providing even the basics of a national health system. Several prominent psychologists who themselves have never been engaged in the direct delivery of human services, Albee, Campbell (see Trotter, 1976), and Humphreys (1973), have thrown their persuasiveness solidly against the inclusion of psychotherapy in a national health insurance program. They argue that such a service cannot be financed or monitored, that it is a "subsidy of the rich by the poor," or that the insurance benefit would be of doubtful value in the overall health of the American people. Others, principally the author and his colleague (Cummings, 1975; Cummings & Follette, 1976), have taken the opposite stance, based on 20 years of providing mental health services within a comprehensive, prepaid health plan. They have found that not only can psychotherapy be economically included as a prepaid insurance benefit but also failure to provide such a benefit jeopardizes the effective functioning of the basic medical services, because 60% or more visits to physicians are by patients who demonstrate an emotional, rather than an organic, etiology for their physical symptoms.

To summarize the above-mentioned series of articles by the author and his colleague, it was found that providing psychotherapy was not only economically feasible, in that the cost of the psychotherapy was more than offset by the savings in medical visits, but also through an 8-year follow-up it was demonstrated that the service was therapeutically effective in maintaining the emotional well-being of the patient for years after the psychotherapy had been provided. A cost–therapeutic-effectiveness index emerges, with the inescapable conclusion that it is not the provision of a mental health component that determines optimal cost–therapeutic effectiveness, but the manner in which psychotherapeutic services are delivered. Unfortunately, proponents of the inclusion of psychotherapy in a national health insurance program have often misread the so-called "Cummings–Follette effect" to be valid even when psychotherapy is delivered in strictly traditional ways, which is definitely not the case. And even more unfortunately, very little attention has been paid to the actual delivery modalities that would render a mental health benefit cost-effective and therapeutically effective, not only within a national health insurance program but within any comprehensive, prepaid health system, whether public or private.

In the brief space allotted, this article attempts to tantalize the reader with the following conclusions, which have emerged from 20 years of experience in providing psychotherapy within a prepaid, comprehensive health plan of several million subscribers: (a) All persons presenting themselves with emotional complaints and problems in living can be treated immediately with psychotherapy without preselection criteria; (b) for 85% of these unselected persons, active, innovative short-term psychotherapy is more effective than long-term psychotherapy; (c) for 5%–6% of these patients, long-term psychotherapy will actually be deleterious; and (d) by providing short-term therapy as the treatment of choice for 85% of all patients seen, long-term psychotherapy becomes economically feasible for the 10% of the patients for whom long-term psychotherapy is necessary and most effective.

OTHER MODALITIES

Before proceeding to the topic of short-term psychotherapy, it is important to touch on two other modalities under serious consideration by various proponents. The first of these is the ominous plan by some segments of organized psychiatry to "remedicalize" psychotherapy. Under such a proposal, a national health insurance program or any health system, public or private, would insure only the organic brain syndromes and functional psychoses, excluding the psychoneuroses and character disorders as being outside the definition of insurable illness. This proposal would reduce the cost of providing psychotherapy by drastically reducing the number of persons eligible. It would further guarantee income to psychiatrists who, as medical practitioners, would be the only persons eligible to provide what is then defined as a medical service. This obviously leaves psychology in a vulnerable position, but even more important, it deprives the majority of Americans suffering from emotional distress of access to treatment.

Of demonstrated effectiveness are the community mental health centers, whose primary limitation is that of cost. Various audits have revealed the cost per unit of service to range from about $60 to a staggering $345 in one center, with a modal cost per unit of service of around $75 to $80 as representative of most centers. Despite the potentially inordinate cost, the National Institute of Mental Health (NIMH) continues to champion the community mental health center concept as the mainstay of the mental health delivery system under a national health insurance program. This is understandable, since NIMH spawned the community mental health center movement; but most authorities have retrenched from the overly ambitious goal of the original Kennedy plan that there eventually be a mental health center in every community. The present author believes that because of their relative effectiveness, the inordinate cost of the centers can still be justified in underserved areas of the nation under a national health insurance program.

A BRIEF HISTORY OF SHORT-TERM PSYCHOTHERAPY

The concept of brief psychotherapy is not new and may be said to date back to Alexander and French (1946). Unfortunately, these authors conceived of the process as a short form of orthodox psychoanalysis, and they touched off such a furor that short-term psychotherapy was plunged into general disrepute. It was not until the classic study of Malan (1963) that brief psychotherapy received unbiased research attention. Perhaps prompted by the necessity to provide mental health services under Britain's national health system, Malan examined the traditional attitudes of psychotherapists toward brief psychotherapy and found them to be mostly in the nature of unjustified prejudices. He found that properly selected patients could achieve long-lasting benefit from brief psychotherapy and that short-term treatment often resulted in major changes in the person's symptoms, relationships, and even life-style.

In the United States the work of Malan (1963) was essentially ignored. Clinics continued the attempt to provide long-term psychotherapy for everyone, and waiting lists of 6 months were standard and 1 year, frequent. The dropout rate was high, but this was accepted as inevitable. The emergence of crisis centers, partly as an effort to provide immediate, brief care to cases regarded as emergencies, did little to alter the prejudice for long-term psychotherapy. It was only conceded that brief therapy might be useful in crisis situations, but it was superficial, supportive, and lacked the dynamic elements that could only take place within the context of long-term treatment. In his most recent studies, Malan (1976) demonstrates what some clinicians have known for some time: Brief psychotherapy can be active and have all the elements of depth attributed to long-term therapy, including the resolution of unconscious conflicts and the analysis of resistance and transference. Unfortunately, Malan (1976) still employed selection criteria for those patients undergoing brief, rather than long-term, therapy. Such selection criteria have been dubbed by Kissen, Platz, & Su (1976) "exclusion criteria," in that they serve as an adverse selection for ethnic minorities, the underprivileged, and the aged.

THE KAISER PERMANENTE STUDIES

Before the first Malan report (1963), and between that and the second report (1976), the work at Kaiser Permanente was demonstrating that psychotherapy could be provided as an insurance benefit to everyone, without preselection criteria. Kaiser Permanente experimented with a number of attempts to provide long-term therapy for all its members who manifested emotional distress. This effort began with an initial bias that short-term psychotherapy is not as effective as long-term psychotherapy. It was additionally burdened with the discovery that providing easily available comprehensive health services as part of a prepaid plan fostered the somatization of emotional problems, with the consequent overutilization of medical facilities by patients who had no physical illness. The Kaiser Permanente effort caused a number of problems (which were present in most traditional clinics of the time); these problems included a long waiting list, a high dropout rate, and an only partially successful attempt to reduce the ever-growing waiting list by providing crisis intervention. It was not until a series of evaluative studies were begun, spanning 15 years, that an efficient, cost–therapeutically effective treatment system emerged. The following is a brief summary of this research.

In the first of a series of investigations into the relationship between psychological services and medical utilization in a prepaid health plan setting, Follette and Cummings (1967) compared the number and type of medical services sought before and after the intervention of psychotherapy in a large group of randomly selected patients. The outpatient and inpatient medical utilization for the year prior to the initial interview in the Department of Psychotherapy, as well as for the 5 years following, was studied for three groups of psychotherapy patients (those who had one interview only, those who underwent brief therapy with a mean of 6.2 interviews, and those who received long-term therapy with a mean of 33.9 interviews) and a control group of matched patients demonstrating similar criteria of distress but not seen in psychotherapy in the 6 years under study. The findings indicated that (a) persons in emotional distress were significantly higher users of both inpatient and outpatient medical facilities as compared to the health plan average; (b) there were significant declines in medical utilization in those emotionally distressed individuals who received psychotherapy as compared to a control group of matched emotionally distressed health plan members who were not accorded psychotherapy; (c) these declines remained constant during the 5 years following the termination of psychotherapy; (d) the most significant declines occurred in the second year after the initial interview, and those patients receiving one session only or brief psychotherapy (two to eight sessions) did not require additional psychotherapy to maintain the lower level of utilization for 5 years; and (e) patients seen 2 years or more in regular psychotherapy demonstrated no overall decline in total outpatient utilization, inasmuch as psychotherapy visits tended to supplant medical visits. However, there was a significant decline in inpatient utilization in the long-term therapy group, from an initial hospitalization rate several times that of the health plan average to a level comparable to that of the general adult health plan population.

In a subsequent study, Cummings and Follette (1968) found that intensive efforts to increase the number of referrals to psychotherapy by computerizing psychological screening, with early detection and alerting of the attending physicians, did not increase significantly the number of patients seeking psychotherapy. The authors concluded that in a prepaid health plan setting already maximally employing educative techniques for both patients and physicians and already providing a range of prepaid psychological services, the number of health plan subscribers seeking psychotherapy reaches an optimal level and remains fairly constant thereafter.

In summarizing 16 years of prepaid experience, Cummings and Follette (1968) demonstrated that there is no basis for the fear that an increased demand for psychotherapy will financially endanger the system, for it is not the number of referrals received that will drive costs up but the manner in which psychotherapy services are delivered that determines optimal cost–therapeutic effectiveness. The finding that one session only, with no repeat psychological visits, can reduce medical utilization by 60% over the following 5 years was surprising and totally unexpected. Equally surprising was the 75% reduction in medical utilization over a 5-year period in those patients initially receiving two to eight psychotherapy sessions (brief therapy).

In a further study, Cummings and Follette (1976) sought to determine in an 8-year telephone follow-up whether the results described previously were a therapeutic effect, the consequence of extraneous factors, or a deleterious effect. It was hypothesized that if better understanding of his or her problem had occurred in the psychotherapeutic sessions, the patient would recall the actual problem rather than the presenting symptom and would have both lost the presenting symptom and coped more effectively with the real problem.

The results suggest that the reduction in medical utilization was the consequence of resolving the emotional distress that was being reflected in physical symptoms and visits to the doctor. The modal patient in this 8-year follow-up may be described as follows: He or she denies ever having consulted a physician for the physical symptoms for which he or she had been originally referred. Rather, the actual problem discussed with the psychotherapist is recalled as the reason for the "psychiatric" visit, and although the problem is resolved, this resolution is attributed to the patient's own efforts and no credit is given the psychotherapist. This affirms the contention that the reduction in medical utilization reflected the diminution in the emotional distress which had been expressed in symptoms that were presented to the physician.

COST–THERAPEUTIC-EFFECTIVENESS RATIO

Demonstrating that savings in medical services offset the cost of providing psychotherapy answers the question of cost effectiveness, but the services provided must also be therapeutic, that is, they must reduce the patient's emotional distress. That both cost *and* therapeutic effectiveness were demonstrated in the Kaiser Permanente studies was attributed by the investigators to the therapist's expectation that emotional distress could be alleviated by brief, active psychotherapy that involved the analysis of transference and resistance and the uncovering of unconscious conflicts, and had all the characteristics of long-term therapy except length. Given this orientation, it was found over a 5-year period that 84.6% of the patients seen in psychotherapy chose to come 15 sessions or less, with a mean of 8.6, and rather than regarding these as "dropouts" from treatment, it was found on follow-up that they had achieved a satisfactory state of emotional well-being that continued to the 8-year follow-up. This finding is in total agreement with Malan's (1976) Tavistock studies, with the exception that Kaiser Permanente used no preselection criteria but saw every patient who presented him/herself for treatment without regard to such factors as age, motivation, or duration and severity of symptoms.

The serendipitous finding that therapeutic outcome correlates highly with reduction in medical utilization is understandable in view of the earlier findings that in a prepaid, comprehensive health system the physician's lack of empathy for symptoms of emotional distress encourages the patient to somatize the distress, for which the reward is the physician's interest and attention. Complaining to one's physician that "my boss is on my back" usually elicits impatience from the medical doctor, whereas a low back pain results in X-rays, laboratory visits, consultations with specialists, and return visits. But in addition, this finding yields a reliable, quantifiable index of therapeutic effectiveness that does not suffer from the subjectivity of most criteria. By dividing the medical utilization for the full year prior to psychotherapy (as calculated by Follette and Cummings in their 1967 study) by the medical utilization for the full year following the initial psychotherapy visit *plus* the year's number of such visits yields this ratio of cost–therapeutic effectiveness:

$$\frac{\text{Medical utilization for year before}}{\text{Medical utilization for year after} + \text{Number of psychotherapy visits}} = \text{Ratio of cost–therapeutic effectiveness}$$

The higher the ratio, the greater is the effectiveness of therapy. Separate ratios can be calculated for inpatient (hospital) and outpatient utilization, or they can be combined by using a cost-weighting factor for the days of hospitalization.

WHEN IS LONG-TERM THERAPY DELETERIOUS?

At Kaiser Permanente the cost–therapeutic-effectiveness ratios for various populations are these: (a) very brief psychotherapy, comprising 56% of all patients (1 to 4 sessions, with a mean of 3.8), 2.59; (b) brief psychotherapy, comprising 84.6% of all patients (1 to 15 sessions, with a mean of 8.6), 2.11; (c) long-term psychotherapy, comprising 10.1% of all patients (more than 16 sessions, with a mean of 19.2), 1.14; (d) "interminable" psychotherapy, comprising 5.3% of all patients (with special characteristics described below and with a mean of 47.9 sessions per year), .91; and (e) a matched control sample of patients in distress not receiving psychotherapy, .88. The "interminable" patient, though reducing inpatient utilization from several times that of the health plan average to average, merely supplanted frequent outpatient medical visits with weekly psychotherapy, resulting in a cost–therapeutic-effectiveness ratio not significantly better than that of the control group. This population became a concern of the researchers that was the basis for further investigation. In studying the clinical characteristics of these patients, it was found that they manifested a pan-anxiety and closely fitted the diagnostic entity of pseudoneurotic schizophrenia. Once this population and its characteristics were identified, the researchers undertook the broader problem of how to provide a cost–therapeutically effective treatment.

Beginning with an understandable but unwarranted preconception, it was postulated that increasing the intensity (frequency) of the treatment would bring the psychotherapy of these "interminable" patients to an early and successful conclusion. Further defined, the problem seemed to be one of finding the optimal increase in intensity that would prove cost–therapeutically effective. Therefore, a new group of patients presenting themselves for psychotherapy, who demonstrated all of the characteristics of the "interminable" subgroup, were divided into once-a-week, twice-a-week, and three-times-a-week psychotherapy. All had the same diagnosis, and there was an attempt to match them on demographic characteristics. The outpatient and inpatient medical utilization of these patients was studied for the year before and each of the two years following the initial psychotherapy visit. There were 23 patients; 2 withdrew from the clinic prior to the conclusion of the research, leaving 21 experimental patients. This was the sum total of such patients who presented themselves for psychotherapy during a 6-month period. None were excluded, except the 2 aforementioned patients who left the clinic. Since that time a replication with a larger sample was begun, and preliminary results are comparable to those reported here.

Although the investigators anticipated a dramatic initial rise in combined utilization (medical plus psychotherapy visit) because of the doubling and tripling of the frequency of psychotherapy visits, they were not prepared for (a) a concomitant rise in outpatient medical utilization with (b) a failure to rapidly conclude psychotherapy, even within the 2 years of the study. Further, the largest concomitant increase in outpatient medical utilization was demonstrated by the three-times-a-week psychotherapy patients, with the lowest outpatient medical utilization being found in the one-time-a-week psychotherapy patients. As can be seen in Table 1, the combined (outpatient medical *plus* psychotherapy) utilization strongly suggests that a different method of managing and treating these patients may be indicated.

In studying the data it was observed that 2 patients, one each in the two-times-a-week and three-times-a-week psychotherapy groups, had failed to keep a majority of their appointments, and this resulted in an average number of psychotherapy visits even below the average for the one-time-a-week psychotherapy group. Surprisingly, these 2 patients had the lowest outpatient medical utilization. The question remained whether these 2 patients just generally did not seek physician visits or whether the planned reduced frequency of psychotherapy visits resulted in the reduction in outpatient medical utilization (all doctors' visits other than psychotherapy).

Table 1. *Averages of Outpatient Medical Visits Only, Psychotherapy Visits Only, and Combined Averages (Outpatient Medical plus Psychotherapy Visits) for the "Interminable" Subgroup Under Three Conditions of Pyschotherapeutic Frequency for the Year Before and the 2 Years After the Initial Psychotherapy Visit*

Condition	No. of Patients	1-B[a]	1-A[b]	2-A[c]
Outpatient medical visits				
One time a week	8	11.2	6.5	7.2
Two times a week	6	12.4	15.1	15.6
Three times a week	7	11.8	18.2	17.4
Psychotherapy visits				
One time a week	8	—	39.3	41.7
Two times a week	6	—	77.2	78.6
Three times a week	7	—	117.9	114.3
Combined outpatient medical and psychotherapy visits				
One time a week	8	11.2	45.8	48.9
Two times a week	6	12.4	92.3	94.2
Three times a week	7	11.8	136.1	131.7

[a] 1-B = One year before initial psychotherapy visit.
[b] 1-A = One year after initial psychotherapy visit.
[c] 2-A = Two years after initial psychotherapy visit.

The investigators decided to initiate drastically curtailed frequencies of psychotherapy visits in the same patients who had been seen once, twice, and three times a week. Beginning in the third year *after* the initial psychotherapy visit, and with the cooperation of the psychotherapists, the patients were seen at 30-, 60-, and 90-day intervals. Because of therapists' resistance, less than half of the patients were placed in the new spacing, leaving the remainder to serve as a contrasting group. Again, to the surprise of the investigators, the drastically reduced frequency of psychotherapy visits resulted in significantly reduced outpatient medical utilization (all doctor visits excluding psychotherapy), with the 30-, 60-, and 90-day frequencies being equally effective, perhaps because the patients were essentially permitted to self-select the exact curtailed frequency. These results are shown in Table 2.

Table 2. *Averages of Outpatient Medical Visits Only, Psychotherapy Visits Only, and Combined Averages (Outpatient Medical Plus Psychotherapy Visits) for the "Interminable" Subgroup in Its Third Year After Initiation of Psychotherapy Under Four Conditions of Frequency of Psychotherapy Visits*

Condition	No. of Patients	3-A*
Outpatient medical visits		
1–3 times a week	11	13.7
Monthly	3	5.6
Bimonthly	3	5.0
Quarterly	4	5.8
Psychotherapy visits		
1–3 times a week	11	64.8
Monthly	3	10.2
Bimonthly	3	5.1
Quarterly	4	3.6
Combined outpatient medical and psychotherapy visits		
1–3 times a week	11	78.5
Monthly	3	15.8
Bimonthly	3	10.1
Quarterly	4	9.4

*3-A = Third year after initiation of psychotherapy.

SUMMARY

A decade and a half of clinical experience and research at Kaiser Permanente has demonstrated that not only can psychotherapy be economically provided in a comprehensive, prepaid health system but failure to do so places a cost burden on medical facilities by the 60% of the physician visits made by patients who demonstrate emotional rather than organic symptoms. Reduction in medical utilization by such patients correlates with effective therapy, rendering a quantifiable measure of therapeutic outcome. Effective treatment must demonstrate both economic feasibility and therapeutic success, and a method of eliciting a cost–therapeutic-effectiveness ratio is described.

The Single-Session Misunderstanding

At Kaiser, we found that many patients benefited from a single session of therapy, and this is reported in the 1967 and 1968 articles. When Moshe Talmon came to Kaiser to do his internship, he took this idea of "single session" psychotherapy and later expanded it into his book on this subject. Of course, this can be misleading, even though there is legitimacy to the fact that a single session can be quite beneficial for certain people. Unfortunately, some psychologists started warning our colleagues that managed care would be expecting therapists to have single-session treatment strategies. Indeed, sometimes there are single-session treatments that can be the right thing for some patients, but this should not be interpreted too broadly. It is for those who choose a single session that the benefits can be significant.

Bernard Bloom also developed a single-session psychotherapy, except that sometimes his sessions lasted as long as five hours! I question whether one can call five hours a single session.

{ 6 }

THE ANATOMY OF PSYCHOTHERAPY
UNDER NATIONAL HEALTH INSURANCE

ABSTRACT: *Experience has demonstrated that when all barriers to medical care are removed, the medical model encourages somatization, and medical facilities become overburdened by the 60% of physician visits that are from sufferers of emotional distress rather than organic illness. When psychotherapy is properly provided within a comprehensive health system, the costs of providing the benefit are more than offset by the savings in medical utilization. Furthermore, it is not the provision of a psychotherapy benefit that can bankrupt a system, as has occurred in a number of programs, but the manner in which the service is delivered that makes the difference for cost–therapeutic effectiveness. Finally, cost-therapeutically effective programs can be developed for problems in living that traditionally have been regarded as too resistant and, therefore, too costly to be insurable. The implications for national health insurance are that the inclusion of an appropriate, realistic psychotherapy benefit is both essential and economically feasible.*

As THE CARTER administration evidences serious concern for the mental and emotional well-being of the American people, there is occurring within the larger context of the pros and cons of national health insurance a heated debate as to whether any national health scheme can feasibly include a mental health component. The dubious experiences of Medicaid, Medicare, and CHAMPUS have left some members of the Congress with the conclusion that the inclusion of a mental health provision in whatever national health system is eventually enacted would overinflate what is already contemplated to be a staggering price tag to provide even the basics of national health insurance. Several prominent psychologists, including two past presidents of the American Psychological Association, who have never been engaged in the direct delivery of human services (Albee, 1977; Campbell, cited in Trotter, 1976; Humphreys, 1973), have thrown their persuasiveness solidly against the inclusion of psychotherapy in national health insurance. They argue that such a service cannot be financed or monitored, that it is a subsidy of the rich by the poor, and that the insurance benefit would be of doubtful value to the overall health of the American people. Others, principally myself and my colleague (Cummings, 1975, 1975; Cummings & Follette, 1976), have taken the opposite stance based on two decades of providing mental health services within a comprehensive, prepaid health plan. We have found not only that psychotherapy can be economically included as a prepaid insurance benefit but also that failure to provide such a benefit jeopardizes the effective functioning of the basic medical services, since 60% or more of the physician visits are made by patients who demonstrate an emotional, rather than an organic, etiology for their physical symptoms.

Despite extensive misquotations to the contrary, Follette and I have never advocated mere across-the-board inclusion of traditional delivery modalities of mental health services into public or third-party payment structures. Rather, we have argued that for psychotherapy to be cost-therapeutically effective, considerable clinical research is necessary before abuses are minimized, therapeutic benefits are maximized, traditionally underserved groups are reached, and deleterious effects are eliminated. It is by addressing the problems confronting the delivery of psychotherapy under public and third-party payment that the anatomy of psychotherapy under national health insurance will be developed and accepted as efficacious by the Congress and the consumer. The failure by the mental health professions to take a proactive research stance may result in the elimination of mental health services from national health insurance or, even worse, may result in the provision of an ineffective token benefit that will only underscore the argument that psychotherapy is an unnecessary service. Before proceeding to this basic issue, it is important to examine arguments made by the opponents of psychotherapy's inclusion in national health insurance, inasmuch as they have presented some warnings that have rightfully commanded the attention of consumer groups and the Congress.

WARNING: THE REVERSE ROBIN HOOD PHENOMENON

The fact that, traditionally, psychotherapy was sought by the more affluent sectors of our society while the underprivileged tended not to utilize such services has prompted some critics, such as Campbell (cited in Trotter, 1976), to view the inclusion of psychotherapy in national health insurance as regressive taxation or, even more harshly, as a "subsidy of the rich by the poor." Simply stated, this view holds that by taxing all of the American people to provide a benefit applicable to a select segment such as the upper-middle class, the benefit is being paid for by the poor, who are least likely to utilize the service and are least able to afford the subsidy. By itself, this position is not totally persuasive, because, as Campbell would be the first to admit, many of our most valued institutions are financed by regressive taxation. The state university system is a case in point. No one would seriously argue the elimination of the state university, but many are striving to make the university more accessible to eligible persons from groups that have traditionally underutilized it. The same would hold true for a mental health benefit if, in fact, it were a valuable service to all of the segments of our population who are at risk.

Since medicine in the United States was originally dispensed under the principle that services to the poor are provided by soaking the rich, it is curious to find mental health subject to a reverse Robin Hood phenomenon. Of the recent rash of so-called abuses that have come to light, two may serve as startling examples of the kind of facts that render the Congress uneasy and that ought to serve as warning signs to the profession that restraint and caution are indicated. According to the U.S. Civil Service Commission (1976), under the Blue Cross and Blue Shield Federal Employees Health Benefits Program in the Washington, D.C., greater metropolitan area, for the years 1971, 1972, and 1973, 2.3% of those seeking psychotherapy exceeded outpatient costs of $10,000 each per year and accounted for approximately one fourth of the total annual psychotherapy dollar. Furthermore, these same 2.3% of utilizers in the District of Columbia area accounted for 66% of the *national* figure spent by Blue Cross and Blue Shield for the over-$10,000-per-year utilizers in the Federal Employees Health Benefits Program during this same 3-year period. For psychotherapy to cost over $10,000 per year, one must visit a psychotherapist no less than four times a week for an entire year at $50 per session. One may speculate that Washington is a fertile area for the young psychiatrist who wants a job for 2 or 3 years so as to complete a training analysis at taxpayer expense and then leave Washington for an originally intended private practice, but this is only speculation. This experience prompted Aetna in 1974 to severely limit its psychotherapy benefit and resulted in Blue Cross/Blue Shield's initiating a troublesome claims review that threatens the confidentiality of the therapist–client relationship, the latter in the interest of determining the variables in the apparent overutilization.

The second example is from an unpublished study by Elpers (1977), available through the Orange County (California) Mental Health Department. As a county health officer, Elpers compared the allocation of Medi-Cal (California's Medicaid program) money to private psychiatrists with a state formula of county needs based on Medi-Cal caseload. He found that the dollars follow not the need but the number of psychiatrists practicing within a county, since Medi-Cal reimburses the practitioner on the basis of number of patients seen. It comes as no surprise that psychiatrists tend to congregate in urban areas; thus Marin County, an affluent bedroom community for San Francisco, received 470% of its "needed" share in 1975, while that same year, rural Lake County, with virtually no psychiatrists, received only 2%. In counties like Marin and San Francisco, the latter having received 271% of its "needed" share in 1975, there is a large supply of psychiatrists, and the competition for patients results in Medi-Cal patients' having no trouble in finding a psychotherapist. In underserved counties, the practitioners tend to shun the Medi-Cal recipient in favor of the higher paying, affluent client.

Such problems notwithstanding, California's Medi-Cal figures reveal that 5% of all recipients utilize psychotherapy. This is two-and-one-half times the national average, thus tending to refute the contention by Campbell (cited in Trotter, 1976) and Albee (1977) that the poor do not seek psychotherapy. In fact, there is reason to believe that the poor are at greater risk and will avail themselves of psychotherapy if it is provided in a manner meaningful to the consumer. Such an example is provided by Kaiser Permanente in San Francisco, which has over the past decades taken meticulous care to provide a consumer-oriented, comprehensive health plan. There, psychotherapy is not merely an upper- or middle-class white phenomenon, and subscribers seeking psychotherapy do so in direct proportion to their occupational class numbers in the health plan population. Additionally, black and Chicano clients in psychotherapy are rapidly approaching figures proportional to the numbers of these ethnic groups in the total health plan population. Utilization by Asian Americans lags behind the proportional figures because of the large Chinese population in San Francisco and its traditional resistance to psychotherapy, but the last few years have seen rapid erosion of that resistance, especially in young persons who not only seek services for themselves but bring their parents in when the latter hesitate to come themselves.

Minority and feminist leaders, as well as consumer advocates, have enunciated the limitations of white, middle-class, male psychotherapists, but in attempting to remedy this problem care must be exercised not to substitute a mischief of a different sort. In stressing the indigenous mental health counselor as an alternative, these leaders are not truly expressing the attitudes of their constituents, for the underprivileged resent (and rightly so) receiving care from paraprofessionals while the more affluent have access to journey-level practitioners. The possible exception may be among Native Americans, where the understandable distrust of the white man's "doctor" is pervasive and deeply rooted. Interestingly, when a group practice retains an appropriate balance of minority and female psychotherapists, the consumer demand for a certain kind of therapist tends to disappear. It is almost as if the client senses the awareness of the institution and is confident that his or her problems will receive the appropriate perspective and proper understanding. The poor, the minorities, and women have an inherent right of access to practitioners who are both aware and experienced, and any proposed national health scheme must take this into account.

WARNING: THE NEW MIND–BODY DUALISM

During the past decade, Albee has demonstrated a propensity to anger clinicians, causing them to overlook his contribution as a critic whose consistent illumination of the flaws and foibles of psychotherapy spurs the serious practitioner to strive to improve the state of the art. Perhaps much of the negative reaction stems from the willingness of the semipopular media to carry Albee's arguments the extra few inches into the realm of absurdity, often beyond his own fondest hopes. Thus, Albee can state that he never advocated suspending all psychotherapy until research can verify the art, that he never pronounced clinical psychology dead, and that he does not believe that all professional societies are conspiracies against the laity, to name only a few excessive positions variously attributed to him in the press. Yet he was the first to point out that psychology does not practice in its own house but in that of medicine. He has tirelessly assailed the medical model and has held steadfastly to the concept that emotional problems are not illnesses but problems in living.

The difficulty with Albee's view is that it would prevent psychology's participation in the treatment process. Interestingly, the same arguments he employs to arrive at such a conclusion also make the case for the inclusion of psychological services within the health model as opposed to the medical model, a distinction Albee fails to make. Many, if not most, physical illnesses are the result of problems in living. The way we live, eat, drink, smoke, compete, and pollute relate inevitably to strokes, heart attacks, cancer, obesity, malnutrition, paralysis, cirrhosis, migraine, suicide, and asthma, to list only a few. The attempt to clearly demarcate psychological problems from physical illness by calling them problems in living is a curious form of mind–body dualism that would bring an immediate déjà vu were it not cloaked in this new terminology and sanctified with the struggle against medical domination of the health field. Psychological services are more than health, but they must be a part of health, if not the overriding principle, if the medical model is not to continue to encourage the somatization of emotional problems. The way we live influences our bodies; conversely, chronic illness and intractable pain create a problem in living. Psychotherapy is a viable form of intervention that can alleviate problems in living and lessen disease, and it belongs in any comprehensive health system until that utopian moment when preventive techniques render it unnecessary.

WARNING: RESEARCH MAY BE HAZARDOUS TO YOUR HEALTH

Historically, studies of the effectiveness of psychotherapy either have suffered from serious experimental flaws or have yielded negative results. A recent and well-executed review by Olbrisch (1977) appears in another section of this issue. If it were taken completely seriously, every practitioner would lock the office and throw away the key. If taken within the perspective that the flawless experimental design is rarely possible in field research with human subjects, it is a valuable document that can motivate clinical researchers to improve and replicate their work.

In making the valid point that clinical researchers demonstrate greater clinical than experimental sophistication, Olbrisch neglects the fact that the critics of clinical practice and research show a shocking absence of tough clinical experience and a lack of appreciation for the limitations of the clinical method. Needy human beings cannot be denied treatment for the sake of experimental purity, and control groups are seldom more than better or worse approximations. With all of its imperfections, we are dependent upon the clinical method, for in spite of the enormous contributions basic research has rendered, the pure experimental method is often helpless in the face of the most pressing human problems. This is not to imply that perfection in design is not the goal of every researcher, but by and large, the clinical method will continue to be ponderous, inefficient, inaccurate, and vulnerable to severe criticism, but by its sheer persistence and response to pressing demands, the weight of clinical evidence will continue to be the primary vehicle through which the field of health progresses.

So as not to belabor the topic, one example must suffice. To date, the definitive experiment upon which the Surgeon General's warning on each package of cigarettes might be based has not been forthcoming. Rather, the warning is the result of the preponderance of clinical evidence, any *portion* of which can and is being refuted by the tobacco industry. In fact, the tobacco industry has produced flawless research which demonstrates that there is no causal link between smoking and lung cancer in humans. Should the American people, as some have done, ignore the weight of 50 years of increasingly sophisticated clinical evidence in favor of the tobacco industry's excellent but unconvincing experiments, such a decision may well be hazardous to their health.

Some patients who are treated for pneumonia die, while others not treated at all recover. Similarly, the successes and failures of problems in living are not immediately discernible, and clinicians would do well to heed the criticisms of the clinical method and work toward increasing the sophistication of their tools. At no time, however, should a clinician be dismayed that no one research project yields a clear answer, for the clinical method is most persuasive in its preponderance of accumulated evidence, knowledge, and experience.

PROPOSED MODALITIES OF DELIVERY UNDER NATIONAL HEALTH INSURANCE

No matter how effective it may be demonstrated to be, it is unlikely that psychoanalysis or any other open-ended psychotherapy benefit will be provided under national health insurance. Where it has been attempted on a large scale, such as in the Federal Employees Health Benefits Program and CHAMPUS as previously noted, the costs have been prohibitive. Aetna responded by severely limiting the benefit, Blue Cross and Blue Shield are looking toward significantly redefining the benefit, and only CHAMPUS has made a conscientious effort to find innovative answers to the problem of cost-therapeutic effectiveness. The experiences with Medicare and Medicaid have only increased uneasiness within the Congress, and as of this point in time, the proponents of the inclusion of psychotherapy in national health insurance will have to demonstrate its effectiveness.

In response, some segments of organized psychiatry are proposing the "remedicalization" of psychotherapy. Under this ominous plan, national health insurance or any other health system, public or private, would insure only the organic brain syndromes and functional psychoses, excluding the psychoneuroses and character disorders as being outside the definition of insurable illness. Under a unique twist to the basic plan, Harrington (1977) would refer all persons with emotional distress, but with no organic brain disease or psychosis, to the community colleges for courses in the art of living. This psychiatric proposal may find a not too distant kinship with the concepts of Albee, who may be somewhat embarrassed by his closeness to the new medical model. Such a plan has appeal because it would reduce the cost of providing psychotherapy by drastically restricting the numbers of persons eligible. It would further guarantee income to psychiatrists who, as medical practitioners, would be the only persons eligible to provide what would be defined as a medical service. This obviously leaves psychology in a vulnerable position, but even more important, it deprives the majority of Americans suffering from emotional distress of access to treatment.

Of demonstrated effectiveness are the community mental health centers, whose primary limitation is that of cost. Various audits have revealed the cost per unit of service to range from about $60 to a staggering $345 in one center, and a modal cost per unit of service of around $75 to $80 is fairly representative of most centers. Despite the potentially inordinate cost, the National Institute of Mental Health (NIMH) continues to champion the community mental health center concept as the mainstay mental health delivery system under national health insurance. This is understandable, since NIMH spawned the community mental health center movement, but most authorities have retrenched from the overly ambitious goal of the original Kennedy plan that there eventually be a community mental health center in every community. I believe that because of their proven effectiveness, community mental health centers (and their inordinate costs) can still be justified in underserved areas of the nation under national health insurance.

A third delivery approach (Cummings, 1975; Cummings & Follette, 1976) insists that psychological services are a basic ingredient in any truly comprehensive health plan. Such a view holds not only that psychotherapy can be economically included as a prepaid insurance benefit but also that failure to provide such a benefit jeopardizes the effective functioning of the basic medical services by the 60% or more of the physician visits from patients who demonstrate emotional, rather than organic, etiologies for their physical symptoms.

THE COMPREHENSIVE HEALTH MODEL

The Kaiser Permanente Health Plan is recognizable by most readers as the prototype of the modern Health Maintenance Organization (HMO). Founded by Henry J. Kaiser just before World War II as a benefit for his employees, the health plan prospered during the postwar period because it offered the public comprehensive care in its own facilities at moderate cost and without the limitations, deductibles, and co-insurances characteristic of most health plans. At the present time, the health plan serves over eight million subscribers in several semiautonomous regions: Northern and Southern California, Portland (Oregon), Hawaii, Cleveland, and Denver. The San Francisco Kaiser Permanente Medical Center is one of a dozen such centers in the northern California region. It is here, in a setting where the clinical psychologist has been the mainstay practitioner, that two decades of pioneering research have been conducted in the delivery of psychological services within a comprehensive health plan. As background, only the briefest summary of several research papers follows.

Beginning with the initial bias that short-term psychotherapy is not as effective as long-term, and burdened with the discovery that providing easily available comprehensive health services as part of a prepaid plan fostered the somatization of emotional problems and the consequent overutilization of medical facilities by patients who had no physical illness, Kaiser Permanente experimented with a number of early attempts to provide long-term therapy for all its subscribers who manifested emotional distress. The problems inherent in most traditional clinics of the time resulted, such as a long waiting list, a high dropout rate, and an only partially successful attempt to reduce the ever-growing waiting list by providing crisis intervention. Following several years on such an unsatisfactory course, a series of evaluative studies were begun that spanned a decade and a half, and during this time an efficient, cost-therapeutically effective treatment system emerged.

In the first of a series of investigations into the relationship between psychological services and medical utilization in a prepaid health plan setting, Follette and Cummings (1967) compared the number and type of medical services sought before and after the intervention of psychotherapy in a large group of randomly selected patients. The outpatient and inpatient medical utilization for the year immediately prior to the initial interview in the Department of Psychotherapy, as well as for the 5 years following, was studied for three groups of psychotherapy patients (one interview only, brief therapy with a mean of 6.2 interviews, and long-term therapy with a mean of 33.9 interviews) and a "control" group of matched patients demonstrating similar criteria of distress but not, in the 6 years under study, seen in psychotherapy. The findings indicated that (a) persons in emotional distress were significantly higher users of both inpatient (hospitalization) and outpatient medical facilities as compared to the health plan average; (b) there were significant declines in medical utilization in those emotionally distressed individuals who received psychotherapy, as compared to a "control" group of matched emotionally distressed health plan subscribers who were not accorded psychotherapy; (c) these declines remained constant during the 5 years following the termination of psychotherapy; (d) the most significant declines occurred in the 2nd year after the initial interview, and those patients receiving one session only or brief psychotherapy (two to eight sessions) did not require additional psychotherapy to maintain the lower level of utilization for 5 years; and (e) patients seen 2 years or more in continuous psychotherapy demonstrated no overall decline in total outpatient utilization, inasmuch as psychotherapy visits tended to supplant medical visits. However, there was a significant decline in inpatient utilization (hospitalization) in this long-term therapy group from an initial rate several times that of the health plan average, to a level comparable to that of the general, adult, health plan population. The authors criticized their retrospective design in its lack of a true control group, and after considerable difficulty and with the unfortunate necessity of denying treatment to needy individuals, they are currently engaged in replicating their work in a prospective experimental design that is responsive to the criticisms of the previous research.

In a subsequent study, Cummings and Follette (1968) found that intensive efforts to increase the number of referrals to psychotherapy by computerizing psychological screening with early detection and alerting of the attending physicians did not significantly increase the number of patients seeking psychotherapy. The authors concluded that in a prepaid health plan setting already maximally employing educative techniques to both patients and physicians, and already providing a range of prepaid psychological services, the number of subscribers seeking psychotherapy reached an optimal level and remained constant thereafter.

In summarizing nearly two decades of prepaid health plan experience, Cummings and Follette (1976) demonstrated that there is no basis for the fear that increased demand for psychotherapy will financially endanger the system, for it is not the number of referrals received that will drive costs up, but the manner in which psychotherapy services are delivered that determines optimal cost-therapeutic effectiveness. The finding that one session only, with no repeat psychological visits, can reduce medical utilization by 60% over the following 5 years was surprising and totally unexpected. Equally surprising was the 75% reduction in medical utilization over a 5-year period in those patients initially receiving two to eight psychotherapy visits (brief therapy).

In a further study, Cummings and Follette (1976) sought to answer in an 8th-year telephone follow-up whether the results described previously were a therapeutic effect, were the consequence of extraneous factors, or were a deleterious effect. It was hypothesized that if better understanding of the problem had occurred in the psychotherapeutic sessions, the patient would recall the actual problem rather than the presenting symptom and would have both lost the presenting symptom and coped more effectively with the real problem. The results suggest that the reduction in medical utilization was the consequence of resolving the emotional distress that was being reflected in the symptoms and in the doctor's visits. The modal patient in this 8th-year follow-up may be described as follows: She or he denies ever having consulted a physician for the symptoms for which the referral was originally made. Rather, the actual problem discussed with the psychotherapist is recalled as the reason for the psychotherapy visit, and although the problem is resolved, this resolution is attributed to the patient's own efforts and no credit is given the psychotherapist. This affirms the contention that the reduction in medical utilization reflected the diminution in emotional distress that had been expressed in symptoms presented to the physician.

Demonstrating, as they did in their earlier work, that savings in medical services offset the cost of providing psychotherapy answers the question of cost-effectiveness, but Cummings and Follette insisted that the services provided must also be therapeutic in that they reduce the patient's emotional distress. That both cost *and* therapeutic effectiveness were demonstrated in the Kaiser Permanente studies was attributed by the authors to the therapists' expectations that emotional distress could be alleviated by brief, active psychotherapy that involves the analysis of transference and resistance and the uncovering of unconscious conflicts, and that has all of the characteristics of long-term therapy except length. Given this orientation, it was found over a 5-year period that 84.6% of the patients seen in psychotherapy chose to come for 15 sessions or less (with a mean of 8.6). Rather than regarding these patients as "dropouts" from treatment, it was found on follow-up that they achieved a satisfactory state of emotional well-being that continued to the 8th year after termination of therapy. Another 10.1% of the patients were in long-term therapy with a mean of 19.2 sessions, a figure that would probably be regarded as short-term in many traditional clinics. Finally, 5.3% of the patients were found to be "interminable," in that once they began psychotherapy they seemingly continued with no indication of termination.

In a recently reported study, Cummings (1979) addressed the problem of the "interminable" patient for whom treatment was neither cost-effective nor therapeutically effective. The concept that some persons may be so emotionally crippled that they may have to be maintained for many years or for life was not satisfactory, for if 5% of the patients entering psychotherapy are in that category, within a few years a program will be hampered by a monolithic case load, which has become a fact in many public clinics where psychotherapy is offered at nominal or no cost. It was hypothesized that these patients required more intensive intervention, and the frequency of psychotherapy visits was doubled for one experimental group, tripled for another experimental group, and held constant for the control group. Surprisingly, the cost–therapeutic-effectiveness ratios deteriorated in direct proportion to the increased intensity; that is, medical utilization increased and the patients manifested greater emotional distress. It was only by reversing the process and seeing these patients at spaced intervals of once every 2 or 3 months that the desired cost-therapeutic effect was obtained. These results are surprising in that they are contrary to traditionally held notions in psychotherapy, but they demonstrate the need for ongoing research, program evaluation, and innovation if psychotherapy is going to be made available to everyone.

The Cost–Therapeutic-Effectiveness Ratio (Cummings, 1979) and the 38 Criteria of Distress (Follette & Cummings, 1967) have proven to be useful evaluation tools at Kaiser Permanente, enabling the San Francisco center to innovate cost-therapeutically effective programs for alcoholism, drug addiction, the "interminable" patient, chronic psychosis, problems of the elderly, severe character disorders, and other conditions considered by many to be too costly and, therefore, uninsurable.

IMPLICATIONS FOR NATIONAL HEALTH INSURANCE

The experiences at Kaiser Permanente demonstrate what has also been found elsewhere: When all barriers are removed from access to medical care, the system will become overloaded with the 60% or more of physician visits by patients manifesting somatized emotional distress. There is every reason to believe this would occur under national health insurance, for the medical model inadvertently encourages somatization. If a patient complains to the physician, "My boss is on my back and it's killing me," a perfunctory, unsympathetic response is most likely. But let the patient unconsciously translate this distress to lower back pain and that patient is immediately rewarded by the physician's attention in the form of X rays, laboratory tests, medications, and return visits. And even worse, temporary disability may be offered which removes the patient from the presence of the hated boss and renders unconsciously mandatory the continuation of the chronic pain as the only possible solution to what originally was an interpersonal problem.

When psychotherapy is properly provided within a comprehensive health system, the costs of providing the benefit are more than offset by the savings in medical utilization. However, this does not mean that traditional delivery modes of mental health services can be parachuted into the system. Such attempts have proven to be near disasters in a number of programs. On the other hand, the uses of artificial limitations and co-insurance are only partial answers, for while controlling costs, therapeutic effectiveness is often sacrificed. The experiences over two decades at Kaiser Permanente indicate that it is not the provision of a psychotherapy benefit that can bankrupt a system, but the manner in which it is delivered. When active, dynamic, brief therapy is provided early and by psychotherapists who are enthusiastic and proactive regarding such intervention, it is the treatment of choice for about 85% of the patients seeking psychotherapy. Such intervention not only yields a high cost–therapeutic-effectiveness ratio, but it is satisfactory to both the patient—in increased emotional well-being—and the patient's physician—in dramatic reduction of somatization and overutilization of medical facilities. Further, by providing such brief therapy, it makes economically feasible the provision of long-term psychotherapy to the approximately 10% of the patients who require it for their treatment to be therapeutically effective.

Finally, cost–therapeutically-effective programs can be developed for problems in living that traditionally have been regarded as too resistant and, therefore, too costly to be insurable. This requires constant research, innovation, and program evaluation, but it is important, because if national health insurance is to meet the emotional needs of all Americans, it is untenable to think of excluding one group or another.

{ 7 }

TURNING BREAD INTO STONES
OUR MODERN ANTIMIRACLE

ABSTRACT: *Addiction and addiction-related problems are currently occupying a significant, but most often unrecognized, portion of psychotherapy and mental health practice. The incidence is increasing rapidly. The medical model inadvertently encourages iatrogenic addiction, and the treatment of addiction by substituting one chemical for another escalates the problem. Traditional psychotherapy, based on the notion that the addictive personality can be altered through insight alone, has had little impact on either the treatment or the prevention of addiction. On the other hand, the mental health movement, in promising a freedom from anxiety that is not possible, may have had a significant role in the current belief that it is a right to feel good, thus contributing to the burgeoning consumption of alcohol and the almost universal prescription of the tranquilizer by physicians. A psychological model of the treatment of addiction*

This article is based on the Presidential Address delivered at the meeting of the American Psychological Association, New York, September 2, 1979.

The psychotherapeutic techniques described were developed by the author and his colleagues at the Golden Gate Mental Health Center, San Francisco, and the Department of Psychotherapy, Kaiser Permanente, San Francisco, during the past 16 years. I am grateful to William T. Follette for his constant support and encouragement throughout that period.

and addiction-related problems can be effective in motivating addicts to alter a life-style. This article presents such a model of intervention, developed over a 16-year period.

WE ARE TOLD in the New Testament (Matthew 4:3) that while Christ was wandering in the wilderness, the Devil tempted Him by saying, "If indeed thou be the Son of God, cast those stones into bread." That would have been the ancient miracle. Let us move forward in time almost 2,000 years to 1975, the last year for which the National Institute of Alcoholism and Alcohol Abuse (NIAAA) and the National Institute of Drug Abuse (NIDA) have figures.

In 1975, alcoholism, its treatment, and its related problems cost the United States $43 billion (National Institute of Alcoholism and Alcohol Abuse, 1978). During that same year, drug abuse and drug-abuse-related problems cost this country $10.5 billion (National Institute of Drug Abuse, 1978), for a combined total of $53 billion, or 2.5% of the gross national product for that year.

Economists have asked how long our society can support such a price before productivity is affected. Many experts think we have already turned that corner. Startling as it may seem, 1 of every 11 adult Americans suffers from a severe addictive problem. Drug addiction is epidemic among teenagers: One of every 6 teenagers suffers from a severe addictive problem. At any given time on our nation's highways, an average of 1 of every 12 drivers is too drunk to drive. We must not overlook the iatrogenic contribution: At any given time, 1 of every 7 Americans is regularly taking a psychotropic drug prescribed by a physician. Worst of all, the overmedication of our elderly is a national disgrace. Often in clinical practice what appeared to be early senile confusion clears up once the elderly individual is removed from mind-altering prescription drugs that have special side effects for older persons, or from several sometimes incompatible medications prescribed by three or four physicians concurrently.

OUR DRUG-ORIENTED SOCIETY

We have indeed become a drug-oriented society. I am not making any judgment about that; this may be good or bad, depending on your perspective. It may be that the mental health movement has promised the

American people a freedom from anxiety that is neither possible nor realistic, resulting in an expectation that we have a right to feel good. We may never know to what extent we ourselves have contributed to the steep rise in alcohol consumption and to the almost universal reliance by physicians on the tranquilizer.

What this translates to is that addictive problems are going to take up more and more of our practice. In a recent survey, 23% of a random sample of psychotherapy patients seen in a large metropolitan mental health center were suffering either from addictive problems or from emotional problems substantially exacerbated by alcohol or drug abuse, and only 3.5% of these were so identified by their own therapists (Cummings, 1975b).

Our drug-oriented society has spawned new industries, and I will only give you three examples. The "free zone" in Miami is the passageway for contraband from Colombia: Literally pounds of cocaine and tons of marijuana come into Miami daily. It is called a free zone because the authorities are totally helpless to stop the drug traffic, and we see entire boatloads of drugs seized and the seamen deported only to show up again within days with another boatload.

In California, where the giant redwoods used to grow but have now been logged, the five most remote northern counties have experienced an economic depression. A new industry is replacing the lumber industry: the growing of marijuana in 7–10-acre plots deep in the forest and hidden from the narcs (narcotics agents). I had the opportunity to visit one of these marijuana-growing communes recently, something you cannot do alone because the foils, traps, and snares that have been created to fool the narc are as complete as the foils, traps, and snares that are set up in the hills of the rural South where moonshiners are avoiding the revenuer. The marijuana growers even seem to dress and talk the same, but there is one important difference: In the South you seldom see 5- and 6-year-olds stoned out of their minds, like I did in the northern counties of California.

I will mention only one other new industry you may not have heard of: Chronic cocaine use so degenerates the nasal membranes that in California, plastic surgeons are inserting plastic passages in the nostrils of chronic cocaine users who have destroyed their natural passages. I could list many more new industries resulting from society's drug orientation, not the least of which is our multimillion-dollar drug paraphernalia industry.

A PSYCHOLOGICAL MODEL OF ADDICTION

The medical profession is totally unprepared to deal with addiction. The medical model treats addiction to one substance by substituting another substance. In this way we used heroin to cure morphine addiction. We now use methadone to cure heroin addiction, Valium to cure alcoholism, amphetamines to cure carbohydrate and sugar addiction. I would suggest to you that the medical model, which plays a kind of addictive musical chairs, is a total failure because it actually escalates the problem in severity. Attempts to educate physicians about the dangers of substitute addiction or overmedication are difficult, if not often futile. The prescription pad is the number-one item in the physician's armamentarium and is one of the very few truly licensable medical activities.

I would like to present to you a psychological model that has its roots 16 years ago in San Francisco in the treatment of the runaways to the Haight-Ashbury district of San Francisco and the Telegraph Avenue area of Berkeley. At that time I was codirector of the Golden Gate Mental Health Center, a privately financed community mental health agency. I was treating these runaways under California law, which allows teenagers to receive treatment for addiction or sex problems without parental consent, something that could not be obtained in these cases.

In one way I was fortunate to be in San Francisco, because we felt the shock waves of a drug-oriented society fully 10 years before the rest of the nation. You may laugh at what happens in California, but whether you talk about the patio, the barbeque pit, the divorce rate, the hot tub, the cocaine party, or Levis, today's California fad becomes commonplace throughout the nation within 5–15 years. The drug cult and the waves of drug taking we saw in San Francisco in the mid-1960s are now commonplace across the land.

What I would like to do is describe a treatment approach that began some 16 years ago and introduce it by some formal comments about the causes of addiction. We just do not know what they are. We know a lot about addiction, none of which satisfactorily explains causality, but the interesting thing is that one does not need to know cause in order to intervene. There is a growing body of evidence which indicates that some people are born with a genetic predisposition to become addicted (Kandel, 1976). For others it is congenital and in utero; for example, very small amounts of alcohol imbibed by its mother during certain months of pregnancy predispose a child to alcoholism

(Julien, 1978). So compelling is this evidence that a couple of years ago, the Food and Drug Administration considered requiring a label on bottles of alcohol stating that even small amounts of alcohol are dangerous to pregnancy. This would have been a very unpopular move, and I think that is why it was dropped. There is alcohol and drug addiction that is acquired (Blum et al., 1972; Peele & Brodsky, 1975). These causes are difficult to demonstrate, and the bottom line has yet to be written in any of them. Apparently, some people must have had a genetic predisposition, because the first time they took a glass of beer at the age of 11, they were alcoholics. Others seem to acquire the addiction. There is no question that the frequent ingestion of any addictive substance is sufficiently reinforcing so that everyone takes the risk of addiction. Yet not everyone becomes addicted, even children born of women who are heroin addicts. Although 92% of these infants show severe withdrawal upon birth, 8% do not, and the presence or absence of withdrawal has nothing to do with the amount of heroin the mother has taken. These are all questions for which we do not have the answers, so in treating my clients, I tell them the answers don't matter. In our program we stress the concept that addiction is something for which the individual can and has to take responsibility. I give the following example to my clients: We do not know what causes diabetes. We know it is a failure of the isles of Langerhans in the pancreas to produce insulin, but why one person's isles of Langerhans fail and another's do not is irrelevant to treatment. Some families seem to be predisposed to the disease, and others do not; in many cases individuals seem to acquire it through prolonged obesity. In any case, the answer is abstinence from sugar. The first, first, first thing one must do when confronted with an addict is convince that person that the prerequisite intervention in addiction is abstinence from the chemical to which one is addicted.

In our program we stress that the concept of addiction as a disease is useless because it implies that one is helpless and cannot do anything about it. We say that least important of all is the debate over what is habitual and what is addictive. The medical definition of an addictive substance has to do with whether or not physical withdrawal occurs when a person is deprived of that chemical. I submit to you that the physical withdrawal from heroin is 72–90 hours. The psychological withdrawal is the rest of your life. The same thing is true with alcohol, amphetamine, tranquilizer, or barbiturate abuse: The psychological reinforcement is the crucial factor. An excellent example is the history of thousands of heroin-addicted combat troops in Vietnam who readily gave up their narcotics use once they were back home and the psychological factors encouraging their addiction were removed (Peele, 1978). I say to my clients, "Do not ask whether a chemical is addictive or habituating," and they understand when I point out that although cocaine is regarded in medicine as not addictive, it is so highly reinforcing that cocaine dependency will not be abated even though the drug costs $2,500–$3,000 an ounce, will burn out your nasal passages, and produces such behavioral side effects as paranoia and grandiosity.

I would like to give a fascinating example of "addiction" in a hospital during the days when alcoholics were placed in locked wards. In this instance the hospitalized moved their cots into the bathroom while the staff looked on, baffled. After several days it was found that these alcoholics had substituted water for alcohol. If one drinks eight gallons or more of water per day, the pH level of the blood is altered and one becomes intoxicated. The consequence of this was that the patients had to move their cots to the bathroom to be near the spout and the toilet, because eight gallons of water per day results in constant drinking and urinating. So I say to my clients, "Do not ask me about what is addictive and what is not. If you are an addictive personality, you can even get addicted to water."

So it is irrelevant whether addicts lack endorphins, the natural substances in the brain that mitigate pain and help us survive unpleasantness, and whether this is genetic, in utero; or acquired. I now want to describe to you how we treat addiction, a method that after several years of trial at the Golden Gate Mental Health Center became the backbone of the addiction treatment program at Kaiser Permanente in San Francisco, and one that is used in several other programs throughout the United States (Cummings, 1969, 1970).

I tell my clients that addiction is not merely popping something into one's mouth but a constellation of behaviors that constitute a way of life. An addict can be likened to an unfinished house that has only an attic and a basement. When one falls out of the attic, one falls all the way down to the basement because there are no intervening floors to stop the fall. My addicts know exactly what I mean, because they know only two moods: elation and depression. They do not know what normal is. They do not experience the limited, normal mood swings common to other persons, because when they start to fall out of the attic, they run quickly to the bottle, the pill, the needle, anything to prevent falling clear down to the basement. So, indeed, the first thing we have to teach them is how to build a floor in that house, because you cannot live just in elation or depression. As one philosopher put it, those who are chronically depressed are damned to pursue pleasure constantly for the rest of their lives.

I remember that during the early days in the Haight-Ashbury, adolescent runaways came to me because they did not want to go to the city clinics, which were required to report addiction. Many got their money from Philadelphia, or Atlanta, or wherever their parents would send the money on the promise they would not come back home and embarrass the family. Others, both girls and boys, sold their bodies on the street to make their bread; still others stole or sold dope. At that time I realized what it costs to keep a habit going, and this is where the title of my address comes from. Using the vernacular I learned from my teenage runaways 15 or 16 years ago, it takes an awful lot of bread to make a stone. This is our modern antimiracle.

In the beginning I treated addiction in the traditional, ineffective fashion, using the premise that one need not confront and prohibit the addictive behavior; through insight and understanding the client will come to lose the compulsive craving. This was before I recognized that addicts are extremely adept at playing this psychotherapy game and do not need the collaboration of an incompetent therapist to perpetuate their addiction under the guise of seeking help. I will never forget the time a young man in one group said to me, "Nick, you are never going to help us as long as we are hitting." I asked what he meant and he wisely indicated that "whether we see you once a week, twice a week, three times a week, or every day, hitting is so pleasurable, we can wipe out all the psychotherapy you give us with one pill or a touch of the needle." He was right, and for the first time in my professional career I learned that all insight is soluble in alcohol or drugs. So in that group we made a commitment to total abstinence for a period of three months. They all agreed but came in the following week and tried to talk me out of it. I said no, that we had made a commitment and I insisted we honor it. They did, and it was the first group of teenage runaways that I was able to help not only to give up drugs but also to become reconnected to life. After that I began to develop with these and other teenagers a system of treatment wherein the client earns his or her way into the treatment situation and continues to earn a place in that treatment situation by making gradual steps agreed on in advance. Failure to meet agreed-on standards results in various degrees of exclusion, and finally one may be thrown completely out of the program. This is why Wolfgang Lederer, seeing a demonstration, named it *exclusion therapy*. I did not like the name at first, but I have since come to regard it as a proper title based on truth in packaging. We anticipated therapeutic contracts before these became popular or standard, and today I make a detailed contract with every client very early in our sessions. As I show below, the technique is a combination of (a) therapeutic contracts, (b) reality therapy, (c) operant conditioning, (d) insight therapy, (e) brief psychotherapy, (f) communication theory employing the double-bind and paradoxical intention, and (g) group therapy, all melded into a system of "psycho-judo," wherein the addict's own massive resistance is used to propel him or her toward giving up the addictive life-style. Although individual sessions are used to establish a transference and to motivate the client toward health, the job really gets done in the group sessions. Group therapy is essential for these persons who, as teenage or adult addicts, are fixated at the adolescent level of rebelliousness and acting out. At this level peer pressure has its greatest impact, and the newfound peer pressure toward health of the group is the ultimate ingredient in solidifying a determination to clean up.

INTERVENTION PHASE 1: WITHDRAWAL

Addicts do not come to us to be helped for their addiction. They come to us because they are about to lose something or have lost something. It may be a spouse, a job, a driver's license, freedom (threat of jail), or health (e.g., cirrhosis of the liver, esophageal hemorrhaging). Essentially, they come wanting the therapist to bring back the halcyon days when drugs worked and made them feel mellow. The therapist must start with the full realization that the client does not really intend to give up either drugs or the way of life. During the first half of the first session the therapist must listen very intently. Then, somewhere in midsession, using all of his or her rigorous training, therapeutic acumen, and the third, fourth, fifth, and sixth ears, the therapist discerns some unresolved wish, some long-gone dream that is still residing deep in that human being, and then the therapist pulls it out and ignites the client with a desire to somehow look at that dream again. This is not easy, because if the right nerve is not touched the therapist loses the client. Some readers will erroneously regard our approach to treating addiction as harsh or punitive in its stark sense of reality.

Whitaker's (1979) admonition is important here: Because the therapist's distance can be destructive in psychotherapy, we tend to emphasize closeness too much. A good therapist is one who can commingle closeness and distance as is appropriate at the moment. An inept therapist is one who has only one approach, either closeness or distance. Because addictive persons have character disorders, they behave in infuriating ways. To become angry (even unconsciously) at someone with a character disorder results in the forfeiture of the therapist's ability to help. Exclusion therapy provides a time-limited microcosm of the real world that enables the therapist to be close when needed but distant enough to avoid anger when the client behaves in an infuriating manner.

Some will also erroneously prejudge exclusion therapy as manipulative. Haley (1976) pointed out that all good psychotherapists manipulate. The inept therapist is often the one who cannot admit this, so that manipulation is to the benefit of the therapist rather than of the client. As I show below, game playing is a cardinal feature of addicts, whose negative or destructive games must be countered with positive or healthy games.

Once the client is motivated to continue in the first session, I advise my client, to his or her amazement, that I will not make a second appointment until he or she is clean. For the heroin addict this means 3 days, for the alcoholic it means 14 days, for the barbiturate addict it means 10 days, for the amphetamine addict it means 7 days. Most clients today are what I call cafeteria addicts; they take anything placed before them, and while remaining constantly stoned, they pride themselves that they are not really addicted to any one substance. The cafeteria addict is required to stay clean for 10 days, and the withdrawal really drives home the fact that he or she has become dependent on being stoned. I say to them, "I will not even give you a second appointment until you call me up and say to me, 'Nick, I'm clean.'" Because of the addicts' negativism, the refusal to see them sets up a challenge they cannot ignore. They become determined to go clean in order to foil the therapist, who expresses out loud doubts that they can really do it. Heroin addicts are amazed that I will not put them in the hospital. What I do is find a friend who has never been on drugs, and I give that person a crash course in taking care of somebody who is going through withdrawal. Then I call the client and the sitter every two hours, day and night for three days. On each call I have the client tell me what is being experienced, and I tell them exactly what they will feel during the next two hours. This removes the terror from the unknown. Then there comes a point some- where around the 60th or 70th hour when I am able to report to the client that he or she has crested: "From now on, every time we talk you are going to feel a little better. You won't be out of the woods for a cou- ple of more days, but you will feel better every time we talk."

When I am asked why I do not hospitalize patients who are with- drawing, I answer with an axiom: "Degree of pain is directly propor- tional to the proximity of the sympathetic physician. In other words, the hospital is where all the drugs are, and if you scream enough and hurt enough, at 3:00 in the morning some intern or nurse will not be able to resist giving you the needle, and that means if you are on your second day you may have to start at Square 1 again." I say to them, "It hurts more in the hospital because the drugs are there." They hear me.

Addicts use what I call the street-paver syndrome. Have you noticed that when a street is torn up to replace underground utilities, the street pavers put the pavement back, but never at quite the same height? It is either half an inch too low or half an inch too high, so passing cars hit a bump. Similarly, addicts will always comply, but not quite. The heroin addict will demand an appointment one hour before the 72 hours are up. The alcoholic will call one day before the 14 days are up. When the heroin addict calls, I say, "Don't call me now, I can't give you another appointment. You call me in an hour." When the al- coholic calls, I say, "Your time is up at 3:30 tomorrow afternoon." They reply that I am the craziest doctor they have ever encountered, and they slam down the telephone vowing never to call again. One hour or 24 hours later to the moment they telephone. No matter what the therapist is doing, it is imperative that the client be seen that day. I am often scheduled as late as 10:00 or 11:00 at night and must see them after that. The client recognizes the commitment of the therapist and never forgets it. I have clients all over California who shake their heads and say, "My second appointment with that guy was at 1:30 in the morning. How do you turn down a guy like that?"

Our treatment has been devised into a set of easily appreciated and understood axioms that reduce the "analgesic experience," as Peele (1978) has called the life-style of the addict, into easily understood phrases which may seem simplistic but which, to the addict, are like words of wisdom. The addict uses what has been called "the cutoff," a form of denial in which the addict tunes out anything that touches on his or her addiction. These simple axioms have a propensity to break through the cutoff. Scare tactics are counterproductive. Telling an alcoholic that cirrhosis will kill is enough to drive him or her to drink.

When addicts first come in, they are determined not to see you. They are there because their spouse, their boss, their probation officer, their doctor, somebody has said, "You've got to do something about this addiction." They come in determined to convince the therapist that they do not need to be seen. During the course of the first interview, after having ascertained the precious deeply buried wish, I say, "It's a shame that you have this dream, but you are not ready to give up your addiction and I can't see you." The first response from this person who came in determined not to continue is rage and a demand to be seen. Addicts are determined to do the opposite of whatever you tell them, and here is where the double bind is useful. When you tell them you won't see them, they get furious. One must start with whatever the client brings to the first session, so the therapist takes seriously the need to get out of trouble. But the client must be helped to see the long-term problem and that the future under the present life-style is bleak. This is done not by reasoning, which will be tuned out, but by outmaneuvering the negativism. With every intent of helping the client, the therapist suggests possible solutions that can be provided but makes these contingent on fulfilling the required number of days of abstinence. The client is thus placed in another double bind. The therapist states unabashedly that he or she will do everything possible to help the client out of trouble once the addict is truly a client, a status that is not attained until the client has been clean for the requisite number of days and has earned a second appointment.

During this phase the therapist will be confronted with two related games addicts play. The first of these is, "I can quit any time but I don't want to." The therapist agrees that the client is indeed not ready and would not be able to quit even if he or she wanted to, for if the person were truly not an addict, quitting for the prescribed period would be easy. The client digests this as a challenge or counters with a related game: "I cannot quit." The first game is, "I am not really addicted," and the second is, "I am no longer responsible." Using psycho-judo again, the therapist agrees with the client, sighs that the client seems hopelessly addicted or unmotivated, and urges him or her not to really try because it would be an exercise in futility. At this point the client needs an assurance, and the therapist cites one or two examples of successful cases that were similar to the present client but again sighs that this would not seem to apply to him or her.

In the 16 years we have been using this technique, four of five addicts so challenged will respond by meeting the requisite number of days of total abstinence. Of the remainder, about half will call six months to a year later to announce they have fulfilled their required period of withdrawal. We have even had addicts return triumphantly as much as two years later, having carried the therapist's telephone number with them for that entire period.

Once the client returns for the second interview, the successful withdrawal is lorded over the therapist, who immediately concedes having been wrong about the client, congratulates the client on the victory, and admits how delighted he or she is to have miscalculated the strength and determination of the client. At this point the client has had the first experience in self-mastery and has put the first plank in the floor that is to be eventually built between the attic and basement, as discussed above.

On the second appointment the therapist is able to build on the client's feeling of self-mastery and to agree on a contract wherein each succeeding session is dependent on the client's continuing to remain clean. Each session is begun by asking if the client is clean. If not, there is no session that day, and the client returns the following week at the scheduled time. The client is not permitted to telephone, admitting he or she has had a fall, and then not come in. It is part of the necessary procedure that the client take responsibility for the fall and experience the therapist's reaction. The therapist does not disapprove; he or she merely complies with the agreed-on terms. Interesting things happen during this period: The client attempts unsuccessfully to draw the therapist into the kind of struggles he or she has carried on with coaddicts (parents, spouse, boss, lover, friends).

The next task is to motivate the client for the group program of 24 sessions. This requires 4–12 sessions, depending on the individual. The therapeutic contract for the group program involves an agreement to attend all 24 sessions, to be excluded from any sessions prior to which the client has had a fall, and to be permanently excluded on the fourth fall. Furthermore, the client must pay for all subsequent sessions after permanent exclusion. Because of insurance, this will often mean no money or as little as one dollar, but the weekly bill is a regular reminder that the client is a member in exclusion. This has very frequently motivated the client to return and try again, something the excluded addict can do after the 24 sessions have been completed and the group disbands.

At this point a note of caution is important. Some addicts, though the minority, require hospitalization for withdrawal, and it is a matter of considerable expertise to differentiate these. The close collaboration with an internist skilled in the treatment of severe withdrawal is essential. Some alcoholics are on the verge of delirium tremens when first seen. Other alcoholics, as well as barbiturate and Valium addicts, are subject to convulsions on withdrawal. Most of these can be treated without hospitalization by providing the sitter with a "hummer," a dose of the chemical from which the client is withdrawing, to be administered when the client demonstrates signs of impending convulsion. It is important that the existence of the hummer be kept a secret from the withdrawing client, because knowledge of it will surely trigger a convulsion as a means of legitimately obtaining the chemical.

It is interesting that heroin withdrawal, with its severe chills, cramps, and other symptoms, does not present these medical complications. Special mention must be made of Valium withdrawal which persists for as long as six weeks, with recurring waves of severity during which the individual may wander or have convulsions that he or she will not remember. Another drug with a prolonged withdrawal period is methadone, which is given to heroin addicts presumably as an alternative to the isolation and criminal behavior which become so important in the addictive life-style. I have seen the bone aches in methadone withdrawal persist well into the second month.

INTERVENTION PHASE 2: THE GAMES

The 10 members in each group all start at once. There is enough flow that new groups are starting at regular intervals. Once the clients have been motivated to come in, the therapist must bear in mind that they have made a 6-month commitment only, after which it is their fond hope that they will become social drinkers or weekend joy poppers. There is an interesting thing about addiction, and it takes the 24 sessions before these clients realize it. Once addicted, no matter how long one remains clean, the addiction remains at the highest achieved level of tolerance for the rest of one's life. This is very easily demonstrated with "foodaholics." A foodaholic may take 20 years to get to 400 pounds. Once a fat cell is formed, it never disappears. Losing weight makes it empty, but it sits there like a flat plastic bag, waiting to be replenished. The foodaholic can shrink back to 175 pounds, but if he or she begins overeating again it is only a matter of a couple of months before the body reaches its greatest attained weight of 400 pounds, because new fat cells do not have to be created. Something similar seems to happen with the addictions to chemicals. This is most easily demonstrated by a heroin addict who took years to build up a $300-a-day habit. That addict can be clean for 5 or 10 years, but if he or she starts to shoot up again, the $300-a-day habit will resume within a brief time. An alcoholic can build up to a quart a day of bourbon over many years. If that person quits and then starts to drink again, the result will be a quart-a-day craving within two weeks. The more you drink, the more you can because your tolerance goes up, except for Valium. Valium has no overdose level. It is the most commonly prescribed drug in America, with 11 billion tablets consumed in the United States in 1975. The only ways one can die on Valium are to swallow enough pills to choke or to mix Valium with alcohol. Valium is usually prescribed in 5-mg pills. Those who are addicted to Valium (another so-called nonaddictive drug) get 20 or 30 physicians to prescribe these 5-mg pills, and they take 700–900 mg per day. A nurse I worked with was taking 1,100 mg of Valium per day, and it was difficult to believe she could carry on her work. On one hand she was a zombie, and on the other hand all she was doing all day was swallowing pills. Debbie has now been clean for seven years.

Once in the group program, the phase called "the games" begins. All addicts play games. The major game played is "the rescue game." All addicts become the focal point of everybody who has a problem. They are called on the phone day and night by friends who tell them their troubles. They play the rescue game no matter how undeserving the person. They attempt to rescue them because when they themselves mess up and are undeserving, they can then feel entitled to be rescued.

Alcoholics Anonymous (AA) turns a destructive rescue game that enables the person to continue to drink into a positive rescue game called sobriety. I have great respect for AA. In our program, however, our goal is to end the rescue game once and for all and free the alcoholic from having to spend the rest of his or her life going to AA meetings or to a psychotherapist. Addicts play games, and they cannot go from destructive games directly to no games. We spend this phase, Phase 2, in teaching them constructive games.

What are some of the games they play? "The rubber ruler" is one of the most frequent and can take many forms. It can consist of telling the bartender to leave the olive out of the martini, with all kinds of jokes about how many cubic centimeters of gin the olive displaces. The real reason is that after seven martinis, the alcoholic does not want to look at an ashtray and see seven toothpicks, because he or she wants to walk out of the bar and say that only three martinis were consumed.

The foodaholic will believe that the giant-sized bag of potato chips he or she just demolished was only one quarter full, when it was really ⅞ full. The rubber ruler can be either stretched or compressed. An addict will often be convinced he or she has been clean for 1½ months when it has only been about 10 days.

"The vending machine" is an interesting game that alcoholics play. It says, "I have been a good boy, I have been a good girl. Why isn't life making it easy for me?" It begins in childhood, when our parents forgive our F in spelling because we did so well in Sunday school two days earlier, even though the two are totally unrelated. Alcoholics continue such childish expectations and demand miracles after having been dry for two or three weeks. Because they have been good, addicts expect life to open up and give them all they want: a better job, a better lover, freedom from their probation officers, instant health.

Another common game is self-pity, and no addicts will resume their addiction until they first get themselves into the vortex of self-pity that makes the thing possible. Self-pity can be justified by a cross word from a boss, a nagging spouse, or a so-called sick society. All of these become excuses to resume drug activity. In fact, addicts quite frequently precipitate crises in order to justify their addiction, a common ploy being to incite a previously nagging spouse to begin nagging again as an excuse to end a period of sobriety.

In all of these games one sees the addict's careful point–counterpoint in which guilt, justification, absolution, and punishment abound in complex acting-out patterns that assure the continuation of the addictive life-style. From morning-after remorse to contrition when arrested for drunk driving, the addict not only is full of good intentions but manages to suffer in such a way that he or she can continue to view himself or herself as blameless and misunderstood. So the addict settles for what Peele (1978) called "comfortable discomfort." He or she becomes a kind of successful loser who alternates between elation at having fooled the world and depression at the discovery of his or her low self-esteem and lack of self-confidence.

The addict is adroit at playing "the feeling game," so the unwary therapist may be fooled into accepting the counterfeit feelings as genuine insight, just as the addict's friends have been fooled for years. In fact, everyone has had the experience of being shocked to learn that a friend or neighbor who was known for sincerity, concern, and honest feeling turned out to be an addict who had neglected his or her family for years. The therapist would do well to employ only positive changes in behavior over suitable periods of time as the real yardstick to insight or understanding.

"The file card" is an important game because it is an unconscious determination to resume drinking at a certain point in time, or once certain conditions have been fulfilled. In *While Rome Burns*, Alexander Woollcott has one of his characters telephone his hostess of the night before to apologize for missing her dinner party, saying, "On the way to your home I was taken unexpectedly drunk." No one is taken unexpectedly drunk. Rather, one plants a decision in the back of one's mind to the effect that if my wife nags me the 20th time or if my boss makes me work weekends, I deserve a drink. So once the event happens, the addict begins to drink, or pop pills, without having to arrive at any further conscious decisions, in such a way that the file card, once filed, is automatic although forgotten.

Alcoholics are perfectionists. If I were an unscrupulous employer I would hire nobody but primary alcoholics. I would expect them not to work on Mondays because they would be recovering from their hangovers, and they would miss work on Fridays because they could not hold off for the weekend and would begin drinking on Thursday night. But on Tuesdays, Wednesdays, and Thursdays, I would get two weeks worth of work out of them. They are perfectionists, but their perfectionism is part of the game that feeds their life-style and justifies addiction.

INTERVENTION PHASE 3: THE WORKING THROUGH

With the mastery of the destructive games and before the substitution of positive or healthy games, the group members suddenly become zealots. This is "the holier-than-thou stage" out of which many reformed drunks never emerge. It is important that this highly authoritarian outlook be understood and ameliorated, for during this phase the addict becomes merciless toward a fellow group member who may have a fall. Such an outlook toward the world can lead only to new kinds of problems in living.

Once this is worked through, and about halfway through the 24 group sessions, the group members become depressed. They realize there is no short-cut, only hard work ahead. The fanaticism disappears, but so does the enthusiasm that carried the client thus far. It is as if the energy goes out of the group, and each group member settles into a profound depression that places him or her at risk. It is interesting that few clients have falls during this period; most of the falls have occurred in Phase 2, when most of the testing of the limits is being acted out. Furthermore, the therapist's vigilance is alerted at this period, and the group members who have now been working together for several months accept the assurance that once this depression is weathered, better days are coming.

INTERVENTION PHASE 4: SELF-RESPONSIBILITY

In the final phase the client seems to finally accept responsibility. This is in the form of a conviction, heretofore aggressively resisted, which concludes that abstinence is for life, not the six months of the group program. With the acceptance of this fact comes a kind of peaceful resolution with oneself and a sense of mastery.

This phase appears just at the point when the addict despairs that he or she will never emerge from the profound depression. It happens suddenly, and clients describe it as an experience similar to learning to type or mastering a foreign language: Proficiency is preceded by a seemingly interminable period of more or less mechanical struggling. Then one day one is typing or speaking the language. In our case, the intervening floor in the house has been built and the client is no longer subject to panicky mood swings that send him or her scurrying for the bottle, the needle, or the pill.

A key ingredient has been the therapist, whose unrelenting firmness, fairness, and honesty have provided a role model and whose deep commitment and concern have ameliorated the client's chronically low self-esteem and interpersonal distrust, so aptly described by Chein, Gerard, Lee, and Rosenfeld (1964).

SPECIAL CASES

Exclusion therapy is applicable to foodaholics as well as to therapy addicts and compulsive gamblers. These require special therapeutic contracts, but space limitations permit only brief mention of them. Exclusion therapy is not applicable to tobacco addiction.

There are two types of foodaholics: carbohydrate addicts and sugar addicts. The two types of addiction are often mixed in one person, but it is surprising how frequently the pure forms of addiction are found. Since the therapist cannot insist on total abstinence (one has to eat), the client is required to lose five pounds for a second appointment and two pounds per week to qualify for the subsequent sessions. Foodaholics usually insist on losing more than the required amount, a sure sign they will fail, so the therapist must point out, "Even when you are losing weight you insist on gluttony in reverse."

Foodaholics will reach what has been termed in the group a "sound barrier," the weight that the client will seemingly be unable to go below. It was so named because once beyond the barrier it is difficult to recall why it was so difficult, somewhat analogous to what the field of aviation experienced with supersonic flight. The sound barrier is mostly psychological, for the client changes from the psychological outlook of a fat person trying to lose weight to that of a thin person who is still somewhat overweight.

The temporary bouts of hypoglycemia experienced by foodaholics as they lose weight are not restricted to them. All withdrawal results in recurring periods of hypoglycemia, not only because the alcoholic is used to a high quantity of alcohol or sugar in the blood but also because the glycogen function of the liver has been disrupted by prolonged use of a chemical. In fact, the so-called "rush" in drug taking is essentially the result of drugs triggering the sudden discharge of stored glycogen.

It is important that the therapist never recommend a diet to the foodaholic, stressing instead that the client understands his or her body a lot better than the therapist does and has long ago learned what will lead to weight loss. This prevents the game that foodaholics play with their physicians, getting them to prescribe a diet that the patient will effectively sabotage.

In the United States we have unfortunately created a legion of therapy addicts who constantly pursue psychotherapy, individual growth, and every new fad that emerges, in the firm belief, somewhat analogous to the Santa Claus fantasy, that the next encounter will produce the desired insight and state of narcissistic peace. We call these persons couch freaks, growth grogs, or woe-is-me artists. Exclusion therapy is very successful in helping these heretofore repressed individuals realize that the cure for constipation is not diarrhea. Space does not permit an adequate description of the special technique required in these cases.

CONCLUSION

Exclusion therapy is not an elegant theory of the addictive personality or a hypothesis about the cause of addiction. It is a viable system of intervention that has proved successful in a variety of settings in the United States during the past 16 years.

With our own clients at the Kaiser Permanente center in San Francisco we have followed a randomly selected sample over the years and have maintained active follow-up. Of this sample of 639 clients who have been in the program, 73% are living drug-free lives. Of these, 472 have been clean for 5 years, and 123 have been clean for more than 10 years. Almost half of the total sample experienced at least one fall, for which they came to the clinic for several individual sessions. Occasionally, someone requests that he or she repeat the entire group program, and this is granted. Others have entered traditional therapy and gained the kind of insight that was not possible as long as they were drunk or stoned.

If the estimate is correct that 23% of clients seen in psychotherapy are suffering from either addictive problems or emotional problems that are exacerbated by alcohol or drug abuse, then psychotherapists must be prepared to discover, confront, and intervene in these conditions. Medicine has not been successful in meeting the wave of addiction and problems exacerbated by drug abuse because the very nature of the medical model inadvertently encourages either iatrogenic addiction or the substitution of one addictive substance for another. Like the efforts of most workers in the field of alcohol and drug abuse, traditional therapy, based on the assumption that insight must precede abstinence, is even worse than no intervention inasmuch as it kindles the addict's fantasy that something will happen for him or her.

In mental health clinics in the San Francisco area, 40% of those seeking psychotherapy are manifesting or hiding alcohol or drug abuse problems, and my own estimates indicate that within a decade, a figure of 40% for the nation as a whole is not to be unexpected. Professional psychology must be prepared to meet this epidemic. The psychological model of intervention remains the most viable, and I hope I have done something in this address to enable psychology to meet the challenge that these problems will continue to present in even greater degree in the future.

{ 8 }

The General Practice of Psychology*

Psychology has developed a variety of specific techniques which are applicable to specific emotional problems, thus enabling brief psychotherapy to be particularly effective. In the past it was said that therapist and patient had only one chance to solve present and future emotional distress, a criterion applied to no other form of intervention. By combining dynamic and behavioral therapies into intervention designed to ameliorate the presenting life problem, using a multimodal group practice, professional psychology can define its own house in which to practice. This general practice of psychology postulates that throughout the life span the client has available, brief, effective interventions designed to meet specific conditions as these may or may not arise. When such techniques are available, brief psychotherapy is the treatment of choice for about 85% of those seeking help, leaving long-term therapy for those clients who are best benefited by a protracted intervention.

HISTORICALLY, PSYCHOLOGY HAS been a research-based profession. It has a history of innovative application of research findings and develop-

* With Gary R. VandenBos.

ment of new treatment and prevention strategies, while rigorously evaluating these advances. But psychology has given away most of its knowledge. No other profession has given away so much, so often, and so freely.

It is paradoxical that, although psychology has contributed so much over the last 80 years to ophthalmology, neurology, medicine, education, and mental health, professional psychologists face continued difficulty gaining appropriate independent recognition. Psychology has put up the frame of its house but has forgotten the siding and roof.

This article is a beginning attempt to complete psychology's own house. Only when we have our house, and practice in it, will we obtain our appropriate recognition. We intend to present a model for the general practice of psychology or, more accurately, the group practice of psychology. Before describing such a model, we will review 20 years of research on treatment that has convinced us of the clinical effectiveness and economic efficacy of active, brief psychological intervention. We will then discuss the implications of short-term treatment for the diagnostic process, the concept of "cure," and the delivery of psychological services. As an illustration, we will present a case history. Finally, we will present the group practice model, its rationale, and range of services.

Short-Term Psychological Intervention: Beneficial and Cost-Saving

Psychological services are valuable, necessary, and effective. Psychotherapy can be economically provided, and failure to provide such services jeopardizes the effective functioning of basic medical services. However, to deliver psychological services effectively and economically, the traditional techniques, concepts, and organization of service delivery must be reexamined.

It is economically unfeasible to provide long-term psychotherapy to all patients. More important, it is a misallocation of treatment resources. Not everyone wants it, needs it, or would accept it. Even when psychotherapy is offered by highly competent psychotherapists, who make the process understandable and the benefits clear (a process well illustrated in Karon and VandenBos, 1977), many patients do not choose long-term treatment for a host of reasons.

At Kaiser Permanente a series of investigations on the effectiveness of psychological services within a prepaid health plan, including its impact on medical utilization, have been conducted. Follette and Cummings (1967) compared the number and type of medical services sought before and after the intervention of psychotherapy in a large group of randomly selected patients. Four groups of patients were studied. These included patients who (a) had a single psychotherapeutic session, (b) underwent brief therapy, averaging 6.2 sessions, (c) received long-term therapy, averaging 33.9 sessions, or (d) served as a matched control group, demonstrating similar distress but not seen in psychotherapy. The findings indicated that (a) persons in emotional distress were significantly higher users of both inpatient and outpatient medical facilities compared with the health plan average, (b) significant declines in medical utilization were manifested in all three groups of emotionally distressed individuals who received psychotherapy compared with the control group, and (c) these declines remained constant during the 5 years following the termination of psychotherapy, without additional psychotherapy being required to maintain the lower level of medical utilization.

In a subsequent study, Cummings and Follette (1968) found that despite intensive efforts to increase the number of referrals to psychotherapy, the number of health plan subscribers seeking psychotherapy reaches a level and remains fairly constant thereafter. They demonstrated that there is *no basis for the fear* that an increased demand for psychotherapy would financially endanger the medical system. In fact, they found that providing psychological services lowers overall costs. In a further study, Cummings and Follette (1976) sought to determine whether the results represented a therapeutic effect, the consequence of extraneous factors, or a deleterious effect. The results suggest that the reduction in medical utilization was the consequence of resolving the emotional distress that was being manifested in physical symptoms.

In the most recent study, Cummings (1977) examined the effect of different frequencies of treatment for the so-called "interminable" patients. Such patients, who represent about 5% of psychotherapy patients, manifest a pan-anxiety and closely fit the traditional diagnostic entity of pseudoneurotic schizophrenia. He found that increased frequency of treatment (i.e., up to three visits per week) was actually deleterious. It led to increased emotional distress and enormous increases in the utilization of medical services. In comparison, schedules of one visit every 30, 60, or 90 days were equally as effective as one per week and far more effective than schedules of several sessions per week.

The results of 20 years of research at Kaiser Permanente suggest that the treatment of choice for all persons presenting themselves with emotional complaints and problems in living is active short-term psychological intervention without preselection criteria. For 85% of these unselected persons, such treatment is more effective than long-term psychotherapy, and for another 5% of patients, intensive long-term psychotherapy may actually be deleterious.

This does *not* mean that long-term psychotherapy is never appropriate or needed. Long-term psychotherapy is a valuable treatment procedure. The policy of providing short-term treatment as the treatment of choice for the vast majority of patients makes long-term psychotherapy economically feasible for the relatively few patients for whom it is necessary and appropriate. But, long-term intensive psychotherapy represents a major commitment of limited resources, and it represents a massive incursion into the patient's life. Long-term psychotherapy, like—to use a medical example—surgery, should not be the initial treatment of choice when less radical interventions could serve as, or even more, effectively.

Brief, active psychotherapy can involve the analysis of transference and resistance, uncover unconscious conflicts, and have all the characteristics of long-term therapy except length. Both behavioral change and resolution of emotional conflict can be accomplished. Such brief treatment is valued by patients because it rapidly and directly addresses their conscious conflicts and behavioral difficulties, and it is of proven value (Karon &VandenBos, 1972, 1975, 1976; Malan, 1963, 1976; Mann, 1973).

RECONSIDERATION OF ASSUMPTIONS

The startling findings of the impact of short-term psychological services on mental health status, as well as the utilization of physical health services, challenges the traditional concepts of diagnosis and "cure." In addition, the use of short-term treatment as the initial treatment of choice challenges the solo practitioner delivery model and beliefs about the lack of specific treatments for specific conditions.

First, we need to reconsider the problem of "diagnosis." Brief psychotherapy is not facilitated by accepting a vague description of the patient's problem or by giving a simplistic DSM-II (or DSM-III) diagnosis, which characterizes the nature of the dysfunction rather than its impact on the person. We believe that central to the initial interview is the establishment of what we call an "operational diagnosis." It stems directly from the question, What brings this individual here today?

Consider the alcoholic husband who sits crying in a psychologist's office, unable to work or function because his wife left him that morning. He states, "It all happened because I drink too much, have for ten years." To simply diagnose and begin treating his alcoholism and reassure him that his wife will return misses what actually motivated him to come to the office. The operational diagnosis would be "reaction to rejection (or loss)," including a resulting inability to act to alter the situation or even to continue routine functioning. This operational diagnosis leads directly to an expanded discussion of his feelings (guilt, concerns about self-esteem, possible fears related to dependency), an assessment of the situation (how does his drinking influence his functioning), and an action plan (to end or control his drinking, to begin communication with his wife, to control anxiety).

The second area that must be reexamined is our own professional conceptualizations of the outcome of psychological intervention. Our concept of treatment outcome might well be termed the "ultimate cure." Any recontact with a former mental health patient is labeled a "relapse" and is viewed as evidence that the earlier intervention was either unsuccessful or incomplete. We usually act as if contact with a professional psychologist is for a single, simple, unified problem and that six sessions will solve everything forever. No other field of healthcare holds this conceptualization of treatment outcome.

A patient sees a physician, for example, because of headaches. On the first visit the physician may find that it is related to a sinus condition. With treatment, the symptoms disappear. Three months later the patient may return with the same symptoms. This time the physician may determine that it is related to a beginning high blood pressure condition. Treatment may eliminate the symptoms. Three months later the patient may again return with headaches. This time the problem may be tension. The symptoms are the same, and the site of the symptoms is the same. In each case the physician may have properly diagnosed, treated, and cured the problem. In such a case, the return is not viewed as a relapse, nor is it viewed as ineffective or incomplete treatment. However, in psychology, both the patient and doctor seem to have one chance. Another view is possible. We now think in terms of "amelioration" rather than "cure." This is more realistic and humane.

The third area that needs reexamination is the conceptualization of the "ideal" therapist. The notion of the "perfect psychologist" grows out of the way we train our students and the way psychological services are delivered. Psychology, as a part of and growing from the mental health field, generally operates on a "one practitioner/one theory" model. We assume every psychologist should be able to treat any patient and any problem. As a result, patients get whatever psychological intervention the therapist was trained to provide, regardless of the nature of the problem or the efficacy of the given technique with that problem. Fortunately, most methods of psychological intervention are helpful, if not always the most efficient.

We need to acknowledge that every therapist is not the "right" therapist for every patient or every problem. In addition, we need to acknowledge that different techniques are differentially effective and efficient with different problems and populations. But, the acknowledgement that no one therapist is *the most* appropriate for all tasks challenges us to develop new psychological service delivery models that reflect and build on this fact. The general (group) practice of psychology is one such model.

A fourth factor concerns the lack of attention that psychology has given to the consideration of specific interventions for specific conditions. As a field, we tend to believe that there are no such specifics. Yet there are many instances in which specific interventions are well known. For example, it has long been known that with school phobias it is important to force the child to attend school. It has been demonstrated that dynamic psychotherapy *plus* biofeedback is more effective than psychotherapy alone in the treatment of migraines. Furthermore, pain clinics have demonstrated the value of well-tailored interventions consisting of dynamic intervention and behavior modification to break drug rituals, to help individuals live with chronic pain, and to end the physician habit. Such examples illustrate that specific psychological interventions are feasible and that research must be directed to develop further specific interventions to ameliorate emotional and physical distress.

AN ILLUSTRATIVE CASE

Let us consider a case that illustrates the general practice of psychology using the concepts of operational diagnosis, amelioration, multi-provider delivery system, and specific interventions. The case is not atypical. It illustrates how brief psychotherapy and other psychological services, available periodically on an "as-needed" basis, have had major impact.

Kevin arrived at the general hospital emergency room with a drug overdose. Psychological consultation was immediately requested in the emergency room, as a drug overdose is far more than a medical problem and the earlier psychological intervention is initiated in the total agency contact, the more effective it becomes.

The initial operational diagnosis was "I hurt, stop the pain, make me happy again." At that moment it is easy to convince the patient to undergo detoxification. The initial goal is simply to stop the pain, to get him "clean." The psychology staff, not the medical staff, assumed responsibility for the patient. Rather than admit him, he was treated through a "home detoxification" program.

Under this program, patients are detoxified in their own home over a 72-hour period. During this process the psychologist (and/or succeeding "on-call" therapists) calls the patient every 2 hours, around the clock, to get a report of the current symptoms, provide realistic explanations of current bodily reactions, and inform the patient of what physical reactions might reasonably occur in the next 2 hours. This is reassuring. It takes the "edge" off the terror of the unknown by making the process understandable and predictable.

The program also involves having a drug-free friend stay with the patient during this 72-hour period. This provides a critical measure of social support, someone with whom to talk, and someone to call the psychology center if additional contact is needed. The friend is given a brief period of training. This time is used to determine whether the friend will be a suitable companion during detoxification (i.e., not a substance-abusive personality). In this situation of crisis and pain, patients usually select a truly "clean" friend. The friend's experience of "kicking a habit" is reviewed (e.g., stopping smoking or losing weight). This serves as a model for understanding the patient's withdrawal experience. Of course, it is emphasized that withdrawal from drugs is much, much worse. The friend is prepared for the patient's pleas for a "fix" and told that giving in hurts the patient by returning him or her to "ground zero" of the addiction. Of course, in the case of alcohol or barbituate withdrawal, the friend is provided a "hummer" to use in case of convulsions, although it is emphasized that the patient cannot know the friend has it, as the knowledge can provide a psychological inducement for convulsions.

At Kaiser Permanente we have found that less than one half of 1% of patients experience convulsions during "home detox," a rate lower than that which occurs when detoxification is done in the hospital. Home detoxification is less subjectively painful for patients. In the hospital both the patient and staff are constantly tempted by the ever-present "pain killers." For the addictive personality, the degree of pain during detoxification is directly proportional to the proximity of a "sympathetic" physician.

At the end of the 72 hours, Kevin was seen in the psychology out-patient clinic for an extended intake, covering four sessions. The operational diagnosis was "accepting a 'temporary' new lifestyle, which might be more 'healthy' and happier." These sessions covered material that any good therapeutically oriented intake evaluation would cover: current life situation, immediate concerns, drug history, entire life history, and how the Center could be helpful to him—in other words, a behavioral and psychodynamic assessment.

He was 28 years old. Despite being a college graduate, he had never really been gainfully employed. During the first week of his first job after graduation he panicked and abruptly left work, hitchhiking from Maine to California without even pausing to pick up his possessions. He had existed in the drug culture for 3.5 years without "my feet ever touching ground," doing whatever was necessary to survive. He was a "cafeteria-addict," using whatever drugs were available. He had had emotional difficulties all his life, had an exceptionally poor self-image, and was convinced that no one could ever love or accept him. His object relations were poor. His sexual relations did not begin until college and consisted of getting drunk with skid row bums and performing fellatio on them.

Kevin was aware that drugs had been hurting him, but all he wanted was to get back to the "happy days" when drugs eased the pain and made him feel good. His desires needed redirection in order to really change his life and use of drugs. This required the therapist to redefine the patient's situation and concerns in a way that made sense to the patient and was "solvable" by a treatment plan. Central to this was finding a narcissistic wish, an unfulfilled dream, that might be achieved if a different lifestyle was adopted. The patient was not asked to change forever, only to agree to change for a short period of time. He was told this amount of time is needed for him and the therapist (and later the group) to "dig" inside him to find the "right" lifestyle for him. This keeps the process a collaborative one and keeps the task achievable.

Kevin was invited to join a group therapy program for drug users. The technique utilized at Kaiser Permanente is called "exclusion therapy." It lasts 24 sessions. This exclusion therapy combines verbal insight therapy, with a schedule of planned covert and overt reinforcements, and a system of exclusion if drugs are used. If the members use drugs, they are excluded for 1 week; with three exclusions, they are removed from that particular group.

With the benefit of this program of social support, benign confrontation, and reinforcement of a drug-free lifestyle, Kevin stopped using drugs for the first time in 3.5 years. He obtained and maintained a job as a laborer. By the end of the group, drug use had a new meaning for Kevin. It was a symptom, a sign that he was trying to escape anxiety—not some vague tension, but anxiety specifically related to pressures to succeed and to the fear of inadequacy. The impulse to use drugs had come to mean that there was "a problem" to discuss, examine, and solve.

Kevin was not cured. In fact, the neurotic aspects of his behavior were just becoming clear to him, but his life had certainly changed. His drug abuse had stopped. He was gainfully employed. He felt better about himself than ever before in his life, both because he was doing things to be proud of and because he had some understanding of his own unreasonable self-criticism.

The initial intervention with Kevin involved 29 contacts. This is more than is typical. However, addiction-related problems are multifaceted and, hence, require longer intervention, although much of it can be done in effective and cost-efficient group settings. It was behaviorally oriented toward ending his drug use, but it also addressed the motivation behind the drug use.

It was more than a year before Kevin returned. He returned in crisis. However, he was still drug-free and functioning adequately in all areas of his life. He had renewed doubts about "being good enough" and feared he would begin using drugs again. Since he was last seen, he had married. The precipitating event for his return was the birth of his son. While he could acknowledge he was "good enough" to have a job and "good enough" to be married, he could not see himself as "good enough" to be a father. These fears were addressed in six individual sessions, which provided an opportunity for emotional growth and insight.

It was more than a year before Kevin was seen again. He returned in an acute anxiety state, again fearing a return to drug use. The precipitant was the purchase of a home which, like earlier "normal" life events, had special symbolic meaning and triggered specific childhood conflicts for Kevin. He was seen for four individual sessions. During this contact it was possible to resolve another portion of his feelings toward male authority figures, this time toward a very successful and somewhat domineering father-in-law.

It was again more than a year before Kevin returned. In the meantime, a second child was born, and he had obtained an entrance-level professional job. This time there was marital conflict. Two sources were apparent. Kevin was overidentifying, in a negative manner, with his older child. He feared that his son would grow up to be "a loser" like himself. As a result, Kevin was being overcritical of the son. The couple differed on discipline. In addition, some sexual difficulties were beginning to develop. Kevin was seen for two individual sessions, and marriage counseling with a *different* therapist was recommended. A new "neutral" therapist was important, so that the wife did not feel outnumbered, as if the therapist was the husband's ally. The group practice organization facilitated the referral to a different therapist who specialized in couple work and who began on a positive footing because of the "halo" effect of the positive transference. In an eight-session contact, the marital difficulties were resolved, and Kevin made further growth in relation to his own sexual conflicts.

Kevin returned a year and a half later in a panic. This time the precipitant was an upcoming promotion. The operational diagnosis was "anxiety management." He was seen for two individual sessions to evaluate the situation and place the anxiety in a familiar context. It was suggested he learn an alternative method of relaxing—biofeedback. Ten sessions of biofeedback training were provided, again by a separate therapist within the group practice, who was especially skilled in these techniques.

It would be 2.5 years before Kevin returned. In the intervening time, his wife contacted the Center and was seen for six individual sessions regarding issues of her own. Again, a different therapist saw her. The short-term contact was successful in resolving the conflict. When Kevin returned again, the nature of his fears were similar and again precipitated by success—becoming a landlord. Four individual sessions resolved the fears and facilitated further resolution of the neurotic struggles.

Another year later Kevin returned in a homosexual panic. He had been attracted to a male tenant and feared returning to nonproductive ways of relating, similar to those he had in college. Four individual sessions allowed further growth concerning sexual issues and resolved the fears.

About a year and a half later, Kevin returned for one session. This time there was no problem. He just wanted an "annual mental health checkup" and to report on the good things that were continuing to happen.

Over the course of 9 years, Kevin received 80 sessions of psychological treatment. Thirty sessions were in the first year, and 50 sessions were spread over the next 8 years, an average of 6 per year. With this minimal contact, Kevin had been moved from an almost nonfunctional "derelict" condition to being gainfully employed, vocationally successful, and a successful and happy husband/father. There had been considerable psychological and economical growth. He had received a wide range of services: detoxification, group therapy, crisis intervention, marriage counseling, individual psychotherapy, and biofeedback training. Four different psychologists with different specialized skills and interest had been involved.

The results obtained in this series of repeated brief interventions with Kevin are on a par with those typically expected from continual treatment. Repeated brief interventions can be effective because crises are tremendous motivators for insight as well as behavior change when the therapist is appropriately knowledgeable and skilled at managing the anxiety and using it both to gain insight and to change behavior. Even with schizophrenics, repeated brief, but active, insight-oriented psychotherapy can be as effective and as successful as continuing contact (Karon & VandenBos, 1972). Some patients will accept treatment only when in crisis. At such times they see and want to receive the value of psychological services.

A MODEL FOR THE GENERAL PRACTICE OF PSYCHOLOGY

In light of the earlier discussion, we would like to present a model for the practice of psychology. How would it operate?

First, it would be an interdependent group practice. Currently, most of the so-called group practices are really solo practitioners who share common offices and related expenses. The psychology group would include meaningful weekly case conferences, with required attendance, at which all members would present and discuss cases. Case transfer and/or supervision would be encouraged when one therapist had particular expertise with a given population, type of problem, or technique.

Second, there would be a diversity of theoretical orientation, technical skills, and preferred populations. This recognizes the fact that virtually all approaches have something to offer but that no one can possibly be truly skilled at all techniques. In fact, skill in some clinical procedures is probably negatively correlated with skill in other interventions. Diversity of available resources would assure that treatment would be more likely to serve the unique needs of the patient. Psychotherapy and other psychological interventions would have the highest probability of being useful rather than simply being what the therapist has to offer. Such an organization has many advantages. Psychologists can function in the manner they prefer and with the type of patients with which they work best. But, it would also expand each member's awareness of the range and potential of psychological interventions.

Third, all members would be directly involved in treatment on, at least, a part-time basis. There would be no full-time administrator or supervisor. Professionals who move into such positions quickly lose touch with patients, research on treatment, and treatment innovation. The group would be the equivalent of 6 full-time persons, although from 6 to 12 persons might be needed to obtain 6 full-time members. Four positions would be doctoral level professionals, each with three or four different "mini-specialities" (i.e., populations, type of problems, techniques). In addition, two positions would be psychological service workers with master's degrees, specialized in such techniques as biofeedback and behavior modification.

There are many justifications for such a group practice of psychology. In recent years there has been a tremendous growth in specialized single-service centers. Such centers offer specialized intensive intervention addressed to specific problems, such as drug abuse, alcohol abuse, suicide, rape, runaway, chronic pain, and hypertension. However, there are coordination and efficiency problems with such centers. Likewise, community mental health centers have difficulty controlling costs, and they are more likely to be staffed by generalists rather than specialists. How long will it be before such an unorganized system collapses? The group practice of psychology offers a diverse, effective, and cost-efficient alternative.

There have been recent efforts to increase the training and involvement of primary care physicians in the broad range of mental health problems. Such basic and continuing education of general physicians has been needed, but there are limits to such efforts. A physician can integrate and implement only a limited number of procedures and still be a general medical practitioner. Moreover, if too much continuing education is provided, the problems of resistance to psychological understanding or, alternatively, a total "conversion" to a psychological perspective can occur. Both defeat the purpose of such education. Another frequently discussed "improvement" in the health system is to have a mental health specialist (generally a registered nurse or someone with a master's degree in arts or social work) employed as an "allied health" professional in a general health setting. This is useful, but is is only a partial solution. Such individuals, of necessity, are either generalists or narrowly focused specialists and, of course, have all the limitations of the solo practitioner model.

The "general practice" of psychology model has implications for the training of professional psychologists. It provides an alternative model to the solo practitioner model and, hence, offers alternative conceptualization of collegial exchange and interdependence. It suggests different views of the therapeutic process and encourages diversity of training. Moreover, professional schools of psychology could utilize this type of organization for operating their own outpatient centers, involving senior staff as well as interns. Unfortunately, it is common to find that the innovative professional schools are training their graduates to work with limited populations, with one theory, with one technique, in a solo delivery model.

This model also has implications for national health insurance. Cost containment must, of necessity, be a major consideration in such planning. The general practice model encourages the least radical and less costly intervention and facilitates the use of the most appropriate, effective, and efficient approach to specific problems. Moreover, psychology practice groups could be capitated to provide psychological services to specific areas or populations. Such a use of capitation is performance based and utilizes the profit motive to achieve clinically effective and cost-efficient service. The fee-for-service model encourages prolonged and costly service. Psychology groups could contract with government and private insurance companies to service specific populations.

However, it must be clear what such groups offer to provide, namely, the artful application of scientifically based knowledge and techniques to solve human problems and relieve unnecessary physical and psychological suffering. In the past, the mental health field had promised society too much—a nirvana of total freedom from all anxiety and guilt. This impossible promise is one small causal factor in our society's problems with drugs and alcohol. Some behavior should cause guilt and anxiety. Who wants a guilt-free murderer, rapist, or child molester in the neighborhood? Freud argued that guilt and anxiety are critical to the development of a mature and healthy personality. Psychology can only, and should only, offer aid in the relief of excessive and unrealistic guilt and anxiety which, if unattended to, can cause physical health problems. The group practice of psychology can offer information, technical skills, and assistance in making alternatives "thinkable" and "achievable."

The general practice of psychology is important to mental health as well as physical health. We know that when behavioral and psychological problems are overlooked, the physical system is overloaded and physical problems develop. In a parallel fashion, if our health delivery systems ignore emotional problems, medical services will be inappropriately overutilized.

{ 9 }

THE TWENTY YEARS KAISER PERMANENTE EXPERIENCE WITH PSYCHOTHERAPY AND MEDICAL UTILIZATION: IMPLICATIONS FOR NATIONAL HEALTH POLICY AND NATIONAL HEALTH INSURANCE*

OUT OF NECESSITY, and very early in its experience of providing comprehensive health coverage without the usual limitations, Kaiser Permanente discovered it had to provide mental health services to prevent over-utilization of medical facilities by otherwise healthy persons who were somaticizing. The 20-year clinical and research experience at Kaiser Permanente of providing mental health coverage as part of a comprehensive health maintenance program has a range of implications for national health policy. These implications include cost, utilization, scope of coverage, range of services, access to care, types of providers, and the role of program evaluation/research.

The Kaiser Permanente Health Plan, as the forerunner to the modern Health Maintenance Organization (HMO), was an early pioneer in the provision of comprehensive mental health care as an integral part of a total, prepaid health care delivery system. The HMO concept was born in the Mojave Desert of California during the severe economic depression of the 1930's. After receiving the contract to build the

---

*With Gary R. VandenBos, Ph.D.

aqueduct to Los Angeles from Boulder Dam (later renamed Hoover Dam), a then unknown builder named Henry J. Kaiser experienced difficulty recruiting and maintaining adequate construction crews on the desert. This was due to the total lack of medical care in the desert and a resulting reluctance of workers to move their families there. Upon hearing of this problem, Sidney Garfield, a young physician, offered to provide all of the facilities and services necessary for comprehensive health care, not only for the workers, but also for their families. The cost of this package would be a nickel per employee work hour; there would be no fee-for-service no matter how adverse the experience. A further unique feature was that a significant proportion of effort would be expended to prevent illness, particularly problems such as sunstroke and heat exhaustion, which are perils on the desert.

The arrangement was made and the concept of a capitation to keep people healthy as opposed to a fee to treat the sick was implemented—perhaps out of necessity, perhaps out of Kaiser's ability to recognize a good idea. Seemingly overnight Kaiser built his shipyards during World War II, and brought along Dr. Garfield and a now greatly expanded prepaid health care group. The Kaiser Permanente Health Plan went public on the West Coast following World War II and immediately flourished. Its tremendous acceptance was obviously the result of the Kaiser plan's providing comprehensive treatment for all problems at low subscriber rates, without the exclusions, limitations, co-insurance and other troublesome features common to other health plans at the time. Kaiser Permanente has enjoyed three decades of growth and success to date and is still flourishing.

Today, there are 8.5 million subscribers. Its nearly three dozen hospitals are divided into semi-autonomous regions which, in order of establishment, are: Northern California, Portland (Oregon), Southern California, Hawaii, Cleveland and Denver. These regions enjoy a great deal of independence from each other, but are tied nominally together by the one Kaiser Foundation. This leads to health care delivery (and particularly mental health care delivery) varying considerably in format from one region to the next.

It was nearly 30 years before Dr. Garfield articulated his concept of "health maintenance" in a historic publication. His idea caught the attention of the federal government, and led to legislation to encourage the creation of Health Maintenance Organizations in the United States instead of the traditional fee-for-service health plan reimbursement.

This paper chronicles the 20-year experience in the first, or Northern California region, and particularly the San Francisco facility where the primary research was conducted.

THE BEGINNING OF THE KAISER PERMANENTE MENTAL HEALTH BENEFIT

Kaiser Permanente soon found, to its dismay, that once a health system makes it easy and free to see a physician, there occurs an alarming inundation of medical utilization by seemingly physically health persons. In private practice the physician's fee has served as a partial deterrent to over-utilization, until the recent growth of third party payment for health care services. The financial base at Kaiser Permanente is one of per capitation, and neither the physician nor the Health Plan derives an additional fee for seeing the patient. Rather than becoming wealthy from imagined physical ills, the system could be bankrupted by what was regarded as abuse by the hypochondriac.

Early in its history, Kaiser Permanente added psychotherapy to its list of services, first on a courtesy reduced fee of five dollars per visit and eventually as a prepaid benefit. This was initially motivated *not* by a belief in the efficacy of psychotherapy, but by the urgent need to get the so-called hypochondriac out of the doctor's office. From this initial perception of mental health as a dumping ground for bothersome patients, twenty years of research has led to the conclusion that no comprehensive prepaid health system can survive that does not provide a psychotherapy benefit.

THE NSA PATIENT

Early investigations confirmed physicians' fears they were being inundated, for it was found that 60% of all visits were by patients who had nothing physically wrong with them. Add to this the medical visits by patients whose physical illnesses are stress related (peptic ulcer, ulcerative colitis, hypertension, etc.), and the total approaches a staggering 80 to 90% of all physician visits. Surprising as these findings were 25 years ago, nationally accepted estimates today range from 50 to 80% (Shapiro, 1971). Interestingly, over 2,000 years ago Galen pointed out that 60% of all persons visiting a doctor suffered from symptoms that were caused emotionally, rather than physically (Shapiro, 1971).

The experience at Kaiser Permanente subsequently demonstrated that it is not merely the removal of all access barriers to physicians that alone fosters somatization. The customary manner in which healthcare is delivered inadvertently promotes somatization (Cummings & VandenBos, 1979). When a patient who has not been feeling up to par attempts to discuss a problem in living (job stress, marital difficulty, etc.) during the course of a consultation with a physician, that patient is usually either politely dismissed by an overworked physician or given a tranquilizer. This unintentionally implies criticism of the patient which, when repeated on subsequent visits, fosters the translation of this emotional problem into something to which the physician will respond. For example, the complaint that "my boss is on my back" may become at some point a low back pain with neither the patient nor the physician associating the symptom with the original complaint. Suddenly the patient is "rewarded" with x-rays, laboratory tests, return visits, referrals to specialists and, finally, even temporary disability which removes the patient from the original job stress and tends to reinforce protraction and even permanence of the disability.

Estimates of stress related physical illness are subjectively determined, whereas number of physician visits by persons demonstrating no physical illness can be objectively verified through random samplings of all visits to the doctor. After more or less exhaustive examination, the physician arrives at a diagnosis of "no significant abnormality," noted by the simple entry of "NSA" in the patient's medical chart. Repeated tabulations of the NSA entries, along with such straightforward notations as "tension syndrome" or similar designations, consistently yielded the average figure of 60%.

During the early years of Kaiser Permanente there was considerable resistance to accepting such estimates because it was reasoned that if 60 to 90% of physician visits reflect emotional distress, 60 to 90% of the doctors should be psychotherapists! This fear, as will be demonstrated below, was unfounded, because subsequent research indicated that a relatively small number of psychotherapists can effectively ameliorate these patients.

In an effort to help the physician recognize and cope with the distress-somatization cycle, Follette and Cummings (1967) developed a scale of 38 Criteria of Distress. These criteria do not employ psychological jargon; rather, they are derived from typical physician entries in the medical charts of their patients. The researchers worked back from patients seen in psychotherapy to their medical charts on which the diagnosis NSA had been made. They gathered extensive samplings of typical entries which connoted distress and validated these into the 38 criteria shown in Table 1. Physicians were urged to refer patients for psychotherapy who scored three points or more on this scale as attested by the physician's own medical chart entries.

After expending considerable effort and time validating this scale, it was discovered that emotional distress could be just as effectively predicted by weighing the patient's medical chart. The reason is that patients with chronic illness (or those involved in prenatal care) tend to see a physician in more or less scheduled appointments, while the patient suffering from emotional distress tends to utilize drop-in services, night visits and the emergency room. In the instance of the chronically ill patient, the physician makes each entry in the chart immediately under the one bearing the date of the previous visit, resulting in several visits being recorded on one sheet front-and-back in the medical chart. By comparison, when emotionally distressed persons make nonscheduled visits the medical chart is not available and the physician makes the entry on a new and separate sheet which is later filed in the chart by medical records librarians. Repeating this practice through months and years builds up enormous medical charts, sometimes into the second and third volume.

Once the patient enters the somatization cycle there is an ever-burgeoning symptomotology because the original stress problem still exists in spite of all the physician's good efforts to treat the physical complaints. The patient's investment in his/her own symptom is only temporarily threatened by the physician's eventual exasperation, often accompanied by that unfortunate phrase, "It's all in your head." A new physician within the care system is found, and one whose sympathy and eagerness to determine the *physical* basis for the symptom have not been worn down by this particular patient. The inadvertent reward system continues, as does the growth of the medical chart.

THE EFFECT OF PSYCHOTHERAPY ON MEDICAL UTILIZATION

In the first of a series of investigations into the relationship between psychological services and medical utilization in a prepaid health plan setting, Follette and Cummings (1967) compared the number and type

Table 1. *Criteria of Psychological Distress with Assigned Weights*

One point	Two points	Three points
1. Tranquilizer or sedative requested.	23. Fear of cancer, brain tumor, venereal disease, heart disease, leukemia, diabetes, etc.	34. Unsubstantiated complaint there is something wrong with genitals.
2. Doctor's statement pt. is tense, chronically tired, was reassured, etc.	*24. Health Questionnaire: yes on 3 or more psych. questions.	35. Psychiatric referral made or requested.
3. Patient's statement as in no. 2.	25. Two or more accidents (bone fractures, etc.) within 1 yr. Pt. may be alcoholic.	36. Suicidal attempt, threat, or preoccupation.
4. Lump in throat.		37. Fear of homosexuals or of homosexuality.
*5. Health Questionnaire: yes on 1 or 2 psych. questions.	26. Alcoholism or its complications: delirium tremens, peripheral neuropathy, cirrhosis.	38. Non-organic delusions and/or hallucinations; paranoid ideation; psychotic thinking or psychotic behavior.
6. Alopecia areata.		
7. Vague, unsubstantiated pain.	27. Spouse is angry at doctor and demands different treatment for patient.	
8. Tranquilizer or sedative given.		
9. Vitamin B$_{12}$ shots (except for pernicious anemia).	28. Seen by hypnotist or seeks referral to hypnotist.	
10. Negative EEG.	29. Requests surgery which is refused.	
11. Migraine or psychogenic headache.	30. Vasectomy: requested or performed.	
12. More than 4 upper respiratory infections per year.	31. Hyperventilation syndrome.	
13. Menstrual or premenstrual tension; menopausal sx.	32. Repetitive movements noted by doctor: tics, grimaces, mannerisms, torticollis, hysterical seizures.	
14. Consults doctor about difficulty in child rearing.	33. Weight-lifting and/or health faddism.	
15. Chronic allergic state.		
16. Compulsive eating (or overeating).		
17. Chronic gastrointestinal upset; aereophagia.		
18. Chronic skin disease.		
19. Anal pruritus.		
20. Excessive scratching.		
21. Use of emergency room: 2 or more per year.		
22. Brings written list of symptoms or complaints to doctor.		

* Refers to the last 4 questions (relating to emotional distress) on a Modified Cornell Medical Index—a general medical questionnaire given to patients undergoing the Multiphasic Health Check in the years concerned (1959–62).

of medical services sought before and after the intervention of psychotherapy for a large group of randomly selected patients. The outpatient and inpatient medical utilization by these patients for the year immediately prior to their initial interview in the Kaiser Permanente Department of Psychotherapy as well as for the five years following that intervention were studied for three groups of psychotherapy patients (one interview only, brief therapy with a mean of 6.2 interviews, and long-term therapy with a mean of 33.9 interviews) and a "control" group of matched patients demonstrating similar criteria of distress but who were not, in the six years under study, seen in psychotherapy.

The findings indicated that: (a) persons in emotional distress were significantly higher users of both inpatient (hospitalization) and outpatient medical facilities as compared with the health plan average; (b) there were significant declines in medical utilization by those emotionally distressed individuals who received psychotherapy, as compared with the "control" group of matched patients; (c) these declines remained constant during the five years following the termination of psychotherapy; (d) the most significant declines occurred in the second year after the initial interview, and those patients receiving one session only or brief psychotherapy (2 to 8 sessions) did not require additional psychotherapy to maintain the lower level of medical utilization for five years, and (e) patients seen two years or more in continuous psychotherapy demonstrated no overall decline in total outpatient utilization (inasmuch as psychotherapy visits tended to supplant medical visits). However, even for this latter group of long-term therapy patients there was a significant decline in inpatient utilization (hospitalization) from an initial rate several times that of the health plan average, to a level comparable to that of the general, adult, health plan population.

In a subsequent study, Cummings and Follette (1968) found that intensive efforts to increase the number of referrals to psychotherapy by computerizing psychological screening with early detection and alerting the attending physicians did not significantly increase the number of patients seeking psychotherapy. The authors concluded that in a prepaid health plan setting that already maximally employs educative techniques to both patients and physicians, and provides a range of psychological services, the number of subscribers seeking psychotherapy at any given time reaches an optimal level and remains constant thereafter.

In another study, Cummings and Follette (1976) sought to answer in an 8th-year telephone follow-up whether the results described previously were a therapeutic effect, were the consequences of extraneous factors, or were a deleterious effect. It was hypothesized that if better understanding of the problem had occurred in the psychotherapeutic sessions, the patient would recall the actual problem rather than the presenting symptom and would have lost the presenting symptom and coped more effectively with the real problem. The results suggest that the reduction in medical utilization was the consequence of resolving the emotional distress that was being reflected in the symptoms and in the doctor's visits. The modal patient in this 8th-year follow up may be described as follows: She or he denies ever having consulted a physician for the symptoms for which the referral was originally made. Rather, the actual problem discussed with the psychotherapist is recalled as the reason for the psychotherapy visit, and although the problem is resolved, this resolution is attributed to the patient's own efforts and no credit is given the psychotherapist. This affirms the contention that the reduction in medical utilization reflected the diminution in emotional distress that had been expressed in symptoms presented to the physician.

Although they demonstrated in this study, as they did in their earlier work, that savings in medical services does offset the cost of providing psychotherapy, Cummings and Follette insisted that services provided must also be therapeutic in that they reduce the patient's emotional distress. That both cost savings *and* therapeutic effectiveness were demonstrated in the Kaiser Permanente studies was attributed by the authors to the therapists' expectations that emotional distress could be alleviated by brief, active psychotherapy that, as Malan (1976) pointed out, involves the analysis of transference and resistance and the uncovering of unconscious conflicts, and that has all the characteristics of long-term therapy except length. Given this orientation, it was found over a 5-year period that 84.6% of the patients seen in psychotherapy chose to come for 15 sessions or less (with a mean of 8.6). Rather than regarding these patients as "dropouts" from treatment, it was found on follow-up that they achieved a satisfactory state of emotional well-being that continued into the 8th year after termination of therapy. Another 10.1% of the patients were in moderate term therapy with a mean of 19.2 sessions, a figure that would probably be regarded as short-term in many traditional clinics. Finally, 5.3% of the patients were found to be "interminable," in that once they began psychotherapy they seemingly continued with no indication of termination.

In the most recently reported study, Cummings (1977) addressed the problem of the "interminable" patient for whom treatment was neither cost-effective nor therapeutically effective. The concept that some persons may be so emotionally crippled that they may have to be maintained for many years or for life was not satisfactory, for if 5% of all patients entering psychotherapy are "interminable," within a few years a program will be hampered by a monolithic case load, a possibility which has become a fact in many public clinics where psychotherapy is offered at nominal or no cost. It was originally hypothesized that these patients required more intensive intervention, and the frequency of psychotherapy visits was doubled for one experimental group, tripled for another experimental group, and held constant for the control group. Surprisingly, the cost–therapeutic effectiveness ratios deteriorated in direct proportion to the increased intensity; that is, medical utilization increased and the patients manifested greater emotional distress. It was only by reversing the process and seeing these patients at spaced intervals of once every 2 or 3 months that the desired cost–therapeutic effect was obtained. These results are surprising in that they are contrary to traditionally held notions about psychotherapy, but they demonstrate the need for ongoing research, program evaluation, and innovation if psychotherapy is going to be made available to everyone as needed.

The Kaiser Permanente findings regarding the offsetting medical cost-savings of providing psychological services have been replicated by others (Goldberg, Krantz, & Locke, 1970; Rosen & Wiens, 1979). In fact, such findings have been replicated in over 20 widely varied healthcare delivery systems (Jones & Vischi, 1978). Even in the most methodologically rigorous review of the literature on the relationship between the provision of psychotherapy and medical utilization (Mumford, Schlesinger, & Glass, 1978) the "best estimate" of cost savings is seen to range between 0% (but more appropriate treatment) and 24%.

IMPLICATIONS FOR NATIONAL HEALTH POLICY

The 20-year clinical and research experience at Kaiser Permanente of providing mental health coverage as part of a comprehensive health maintainence program has a range of implications for national health policy. These implications include cost, utilization, scope of coverage, range of services, access to care, types of providers, and the role of program evaluation/research.

In debates about the inclusion of a mental health component in national health insurance the foremost concern is cost. Fear and apprehension abound regarding the possibility of over-utilization, inappropriate utilization, and runaway costs. However, the experience at Kaiser Permanente clearly demonstrates that the inclusion of mental health benefits within a comprehensive healthcare plan will *not* bankrupt the "healthcare financing system." It has been incorrectly argued that mental health services are overly costly and cannot be controlled. Yet, the cost of providing mental health coverage at Kaiser Permanente only increased 3.5% per year between 1959 and 1979, while nationwide general medical costs have increased between 12% and 20% per year (Kiesler, Cummings, & VandenBos, 1979). It has been erroneously argued that utilization rates cannot be predicted, and, hence, that mental health is "uninsurable." However, it has been shown at Kaiser Permanente that utilization rates will rise to a predictable level and remain stable thereafter, despite intense efforts to increase it.

All of the false speculation about mental health coverage has gone on as if there were no data on and/or experience with the delivery of mental health care within large organized systems of care. Even beyond the Kaiser Permanente system, there are considerable data that address these concerns.

Dörken (1977) found that, within the Civilian Health and Medical Program of the Uniformed Services (CHAMPUS), mental health utilization rates overall were less than 2%, ranging from 0.7% to 3.9% for various states. The rates were stable over three separate years. The average length of mental health treatment per actual user in that program was 13.9 visits, and 83.7% of all mental health treatment was completed in 24 or fewer sessions.

It is also important to note an incidental finding by Dörken. Data on "mental health care" which are tabulated by primary diagnostic code can be grossly inaccurate. He found a 50% exaggeration in mental health utilization rates when such tabulation was done, tabulation by service code showed 644,650 mental health visits as compared with 941,755 visits when diagnosis codes were used. This results from routine physical health visits being classified as "mental health care" just because the patient is also receiving mental health care. Tabulation by actual treatment procedure eliminates this error.

Within the Federal Employees Health Benefits Plan it has been found that the utilization of intensive psychotherapy is miniscule, even when such treatment is available through the joint decision of the patient and the therapist (NIMH, 1976). In this particular analysis, 80% of all mental health patients were seen for 20 or fewer sessions.

The utilization of mental health services was studied by Blue Cross of Western Pennsylvania as the benefit was introduced in a particular health care plan (Jameson, Shuman, & Young, 1976). They found a progressive increase in the use of such health services over the first several years, but the utilization rate stabilized at about 1.5% for that particular population.

It has been a recurring finding in the psychotherapy research literature of the past twenty-five years that the average length of outpatient psychotherapy is between 6 and 12 sessions, and that 80% of all mental health treatment is completed in fewer than 20 sessions. Experience in the delivery of mental health services within organized systems of care has repeatedly found that mental health utilization rates and the length of mental health treatment are predictable and stable. Mental health benefits are obviously "insurable."

The experience at Kaiser Permanente suggests that the *failure* to provide mental health services is the factor that actually has the potential to bankrupt the healthcare financing system. When all barriers to access to medical care are removed, the health care system becomes overloaded because 60% or more of all physician visits are being made by patients manifesting somatized emotional distress. The exclusion of psychological services from national health insurance would encourage somatization and expensive over-utilization of general medical services.

Patients with concerns and symptoms related to social, interpersonal, and work difficulties do not tend to receive appropriate and responsive care within general health care systems. A perfunctory and unsympathetic response is most typical. As previously discussed, if the patient, however unconsciously translates this distress into a low back pain, the patient is immediately "rewarded" by the physician in the form of x-rays, laboratory tests, medications, and return visits. Even worse, temporary disability may be offered—which removes the patient from the presence of the stressor and renders unconsciously mandatory the continuation of the chronic pain as the only possible solution to what originally was an interpersonal problem. This is both costly and low-quality care.

Once studies at Kaiser Permanente showed that it was critical to provide mental health coverage, it had to be determined what type of mental health coverage to provide. The Kaiser Permanente experience has shown that when active, dynamic, brief psychotherapy is readily available and provided early in the individual's contact with the health care system by psychotherapists who are enthusiastic and proactive regarding such intervention, it is the treatment of choice for about 85% of the patients seeking mental health care. Such intervention yields a high cost–therapeutic effectiveness ratio, and is satisfactory to both patient and therapist. It dramatically reduces somatization and over-utilization of medical facilities. In the vast majority of cases, the provision of such brief therapy as the initial treatment intervention makes it economically feasible to provide long-term psychotherapy to the approximately 10% of patients who require it for therapeutically effective treatment.

The twenty year Kaiser Permanente experience indicates that mental health benefits should be included in national health insurance, and that the mental health system should emphasize readily available, brief, outpatient psychotherapy. This would make it possible to provide additional, second-level, mental health benefits to patients with certain emotional/behavioral problems, such as substance abuse, which require more extensive measures for treatment to be effective. We believe it is obvious that mere across-the-board inclusion in national health insurance of all traditional mental health service delivery modes (and the routine ways of determining which mode to pay) would be costly and inefficient. Clinical trials and systematic comparison of alternative methods of treatment for particular difficulties would determine what specifiable emotional/behavioral difficulties require more extensive treatment and would be eligible for reimbursement. This is how mental health coverage developed at Kaiser Permanente and continues to evolve.

National health insurance should avoid artificial limitations, upfront deductibles, and constant co-insurance. They are only partial solutions. Moreover, such mechanisms can block appropriate utilization of mental health services and appropriate use can prevent unnecessary medical costs as well as unnecessary human suffering. Rather, NHI should have no separate deductibles and co-payment should gradually increase the longer the patient receives service. The points at which co-payment percentages increase would occur should vary from specific problem to specific problem.

The organization of mental health service delivery at Kaiser Permanente is central to its effectiveness and cost efficiency. Mental health care is readily and directly available. This insures that the most clinically effective service is provided at the lowest possible cost. In order to accomplish this, multiple entry points exist. Early in our experience with mental health care it became clear that if there was only one entry point for gaining access to care, and this point was controlled by one profession with one orientation, mental health care, as well as the entire health care system, would be costly, biased, and nonresponsive. It is inefficient to require that the patient must first secure the "permission" of a primary care provider before seeking mental health services. Such a requirement wastes a medical visit, and primary care providers are not the most knowledgeable professionals to determine whether or not psychological care is indicated. The experience at Kaiser Permanente has shown that there are serious limits to the effectiveness of in-service education of primary care providers concerning the utilization of mental health services. Despite objective evidence that their patients need mental health services and specific recommendations to the physician that a referral should be made, a large percentage of primary care providers do not make needed referrals because of what appear to be professional biases.

The patient at Kaiser Permanente plays a major role in determining what services to seek and when to seek them. Our experience has shown that when the patient believes they should seek psychological treatment it is most cost efficient to allow them to seek such services, knowing that there are checks on the mental health provider. Referral to appropriate services, mental health or otherwise, is, of course, provided when the patient is unaware of the service or its potential value to them. Kaiser Permanente is an efficient health care system because it encourages educated consumers to utilize their knowledge to obtain the most appropriate service to meet their needs. National health insurance should include such cost-efficient mechanisms through freedom-of-choice in the selection of provider provisions.

It should be noted that the American public is far more knowledgeable about mental health problems and mental health resources than often realized. For example, the Survey Research Center at the University of Michigan recently conducted a large-scale nationwide study (Kulka, Veroff, & Douvan, 1979) replicating a 1957 study done for the Joint Commission on Mental Illness and Health. The samples for the two national surveys were independently selected using area-sampling probability methods to constitute representative cross-sections of individuals 21 years of age or older living in private households. It was found that 60% of the respondents had utilized or felt they would utilize mental health services for particular problems. There was a substantial increase in the proportion of the general population who had actually utilized mental health services—from 15% in 1957 to 26% in 1976. Further, there has been a change over the past two decades as to where help for mental health problems is sought. In 1957, 30% of those who had utilized mental health services sought help from their family doctor (or primary care provider); this dropped to 21% in 1976. Concurrently, there has been a dramatic increase in those seeking help from mental health providers, from 28% in 1957 to 47% in 1976. These data suggest two things. First, the stigma attached to having mental health problems and seeking mental health treatment has decreased over the last 20 years. Second, there has been a concommitant increase in the use of providers who are appropriately and specifically trained in the delivery of mental health care. Our 30-year effort to increase the number and quality of mental health services has had a positive effect. These data suggest that a strategy geared toward increasing the amount of advice given by family physicians about emotional and behavioral problems is regressive. Such a policy would tend to push mental health service delivery backward toward an inadequate and inappropriate system of health and mental health care such as that which existed twenty years ago. The public has been educated about mental health care. National health insurance, in order to be cost efficient, should utilize this public knowledge by incorporating multiple entry points into mental health care, just as Kaiser Permanente has been doing for the last twenty years.

Kaiser Permanente learned long ago that in order to provide mental health care in an effective and efficient manner, mental health care must be provided by professionals who are specifically trained to provide such care. While primary care providers are given in-service training to help them identify patients with mental health problems and make needed referrals, mental health care should be provided by fully-trained mental health professionals from the four core mental health professions. National health insurance should take the same course of action. Only those providers who are well-trained specifically in the delivery of mental health care should be allowed to provide and be reimbursed for such services. Standards for reimbursement of mental health services must be dependent on relevant mental health training, not professional degree independent of specialized training and supervised experience. Individuals without adequate professional training, such as general care physicians with a three-day introductory seminar on mental health issues, should not be eligible for reimbursement for the provision of mental health services. In addition, national health insurance should utilize the full range of fully trained mental health professionals to adequately meet the mental health needs of the nation at the lowest possible cost. No one profession, treatment approach, type of service, or system of service delivery is the most appropriate for all patients and all problems. If national health insurance should rely on only one profession or one treatment approach, it would be ineffective, costly, and nonresponsive. We learned this lesson long ago at Kaiser Permanente.

Inappropriate over-utilization of any health service will introduce unnecessary cost to a comprehensive health care system. At Kaiser Permanente a variety of reviews are utilized to monitor health care utilization and eliminate inappropriate over-utilization. This requires that patients who are over-utilizing medical services be identified and targeted for special alternative services which will eliminate their inappropriate over-utilization. Providers who inappropriately prescribe various laboratory testings and other services also need to be identified and provided with appropriate in-service training. Much of this can be done through appropriate management information systems, but multidisciplinary review of the appropriateness of care, both physical health care and mental health care, is also necessary. This serves as a check against inappropriate treatment and runaway costs, as well as serving to educate health and mental health care providers about the appropriateness and effectiveness of alternative health care services. Review of all types of health care delivery should occur under national health insurance after a certain number of visits or a certain dollar amount has been reached. Such reviews should be outcome oriented, consider unintended as well as intended outcomes, and utilize comprehensive objective data when subjective data within the group differ. Multidisciplinary review can be an accountability process, a continuing education process, and a clinical research process. National health insurance should utilize this opportunity.

The effectiveness and efficiency of the Kaiser Permanente health care system is related to the emphasis that is placed on meaningful program evaluation and health system research. National health insurance should incorporate an appropriately designed and utilized system of evaluation and monitoring. Without a meaningful program of research the role and value of psychological services within the Kaiser Permanente system would never have been discovered and refined. The interest of Congress, the executive branch, consumers, and taxpayers coincide in the need for a mechanism to assure appropriate high-quality service for the lowest reasonable price. Well-designed and appropriately utilized evaluation programs should be the core of vital cost-contained and quality assurance measures in national health insurance. NHI must provide for the best currently available treatment, yet it must be designed to facilitate innovation and incorporate change. This can best be accomplished by a system that emphasizes a range of alternative services, providers, and modes of delivery, assesses their intended and unintended outcomes in a comparative manner, and uses the feedback to produce appropriate change in the system itself. It is rare that a federal program is initiated with appropriate and comprehensive evaluation components designed as an integral aspect of the program, but national health insurance will be costly and ineffective if it does not include such a mechanism.

An evaluation/accountability/research component must be an integral part of any national health insurance structure. First, such an evaluation unit must be relatively autonomous. Second, the director of the evaluation unit must have an influential position within the health system and the ability to help modify the system. Third, the major directors of the evaluation unit must be broadly representative—no one profession, intervention strategy, or priority should dominate it. Fourth, the priorities and goals of the national health insurance system must be prospectively articulated. Fifth, the goals of the system must be stated in measurable clinical and behavioral outcome terms. Sixth, such program evaluation, health services research, and clinical research must be a continuous process. Seventh, the results must be publicly discussed and, when appropriate, the health system must be changed. A properly designed and funded evaluation component would pay off in dollars and cents by only continuing the funding of those services that are demonstrably effective and are provided in a cost-efficient manner.

SUMMARY

The experiences of Kaiser Permanente demonstrate that, when all barriers to physical health care are removed, the system becomes overloaded with 60% or more of physician visits by patients manifesting somatized emotional distress. When psychotherapy is properly provided within a comprehensive health system, the costs of providing the benefit are more than offset by the savings in medical utilization. The experience of over two decades at Kaiser Permanente indicates that it is not the provision of a psychotherapy benefit that can bankrupt a national health system. Rather, the failure to provide psychological care and/or the failure to appropriately provide it would bankrupt the system. National health insurance must include mental health benefits if the system is to operate on an efficient and effective basis. A system of constant research, innovation, and program evaluation is critical to meeting the health and mental health needs of all Americans.

Paratrooper Psychotherapy

I was a paratrooper in the 82nd Airborne in World War II, and I had made about 13 or 14 jumps behind enemy lines by the time the war was over. One interesting thing about paratroopers was that after about the third or fourth jump, they would get skittish, and when they landed, they would forget all they knew, and get themselves killed or wounded. I was one of several people sent back to the United States to work with the best psychologists and psychiatrists in the country to try to figure out what we could do to help these young men survive.

A training program was established on Long Island, and the best professionals in the country came to work with us—William Menninger, Frieda Fromm-Reichman, Karen Horney, and Patrick Mullaby. I remember Dr. Fromm-Reichman's saying, "It is not the length of the therapy which makes for change. It is the depth." This stuck with me, and I confronted this issue again at Kaiser Permanente. As a result of this training, my job during the war was to help the paratroopers keep their cool when they jumped into enemy territory. This "coaching" seemed to help these young men survive. So this might be called Paratrooper Psychotherapy, just in case someone wants to note yet another psychotherapy method.

I learned that some people could get better very quickly, or at least improve their behavior and functioning to a significant degree, with even a very brief intervention. I accepted this as legitimate, because I had seen it work effectively in helping paratroopers make their jumps.

On one of my last jumps, I was shot, and I lay bleeding in the snow for three days. Someone came by and said of my seemingly lifeless body, "Hey, I think this guy is alive!" I yelled out, "You're damn right I'm alive!" I was shipped back to get medical care and was in the hospital recuperating from my shattered knee and abdominal wounds, when I heard that the 82nd Airborne was going for another jump, and that the plan was to free Buchenwald con-

centration camp. No way was I going to miss this! I used my offi-cer's rank to leave the hospital, and became one of the American liberators of Buchenwald. I was probably the only paratrooper to make a jump with a cane during World War II. I wouldn't have missed that for the world.

{ 10 }

THE HEALTH MAINTENANCE ORGANIZATION

THE CONCEPT OF preventing disease and keeping the person healthy is inherent in the structure of the health maintenance organization (HMO). The HMO differs strikingly from the traditional health insurance plan, which reimburses the physician for treating illness only—a system that might be more properly termed a "sickness plan." In contrast, the HMO receives a capitation—a set monthly sum per subscriber—and in return agrees to care for all the health needs of that subscriber. No fee is paid the physician each time a patient is seen, and all care must be provided within the economics of the capitation. The incentive is toward keeping the person healthy, thereby avoiding costly medical treatment for disease that might have been prevented. From the beginning, the HMO is free to allocate a significant portion of its resources to the maintenance of health through various approaches, such as behavioral health, consumer education and outreach, preventive services such as periodic health checks, program evaluation and innovation, and the abandonment of traditional techniques and personnel, with concern only for effectiveness. To the extent that these efforts are successful, less money will be required for the treatment of chronic and serious diseases, eventually reducing costs to the consumer.

HISTORICAL PERSPECTIVE

Although the term *health maintenance organization* did not come into use until the Nixon administration, during which federal legislation designed to encourage the establishment of HMOs was enacted, the concept was born in the Mojave Desert of California four decades earlier (Cummings & VandenBos, 1981). After receiving the contract to build the aqueduct to Los Angeles from Boulder Dam (later renamed Hoover Dam), a then unknown builder named Henry J. Kaiser experienced difficulty recruiting and maintaining adequate construction crews on the desert. This problem was due to the total lack of medical care in the desert and the resulting reluctance of workers to move their families there. Upon hearing of this problem, Sidney Garfield, a young physician, offered to provide all the facilities and services necessary for comprehensive health care—not only for the workers, but also for their families. The cost of this package would be a nickel per employee work hour; there would be no fee for service, no matter how adverse the experience. A further unique feature was that a significant portion of effort would be expended to prevent illness, particularly such problems as sunstroke and heat exhaustion, which are perils in the desert.

The arrangement was made and the concept of a capitation to keep people healthy as opposed to a fee to treat the sick was implemented—perhaps out of necessity, perhaps out of Kaiser's ability to recognize a good idea. Seemingly overnight, Kaiser built his shipyards during World War II and brought along Dr. Garfield and a now greatly expanded prepaid health care group. The Kaiser Permanente Health Plan went public in 1945 and flourished immediately. Its tremendous acceptance was obviously because the Kaiser Plan provided comprehensive treatment without the exclusions, limitations, co-insurance and other troublesome features common to other health plans at the time. Kaiser Permanente has enjoyed four decades of growth, with nearly 10 million subscribers and 40 hospitals in California, Hawaii, Cleveland, Denver, and Washington, D.C.

As health costs began to escalate alarmingly in the 1970s, Garfield's concept of health maintenance caught the attention of the federal government and led to legislation aimed at encouraging the creation of health maintenance organizations in the United States instead of the traditional fee-for-service health plan reimbursement. Since that time, many HMOs have been established, but on a more modest scale than Kaiser Permanente. In fact, the subscriber population of the Kaiser

Plan still exceeds the combined populations of all other HMOs. For this reason, and because only the Kaiser Plan has existed for sufficient time, this chapter will discuss the Kaiser Permanente experience.

THE NEW MODEL OF HEALTH CARE DELIVERY

In traditional medical care, developed in the United States over two centuries, demand is regulated by the fee in the marketplace. Because of fees, people tend to put off medical care until they are definitely sick, giving the illusion that well-being is binary—that is, composed of either sick or healthy individuals. As Garfield (1976) has pointed out, however, four groups of individuals comprise an indefinite potential user population for health facilities: the well, the worried well (soma-tocizers and potential somatocizers), the asymptomatic sick, and the definitely sick. The fee is a regulator of demand, but it is not the only regulator. It tends to keep out the well, the worried well, and the asymptomatic sick. It may also keep out some definitely sick people who cannot afford the fee. For others, entry into the system is eco-nomically traumatic. For these reasons, a variety of prepaid health plans have been developed, all designed to reduce or eliminate the personal fee as a barrier to the sick in receiving treatment.

Once "sickness plans" eliminate the personal fee, something very in-teresting happens. The entire range of potential users enters the arena: the well, the worried well, the asymptomatic sick, and the definitely sick. The well and the worried well begin to compete with the sick on a first-come–first-served basis, causing an inevitable overloading of medical facilities, with reduced quality and efficiency. Physicians, who are trained to find disease, are frustrated as they strive to find sickness in the worried well, who now are beginning to squeeze out the sick in the competition for care.

Garfield, Collen, Feldman, Soghikian, Richardt, and Duncan (1976) identify four serious problems resulting from the impact of the well plus the sick once personal fees have been eliminated as a factor: (a) it overloads the relatively inelastic sick-care delivery system, causing a backlog of unavailable services and the inevitable queuing that has ac-companied free care; (b) the large number of well people that get into the system, by usurping the physician's time, act as a barrier to the entry of the sick—the reverse of what was intended by eliminating fees; (c) with this altered demand, instead of caring for the sick, physicians are spending a large portion of their time trying to find something wrong with well people, and they are doing this with techniques they learned for diagnosing sick people; and (d) the impact of the relatively unlimited amount of uncertainty demand on the limited supply of physicians inevitably creates inflationary costs.

To meet these serious problems, Garfield, Collen, Feldman, Soghikian, Richardt, and Duncan (1976) designed a system in which health testing is the key to matching the sick to the sick care system and the well to alternate systems that best meet their needs. This health testing combines a detailed automated medical history with comprehensive panels of physiological and laboratory tests administered by nonphysicians, a physical examination by a nurse practitioner, computer processing of results, and a physician review. This health testing has proved to be an effective way of separating demand into its component parts and matching each user with the appropriate care system, as illustrated in Figure 1.

The well and the worried well are directed into the health care system—a new concept designed to enhance health and to keep healthy people well. It is conducted by nonphysician personnel, ranging from educators to nurse practitioners and psychologists. The worried well receive definite guidance on maintaining well-being without overloading physicians by forcing them to try to find something wrong with people who are actually well. Those who have somaticized their concerns and their emotions are directed to the mental health service to see a psychologist. In all instances, the well and the worried well are kept out of the sick care system, where they would be mismatched.

The asymptomatic sick are directed to a system of preventive services, again conducted by nonphysician personnel, who are guided by computer-provided advice rules, with follow-up printouts of pertinent data sent to the patients' physicians. This obviously relieves the physician of many routine visits. Finally, the definitely sick are directed to the sick care system, where the physician's techniques to diagnose and treat disease are applied appropriately, and where the physician is now freed to devote the resources of the system only to the sick.

Figure 1. New Medical Care Delivery System

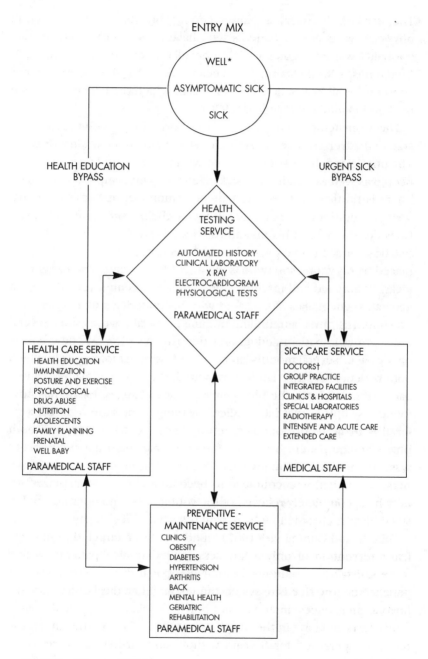

ENTRY MIX

WELL*

ASYMPTOMATIC SICK

SICK

HEALTH EDUCATION
BYPASS

URGENT SICK
BYPASS

HEALTH
TESTING
SERVICE

AUTOMATED HISTORY
CLINICAL LABORATORY
X RAY
ELECTROCARDIOGRAM
PHYSIOLOGICAL TESTS

PARAMEDICAL STAFF

HEALTH CARE SERVICE
  HEALTH EDUCATION
  IMMUNIZATION
  POSTURE AND EXERCISE
  PSYCHOLOGICAL
  DRUG ABUSE
  NUTRITION
  ADOLESCENTS
  FAMILY PLANNING
  PRENATAL
  WELL BABY

PARAMEDICAL STAFF

SICK CARE SERVICE
  DOCTORS†
  GROUP PRACTICE
  INTEGRATED FACILITIES
  CLINICS & HOSPITALS
  SPECIAL LABORATORIES
  RADIOTHERAPY
  INTENSIVE AND ACUTE CARE
  EXTENDED CARE

MEDICAL STAFF

PREVENTIVE -
MAINTENANCE SERVICE
CLINICS
  OBESITY
  DIABETES
  HYPERTENSION
  ARTHRITIS
  BACK
  MENTAL HEALTH
  GERIATRIC
  REHABILITATION
PARAMEDICAL STAFF

*Includes Worried Well   †Solo or Group Practice

PREVENTION AND MENTAL HEALTH

The startling discovery at Kaiser Permanente that up to 60% of all physician visits are by patients who have no significant physical abnormality was first thought to be a peculiarity of the HMO (Follette & Cummings, 1967). Eventually, it became clear that this figure is rather constant for all health delivery systems in which the barrier of the fee has been eliminated (Garfield, 1976).

The mismatching of the well and the worried well with the sick care system inadvertently rewards the somaticization of emotional distress. The physician who is overburdened with trying to find disease in well people as well as treating the sick listens only for symptoms of illness. There is no time to heed the patient's emotional distress, so the patient is conditioned to respond with what the physician needs to hear. Consider the man in his mid-fifties who has worked continuously for one boss since his mid-twenties. The boss has retired and has been replaced by his young son, who is impatient to implement a host of new ideas. Frightened and insecure, the middle-aged employee develops a general, vague malaise associated with his underlying anxiety and depression. His physician, finding nothing physically wrong after several visits, grows impatient and ignores the patient's plea, "My new boss is on my back." Several months later, and after several more visits in which both patient and physician feel frustrated, the man complains of a low back pain. Suddenly, the physician's attitude changes, for he has now found a symptom that has medical meaning. X rays are ordered, a referral is made to orthopedics, return visits are scheduled, and both physician and patient have now forgotten that the original complaint was, "My new boss is on my back." If the physician signs sick leave papers, the patient is encouraged to become a chronic somaticizer, for now he is completely relieved of the young boss who does not understand him. A chronic low back pain is a small price to pay.

Follette and Cummings (1967) found that brief, targeted psychological intervention of only a few sessions aided such patients to find more satisfactory solutions to their emotional distress, removed the patient from the sick care system, and reduced medical utilization (defined as all services, including not only physician visits, but also laboratory tests and days in the hospital) by 65% to 75%. Furthermore, the reduction persisted for 8 years without any further recourse to somaticization or recurrence of the emotional distress (Cummings & Follette, 1976). An intensive outreach program designed to transfer the patient with emotional distress from the sick care system to the preventive mental health system did not inundate the mental health system with patients, as had been feared would be the case (Cummings & Follette, 1968). Furthermore, when given a choice, 85% of patients chose short-term rather than long-term psychotherapy, with equally efficacious results (Cummings, 1977).

The Kaiser Permanente series of researches into the effect of psychological intervention on medical utilization (as summarized by Cummings, 1977) have been replicated 24 times, with similar results (Jones & Vischi, 1979), despite the wide variation of delivery systems and geographic locations in which the replications occurred. Mechanic (1966) has demonstrated that emotional distress can have a direct causal relationship to illness, either as a direct contributor or as an inhibitor to recovery. Schlesinger, Mumford, and Glass (1980) found that in the airways diseases, hypertension, ischemic heart disease, and diabetes, psychological intervention reduced medical utilization by increasing compliance to required medical regimens. The conclusion drawn from these studies is that by adding to the somaticizers of emotional distress those patients whose recovery can be enhanced by psychological intervention, up to 90% of physician visits are by persons who could benefit from brief psychotherapy—whether they are the worried well, the early sick, or the definitely sick.

Automated Multiphasic Screening

The heart of the HMO delivery system—which separates at entry the well, the worried well, the asymptomatic sick, and the definitely sick into the health care, preventive care, and sick care systems—is automated multiphasic screening administered as a periodic health check. Breslow (1973), who was the first to use the term *multiphasic screening*, has reviewed its evolution from a single-test procedure to the present complex automatic multiphasic services. In the decade spanning the late 1940s to the late 1950s, three pioneers can be identified: Breslow in California (Canelo, Bissell, Abrams, & Breslow, 1949), Ryder and Getting (1950) in Massachusetts, and Petrie in Georgia (Petrie, Bowdoin, & McLaughlin, 1952). In 1951, Collen first employed multiphasic screening as part of a periodic health examination within an organized group practice—in this case the Kaiser Permanente HMO (Collen & Linden, 1955). In 1964, that system was computerized into an automated multiphasic screening (Collen, 1966).

The health testing service at Kaiser Permanente includes a comprehensive automated medical history, 28 computerized laboratory tests, a 155-item automated psychological questionnaire designed to diagnose emotional distress, a physical examination by a nurse practitioner, and follow-up computer printouts to the patient's own physician. The automated test equipment and the computer determine automatically whether there is sufficient likelihood of disease being present to warrant further diagnostic testing. Advice rules, on printouts, determine the assignment of each patient to the health care system, the preventive care system, or the sick care system. Several studies have demonstrated that this automated multiphasic system, using no direct physician services, is as effective in diagnosis as are systems employing varying amounts of costly physician time (Collen, 1973; Cutler, 1973; Dales, 1973; Ramcharan, 1973).

Because the HMO must remain committed to program evaluation and to a constant monitoring of effectiveness in order to survive economically, the automated multiphasic screening service has provided a wealth of research data. Stored in the computer are hundreds of thousands of protocols of well patients who subsequently developed disease. Beyond the importance of early detection, these data provide the opportunity to compare those who develop disease with those who do not. Hundreds of studies have been conducted, with many more in progress or planned, and only a few examples can be cited here. Nonetheless, these studies revealed the importance of psychological, environmental, and lifestyle factors long before it was popular to devote attention to such factors.

In one study, patients who suffered a myocardial infarction were compared with their "normal" multiphasic health checks, which had preceded the infarction by an average of 16.8 months (Friedman, Ury, Klatsky, & Siegelaub, 1974). The automated psychological questionnaire revealed a specific pattern of anxiety and depression, which was absent in the control group and was predictive of myocardial infarction. This pattern was also predictive of whether the person suffering the event would be a slow or fast recoverer. Once the event occurred, however, all patients demonstrated enough emotional distress to render their test protocols indistinguishable. This study illustrates not only the importance of psychological distress in myocardial infarction but also the need to have psychological data before the onset of an illness. Finally, it illustrates the kind of innovative research that is possible with an ongoing program of extensive multiphasic health screening.

By using automated multiphasic screening information Dales, Friedman, Ury, Grossman, and Williams (1978) were able to expand the list of lifestyle patterns that lead to subsequent cancer of the colon. In addition to confirming the importance of high fat and low fiber in the diets of persons developing colorectal cancer, it was found that prolonged cigar smoking in men and nulliparity in women are also risk factors.

Reports that vasectomized men are prone to suffer much more subsequent disease prompted Kaiser Permanente to reexamine their benefit of providing vasectomies upon request. In a study of 4,385 men who indicated in their multiphasic screening that they had had vasectomies, the computer provided three exact matches for each, or 13,155 men who had not been vasectomized (Petitti, Klein, Kipp, Kahn, Siegelaub, & Friedman, 1982). Comparisons of their health histories over several years revealed no evidence that vasectomy leads to disease in humans. Therefore, provision of vasectomy as a covered benefit continues.

Another study, designed to test side effects and improve effectiveness, investigated the oral contraceptive services. It was found that serum cholesterol levels in women depend on the formulation of the oral contraceptive used (Bradley, Wingerd, Petitti, Krauss, & Ramcharan, 1978). Also, the risk of vascular disease in women taking oral contraceptives was found to be present if the woman smokes cigarettes (Petitti, Wingerd, Pellegrin, & Ramcharan, 1979). Therefore, a program strongly urging such women not to smoke was begun.

Lech, Friedman, and Ury (1975) compared heavy users of prescription drugs with light users and found that the former experienced almost four times the number of adverse reactions. Among the heavy users were many individuals with emotional problems that appeared to contribute to symptoms and requests for drugs. Such patients consult several physicians concurrently and tend to use emergency and drop-in services, where records of prescriptions written by other physicians are not immediately available. As a result of this study, Kaiser Permanente made the patients' prescription drug histories available to physicians on a computer terminal.

Because of the high cost of alcohol- and tobacco-related illness, numerous studies have been conducted on the mortality rate among heavy users of these substances. Besides confirming previous findings, these studies have delineated guidelines for use by physicians and other health personnel in treating such users within a variety of illnesses and conditions. Most notable are the 10-year study of alcohol mortality (Klatsky, Friedman, & Siegelaub, 1981) and another longitudinal study of middle-aged smokers (Friedman, Dales, & Ury, 1979). As a result of these studies, stop-smoking clinics and alcohol and drug abuse programs have been established as part of the HMO.

CONSUMER EDUCATION

Integral to the concept of maintaining subscriber health is the ongoing, effective education of the consumer. This educational effort must respond not only to the immediate concerns of the patient but also to the long-range dissemination of health information. Part of the latter is accomplished by publication of a monthly magazine, attractively prepared and sent to all subscribers. It highlights various health issues and focuses on prevention and early self-detection of disease. Health exhibits provided in the Kaiser Permanente system's many hospitals are well attended. One study demonstrated that three-dimensional and multimedia presentations that give a positive view of health encourage visitors to accept personal responsibility for their own well-being (Collen & Soghikian, 1974).

Much of the immediate health education is provided through the services of nurse practitioners who provide 24-hour coverage as "advice nurses." Responses are given to telephone inquiries on whether the caller's symptoms warrant coming into the medical center or whether there is something that the patient may more properly do at home. The patient is given practical, effective advice that insures quality care and reassures the worried caller. If the advice nurse on duty is not able to deal with the problem, there is immediate recourse to consultation with the physician specialist on call. In addition to providing quick response to the patient day or night, the use of the nurse practitioner saves costly physician time.

Patients often need to be educated regarding the proper use of medication or the need for cooperation with prescribed regimens. Griffith and Madero (1973) and Soghikian (1978) found that compliance by patients suffering from such conditions as hypertension was increased by a well-structured program of nurse-educator intervention.

In a 4-year study employing nurse practitioners, rather than physicians, to conduct routine physical examinations, it was expected that the substitution of nursing personnel would reduce costs, but the finding that patient compliance was 90% because of the nurses' use of educative techniques was surprising. Also, patient satisfaction equaled that found with physician evaluation. Most important, however, the approach freed the sick care system of the well patients and improved the waiting list for physician appointments from 6 weeks to a few days (Feldman, Taller, Garfield, Collen, Richart, Cella, & Sender, 1977).

In summarizing the educational aspect of the HMO delivery system, Collen, Feldman, Soghikian, and Garfield (1973) state that once the educational need is integrated into the delivery of medical care, it can be handled completely by nonphysician personnel. It has become an essential adjunct to the management of care as prescribed by the physician and an imperative in the health maintenance of all people—sick and well.

Somatizers or Not Somatizers

In the early years at Kaiser, we worked with people whom most would call somatizers, and all of them were getting some kind of biological treatment. That is, they had various stresses in their lives, and they somehow converted those stresses into bodily symptoms. I will assure you that almost any major medical symptom can be a result of stresses or underlying psychological issues. When we came in with behavioral interventions, the symptoms often went away and the patient didn't need the doctor anymore.

We've since learned that if you take sufferers of the five major illnesses that account for 40 percent of health-care dollars in the 20- to 60-year-old group—such as asthma, diabetes, and heart disease—and apply behavioral techniques, the result is tremendous medical cost offset. One major reason is a substantial increase in compliance with the medical treatment.

We learned that it was irrelevant whether the people had real diseases or were somatizing. We got them better anyway. And none of these people were denied treatment. It wasn't a situation where we had a screening and said, "You are a somatizer, and you don't get to see the doctor." This was not how they were treated. These people were never deprived of medical interventions. In fact, they were given medical interventions they probably didn't need, because they were using the medical system as a means to help them with their psychological issues.

1985–1997
The Era of Managed Care

A Commentary by Nick Cummings

B Y THE MID-1980s, it was apparent to me that the cottage industry, which constituted a fractionated and disorganized non-system of healthcare (to use Senator Edward Kennedy's terminology in a personal communication, April 1976), was about to industrialize. Evidence was mounting regarding the need for organized settings in mental healthcare, and such was the specific conclusion of the government-convened Bethesda Consensus Conference in 1980. Soon there would be the results over seven years of the HCFA Hawaii Medicaid Project. The study, which involved 36,000 Medicaid recipients and 90,000 federal employees, showed that traditional therapy increases costs and yet is less effective therapeutically than are targeted, focused interventions in an organized setting. All of this was several years before the term "managed care" was coined.

In the five years from 1985 through 1990, the solo practice of psychotherapy was experiencing an even greater boom than it had during what I have termed the "golden age," which preceded. The Congress enacted Diagnosis Related Groups (DRGs), which very quickly tethered medical and surgical costs. Hospitals, used to the reimbursement of costs plus 15 percent, found it difficult to remain solvent and many closed their doors. Most, however, were acquired by proprietary health companies that converted the as many as 50 percent empty medical and surgical beds to psychiatry, where there were no DRGs. They huckstered inpatient programs in adult and adolescent psychiatry and chemical dependency, and psychiatric hospitalization became a growth industry on Wall Street. Psychologists in solo practice benefited from the economic outflow from this psychiatric inpatient boom, and experienced the highest private-practice revenues in their history. In such a setting, my predictions that the solo practice of psychotherapy was an endangered species, that psychological incomes would be substantially reduced, and that what was later to be named "managed care" would control healthcare, constituted not only an unpopular message, but an unbelievable one.

Although I accurately predicted how events would unfold, I drastically underpredicted the magnitude. I foresaw that managed care would be a 25-million-covered-lives industry. I indicated that I would form the first behavioral care carve-out, American Biodyne, and would cap it at 500,000 covered lives. It would serve as a model for psychologists to visit and emulate by creating the other 49 "Biodynes." In this way, the profession would own the new industrialization of healthcare, not business interests, thus maintaining its clinical integrity. This future was clear to me, and being regarded by my colleagues as paranoid for thinking that solo practice was in danger, and grandiose in my belief that I could form a company with half a million enrollees, was surprising and distressing. It was probably the first time in the history of commerce that someone created a new industry and was willing to give the "black box" away to his colleagues in the interest of furthering the profession, to say nothing of saving it. While no one believed me or accepted my offer, by 1998, the managed-care industry had captured 75 percent of the insured market, represented 160 million covered lives, and was rapidly gobbling up Medicaid and Medicare.

I kept my promise for two years by capping Biodyne at 500,000 covered lives, a figure that was quickly achieved in the company's first year. Then, as I saw business interests, not psychologists, emulating the model, I removed my foot from the brake, and in the ensuing five years, the company grew to 14.5 million covered lives. The profession of psychology, finding itself no longer in charge of its own practice patterns, emerged from several years of denial and plunged into unmitigated rage. It absolved itself of all responsibility for its self-imposed myopia, declared itself a victim, and demonized managed care. To this day, the leadership in professional psychology refuses to recognize its own failure to foresee the industrialization of healthcare and to prepare appropriately for it. It is still intent upon righteously repealing an evolutionary process.

While psychotherapists were reaping a financial bonanza, the inflationary spiral in mental health/chemical dependency (MH/CD) escalated to an annual rate of 16 percent, and was continuing to rise when healthcare costs in general were 12 percent and dropping. For the first time in history, the inflation in healthcare was being driven by MH/CD. What did psychology do in an attempt to halt the inflation in its own services? Nothing, of course. The desperate response by the insurers was to drop MH/CD as a covered benefit in health insurance. This trend was mushrooming and threatening to wipe out the psychotherapy benefit that had been expanded over many long, difficult years. The behavioral health carve-out went at risk, guaranteed that the capitated cost would not rise, and saved the MH/CD benefit from extinction. Has psychology, in its rage, recognized that if it were not for managed care, there would be no private practice at all?

By 1997, inflation in MH/CD was at an annual rate of 4.4 percent, close to that of healthcare in general. This rate of inflation was the lowest since 1960, and clearly the healthcare system had been saved from bankruptcy. The winners in all this were those who pay the bills: the employers and the government—and ultimately the consumers and taxpayers, who really pay the bills. The unequivocal losers have been the practitioners, who not only have had their incomes curtailed, but also have lost control of their own practices. And among these, the most affected are the younger practitioners, who were prevented from receiving the training appropriate to the new era, and were further discouraged from tailoring their practices to meet the exigencies of industrialization. The APA governance is still dominated by an old guard of independent practitioners who would rather see the demise of solo practice than change. This old guard has made managed care politically incorrect and thus has created a climate in which anyone disagreeing with it can never be appointed to APA boards and committees or be elected to office. It justifies its management and filtering of the information that practitioners receive from the APA, and also makes certain that the advocates, lobbyists, and staff officers who are hired are those who will tell them what they want to hear: "Managed care is about to be vanquished." The APA leadership has been screeching to the choir, and will probably remain on a collision course with reality until the younger psychologists demand otherwise.

What does the future portend? No industry grows as fast as managed care has grown without making mistakes. It not only has pushed aside the practitioners who attempted to stop it, but it has lost its clinical focus and so is not doing the best it can for patients. So there will be regulation and evolution. The regulation will be analogous to the mandating of seat belts, air bags, and catalytic converters for cars, not the elimination of the automobile industry. Abuses will be addressed, but psychologists have confused patient rights with practitioner concerns, so reforms will be confusing and acrimonious. Now that the industrialization of healthcare has occurred, we will never return to being the cottage industry that psychotherapists recall so nostalgically. But what we now see as managed care will have little resemblance to what will evolve over the next decade.

Managed care affected medicine much sooner than it did psychology, resulting in an earlier acculturation of the medical profession. The first result of this is a difference in the expectations and aspirations of students currently entering medical school. Such changes in future students who elect to become professional psychologists will be coincidental with the belated retirement of the old guard, and they will realistically demand training programs that are more in tune with the requirements of future practice.

The carve-out has outlived its usefulness, but will struggle to survive and will resist the need to carve in, defined as the integration of behavioral healthcare with primary care. Two outmoded entities, the solo practice of long-term psychotherapy and the behavioral-care carve-out, currently adversaries, will embarrassingly find themselves on the same side as they both oppose such integration. But this integration of behavioral health with primary care is the logical next evolutionary step in healthcare delivery and eventually will take place. It is toward implementing that need to recognize progress that I am currently devoting my writing and professional activities.

{ 11 }

THE DISMANTLING OF OUR HEALTH SYSTEM
STRATEGIES FOR THE SURVIVAL OF
PSYCHOLOGICAL PRACTICE

ABSTRACT: *The growing revolution in health care delivery as a response to needed cost-containment reform is threatening psychology's hard-fought gains. As more and more elements of the health care delivery system are coming under the ownership of giant health corporations, psychology's focus continues to be one of gaining recognition in an outmoded health system. If psychology is to survive, it must develop strategies responsive to the current cost-containment climate. In such an effort psychology has the advantage of having the only natural approach to cost containment: that of identifying the patients who, without being physically ill, account for 60% of all physician visits and moving them out of the medical system into a psychological system that addresses the cause of this somaticization. Traditional psychological practice is both inefficient and ineffective in meeting this need. Psychologists must learn to establish innovative models of mental health care delivery and then, further, learn to market these models. The alternative is for psychologists to become poorly paid and little respected employees of the giant health corporations that will soon own and control most health care in the United States.*

TWO MEN WERE on a mountain trek through the high Sierra Nevada Range of California when they were suddenly accosted by a ferocious grizzly bear. The first man froze in his tracks from fear, whereas the second man began to remove his hiking boots and put on his running shoes. The first man jeered and said, "You don't think that you're going to be able to outrun that bear, do you?" And the second man replied, "I don't have to. All I have to do is outrun you."

Psychologists are ill prepared for the competitive market for their services that lies ahead. It is almost as if we have gravitated to our profession because we eschew anything that has to do with business, anything that has to do with marketing, anything that has to do with merchandising our products. Consequently, psychology is once again in danger of losing out. Before discussing this concern, it may be well for me to review for a moment how this competitive market has come about.

During the Lyndon Johnson administration, the government and the Congress began to fuel a noncompetitive economy, first with the Hill-Burton bill, then with Medicare, then with Medicaid, then on and on. The crucial aspect is that it began to fuel a noncompetitive economy. And the reason why this came about is that at the time the American Medical Association had enough clout to prevent a competitive model from being introduced into federal funding. The rest is history.

The inflation rate of health services delivery grew at several times the inflation rate of the economy as a whole. During that time the government tried in vain to slow down the inflation rate of health services delivery. However, health costs in the United States have now grown to the point where they account for 11% of the gross national product. Those of you who know anything about economics know what a staggering figure we are talking about, because inflationary growth really adds nothing to the economy; rather it subtracts from productivity in a manner that raises the deficit and other economic warnings in our economy.

Finally, after years of the government's attempting alone to slow down the inflation in health costs, the people that pay the bill, the third party payers, said. "This has to come to a halt." And they found their natural allies in the employers, who ultimately foot the bill. Across the United States a powerful consortium began to develop, a consortium of the industrial might of America that included the unions, the farmers, and now the consumers of health services.

For the first time, the health scene is changing. The problem is that it's like the walls of Jericho. The trumpet has been sounded, and the very fabric of our health economy is about to tumble down. I am considerably worried, as well as stimulated, by what the results might be. This time around, competition has been built into the scheme of things. This first casualties of increased cost and competition have been the nonprofit hospitals that were used to cost plus reimbursement: they can no longer make it. And it isn't going to be very long before there will be no more nonprofit hospitals in the United States because they are going out of business or they are rapidly being bought up. In one year, in one state alone, one health corporation bought 27 Catholic hospitals that had been nonprofit for years and converted them to proprietary institutions. In one state, in one year! This is happening all across the land, and the reason I have fears is because corporate. America is going to control the health delivery systems of the United States within a very brief time. Now, you say, "Nick, you were with Kaiser Permanente for 25 years. What's to fear?" Consider the fact that Kaiser Permanente has always been controlled by the providers, so that quality care, the considerations of unrecoverable costs that lead to deficits in a practice have always been in the forefront. The corporations that are now looking at, and buying up, the health delivery systems of America are not provider controlled; they're business controlled. And the providers have very little to say about what is going to happen. I am concerned because the corporations are going to be able to come in with computers, efficiency methods, and management techniques, and they're going to be able to underbid everybody and take over the health system of America. My prediction is that health quality is going to go down, unless we somehow address this issue.

Although, ultimately, the competitive system is going to resolve this issue—because those plans for which quality has been sacrificed are going to lose out in the marketplace—in the meantime, I predict several years of absolute chaos, where the business interests, through the corporation, are going to be at the helm and if it "ain't good for business, it ain't good for the patient." That situation worries me.

PSYCHOLOGY AND THE MARKETPLACE

Psychology is particularly vulnerable because corporate America does not understand psychological services. They think that psychologists are those ethereal social scientists who talk about the human potential movement and self-realization, and psychological concepts are viewed by businesspeople as being as valid as asking "How long is a piece of string?" They don't know when therapy begins and when it ends, what psychologists' goals are and what psychology's product is: so, they're very wary of us. They do understand hospitalization for medical reasons. They know how many days medical procedures take—an apendectomy takes so many days, a hysterectomy takes so many days, a tonsilectomy takes X number of days. With psychotherapy they're terrified that they're opening up an open-ended system. If they could somehow predict actuarially how long therapy would take, they wouldn't mind funding it. Psychologists have not helped them in this task. Psychologists are going to have to market their services. It is that pure and simple.

I want to tell you a little story. For three years I cajoled the American Psychological Association (APA) until it finally formed the Task Force on Future Markets of Psychology. It's a brilliant task force, and it's been doing its job well. It has held workshops in the last two conventions and has stimulated psychologists all over the country to start thinking in terms of the new delivery models. And it did the job so well that the Board of Professional Affairs (BPA) decided it was time the Task Force on Future Markets of Psychology become a standing committee. And so the Task Force was asked to expand its charge, to write the charge up and submit it for approval. And the BPA enthusiastically endorsed the mission and purposes of the new committee, which called itself the Committee on the Marketing and Promotion of Psychological Services (MAPPS), but sent back a letter saying, "Before we endorse you as a standing committee we feel that the term 'marketing' is too ominous and we ask you to find a different word."

I'm reminded that 25 years ago the predecessor to the APA Committee on Health Insurance, on which I was privileged to sit, was told that insurance was not important enough for a standing committee and it was not respectable enough for the committee to bear its name alone. So the name, Ad Hoc Committee on Insurance and Related Social Developments (AHCIRSD), was appointed by the Board of Professional Affairs. Because of its initials, we called it "acurse-ed," and we started the long arduous task of educating the insurance industry about the services psychologists could provide. But before we could do that, we had to convince American psychology that insurance was an important issue.

I could tell you that if that committee had not been formed, if we had not developed the freedom-of-choice legislation that included psychologists in health plans, none of us would be sitting here today as practitioners. The market would have dried up for us, and psychiatry would have owned it all. We are confronted with the same issue today about marketing. I am delighted that the Task Force on Future Markets in Psychology responded to the BPA and said that we want to teach the American psychologist how to market her and his products and we cannot do that unless we use the right word, which is *marketing*.

I'm pleased that in the prior example I gave, which took four years for BPA to come around and acknowledge that insurance was respectable and important enough, this time it only took a couple of weeks. And so we now have the Committee on the Marketing and Promotion of Psychological Services, which should be very active.

We have learned from our past mistakes and our past foot-dragging. We are prepared finally for the 1980s. What do the 1980s portend? The giant health corporations that are buying up health delivery systems don't understand psychotherapy. First of all, they are hiring social workers, because social workers are cheaper than psychologists. And now, they have learned that even cheaper still are mental health counselors with two-year community college degrees.

In one giant corporation I visited, however, I looked at the mental health system and for every psychologist they had on the staff, they had 18 mental health counselors. You haven't heard it all—the pay for both was the same! This, my friends, is the marketplace. Suppose a person wants to buy a pair of shoes. If one store sells inexpensive, low-quality shoes and another sells more expensive high-quality shoes, that person may buy the cheaper pair of shoes unless he or she knows about quality. To get a quality pair of shoes, you must pay the price. We have to educate these giant health systems in quality care. I have been saying for the last three years that we are about to go through a health change. We're going to see a full-scale health revolution in the next two years. And make no mistake, if psychology is not prepared for it, psychologists are going to find their practices drying up.

You may be from states that do not yet have a large number of health maintenance organizations (HMOs) or preferred provider organizations (PPOs). If so, don't sit there complacently. Because of this low HMO and PPO penetration, you are prime targets for the large corporations. Last year, Bryant Welch, a respected friend and colleague, said to me that he was going to fight in the legislature of North Carolina the intrusion of the impending HMOs and PPOs, and I said to him, "Bryant, good luck, but you haven't got a chance." Even the American Medical Association has thrown in the towel after one important test case. The California Medical Association (CMA) went into the legislature to pass rules that would be so stringent that they would make it impossible for PPOs to proliferate. Despite its might, the CMA suffered its greatest legislative humiliation in its entire history. The state legislature not only turned down the CMA's bill, it turned it upside down and passed legislation to facilitate formation of PPOs. So I said, "Good luck. Bryant. If you want to play David and Goliath, fine. But I don't think history will repeat itself this time around. I think David is going to get the stuffing kicked out of him."

Bryant caught me at the APA convention in Los Angeles, and he said, "I have to yield to age over brashness. The HMOs and PPOs have steam-rolled into North Carolina, and I felt that the Sherman tanks had come over me as I tried to stop them." Nobody is going to stop them.

If I don't do anything else. I would like to stimulate each of you to begin thinking about offering your services under a different kind of model than you have been used to doing.

Nobody likes a prophet of doom. I don't want you to say "Nick Cummings thinks we're done for." I don't. I didn't think we were done for 25 years ago when there wasn't a single insurance company in the United States that recognized psychologists, and I don't think we're all done for now. But some of us are going to be done in. I recall a colleague in a state that had low HMO penetration. He had a beautiful practice, a Mercedes, and a beautiful home. He was stimulated by his clients: he loved going down to his office every morning, opening it up, and being his own boss. He said to me, "Nick, this will never happen to me." I saw him two months ago, and he said it seemingly happened over night. "My patients said to me. 'Doctor, I love you, but if I see you, it costs me $80; if I go over to the HMO that I now belong to, it's free.' " And he said, "Within three months my practice literally dried up." It will happen to many psychologists because when everyone in an area has signed up to join an HMO or a PPO, psychologists will no longer have a market.

So, now I want to talk with you about how to market yourselves to PPOs and HMOs and how to form your own PPO.

A MODEL FOR THE FUTURE

Some of you may already know that some colleagues and I have formed American Biodyne Centers. We began in Honolulu, and now we've opened up three centers in Arizona with another 150,000 subscribers (Cummings & Fernandez, 1985). We are marketing in several other states. American Biodyne intends to have one million subscribers this time next year. We do not intend to seal up the market. American Biodyne wants to put centers across the United States, in as many states as we can, as models for the rest of psychology to follow suit. We plan to have 50 centers. My estimate is that there's room in the United States for 2,000 such centers. So we're leaving 1,950 of them for you to found.

Try to do it before you go down to your office one morning and find out you don't have any patients. Don't wait until then, because the old saying, "It's easier to get a job when you still have a job," is also true of marketing. You can't market out of desperation.

How do you market? Only a fool and a few psychologists would ever dream of doing their own marketing. It requires a special talent. You have to hire a marketer. It costs money—anywhere between $2,000 and $5,000 a month—and marketing research will add to that bill. You may say, "No individual private practitioner can afford that!" Of course not. But, we're talking about forming a PPO. You're going to do this with a group of your colleagues, and you're going to have to put up some of your money, because if you can't invest in yourself at this point in time, forget it. Don't wait until your patients dry up. If you do, just close up your office, retire, and go off somewhere fishing. You're going to have to invest in yourself. Biodyne is offering a model we call the Small Intensive Brief Psychotherapy Model of Group Practice (Cummings & Dörken, 1986).

Many psychologists have formed what they call "group practices." Psychologists get together with other psychologists they like and who practice therapy exactly the same way as they do, and then they all go into business together. They get one building, share the telephone, and share a secretary's time. Then they all do the same thing. A group of psychoanalysts are going to get together, a group of Jungian analysts are going to get together, and a group of behavioral psychologists are going to get together.

That is not the kind of model those of us with Biodyne are talking about because that is not group practice. All that amounts to is a group of individual practitioners practicing under one roof and sharing expenses. The model that I'm talking about means that psychologists bring together every orientation and skill in psychology. The model that's going to do the job efficiently is going to be the model that blends all the schools of psychology and psychotherapy into one.

When I went to school, the Freudians didn't talk to the neo-Freudians, and no one talked to the Jungians. The Adlerians and Rankians were around somewhere. Leaders of the various schools said that these schools of psychotherapy could never meld. Psychologists in intensive group practice are going to have to get over the concept of the ideal therapist, that one person who can do all things for all people (Cummings & VandenBos, 1978). Psychologists are going to have to go back to school and they are going to have to learn brief, targeted psychotherapy. The parameters of brief therapy are totally different from long-term therapy. Brief therapy does not mean less therapy; it means more efficient therapy. And what I mean by efficient therapy is *targeted therapy*.

It is a propensity of psychotherapy that every patient who walks into a therapist's office receives the type of therapy the psychotherapist has to offer. If the therapist is a Freudian analyst, he or she does not care what the patient has—alcoholism, marital problems, or job problems—that patient is going to get the couch. If the therapist is a Jungian analyst, the patient is going to paint pictures. If the therapist is a behaviorist, the patient is going to get desensitization. It's not surprising that this is done, but what's surprising to me is that it works. It really works. We help our patients. But the problem is we help them with lots and lots and lots more sessions than might otherwise be needed. When treatment programs are targeted for specific conditions, lo and behold, the patient responds more readily, more efficiently. It is not necessary to limit psychotherapy to 10 sessions, or 20 sessions, or to mandate a 50% co-insurance. The patient looks up and says. "Gee, you know this is great. My problem is solved."

At Biodyne we use over 50 targeted therapies (Cummings, 1983). I ask you, would you go to a physician that treated everybody who came in the door with penicillin, whether one person had a broken leg from skiing or another had pneumonia? Of course you wouldn't. Fifty years ago all physicians practiced in that manner. Physicians had five favorite medications; if one didn't work, they gave the next one. If that one didn't work, they gave the third, and so on until they exhausted their repertoire of five favorite medications. When I was in school, the list of the pharmacopia of the United States was contained in one volume. Now the volumes containing that list would stretch clear across the room. Physicians have literally hundreds of specific treatments for specific conditions. I want all of you to begin to understand that we have far more specific treatment approaches in psychology than most practicing psychologists ever dream of because we are stuck in the rut of doing what we were initially trained to do regardless of the patient's condition.

You have to give up the concept of cure (Cummings & VandenBos,

1978). That concept has held back psychotherapy more than any other concept. George Albee has been chiding us for decades for practicing in the house of medicine. We're finally extricating ourselves from that house, but we still use medicine's concept of cure. And so, psychologists keep patients in treatment until they are sure that every recess of the unconscious has been analyzed as to its conflicts, because both patient and therapist only get one chance. If three years from now the patient has another problem, the psychologist hasn't done the job correctly. This is absolute, sheer nonsense. The only time all of us are going to be free of anxiety is when we're six feet under and there are gravestones over us. And so at Biodyne we employ what we call "brief intermittent psychotherapy throughout the life cycle" (Cummings, 1983). This means that when a patient comes in with a problem, the psychologist takes the problem seriously but not necessarily at face value and he or she treats that problem. When that problem is resolved, the psychologist interrupts treatment. Now, I didn't say "terminates." I said "interrupt" because under this model I see the psychological practitioner behaving like the old-fashioned family doctor. The patient goes to the doctor because he or she has the flu. With treatment, the patient recovers from the flu and stops going to the doctor. The patient does not keep seeing the doctor to keep from catching the flu again. Two years later, the patient may come back with a broken leg. The patient doesn't stay in treatment to prevent something else from happening, and the physician is not deemed to have failed because the patient now has a broken leg. Psychotherapy is the only area of health that I know of where both patients and therapists only get one chance. I have been doing brief intermittent psychotherapy for long enough so that I have seen not only children and grandchildren of my patients, but I've also recently seen two great-grandchildren.

Not long ago, I saw an eleven-year-old and I said to him, "Of all the psychotherapists in San Francisco, why did you choose me to come to with your school problem?" He said, "You're legendary in our home. You saw my great-grandfather and when it was time for me to see somebody I said to Dad, 'Can I go see Nick Cummings?' My father said, 'Of course.' I said, 'How do I get a hold of him?' and he gave me your number and I called you." Two weeks later I saw his older brother.

One of the therapist's problems in doing brief therapy is that the therapist is always having separation anxiety. There's a tremendous turnover of patients because you're terminating constantly, and as a therapist you're always depressed because of separation anxiety. I'm saying to you, under this model we don't terminate. Rather, therapy is interrupted. In putting this model through almost 30 years of experience, given therapists trained in the model, 85% of the patients who come opt for brief therapy. They enter under this model, use it and come back when they have the need. In tracking them for 10, 20, or 25 years, we have found that it takes less time in psychotherapy overall than it would if we kept a patient in therapy twice a week for a year or a year and a half or even eight months. And I could report on case after case that demonstrates this.

So, I say to you, you can free yourself from the concepts of the ideal therapist, where each of us has to be all things to all people. You can free yourself from the concept of cure, and you can free yourself from the troublesomeness of termination.

PARAMETERS OF BRIEF THERAPY

Now, what are some of the parameters of "brief intermittent psychotherapy throughout the life cycle?" Time permits me to discuss only a few of them (Cummings, 1983), and then very briefly.

1. Literally hit the ground running. The first session must be therapeutic. The concept that you must devote the first session to taking a history (a duty performed preferably by a social worker so you won't have to bother) is nonsense. The first session must be therapeutic. Now it's important to know some of the patient's history, but you know, I haven't learned all of the history of some of my patients until they've come back five or six years later. I concentrate on the following items.

2. Perform an operational diagnosis. Now, an operational diagnosis is different from some vague DSM-III (American Psychiatric Association, 1980) psychiatric diagnosis that labels a person. The operational diagnosis asks one thing, "Why is the patient here today instead of last week or last month, last year, or next year?" And when you answer that, you know what the patient is here for. The operational diagnosis is absolutely necessary for you to set about your treatment plan, and it is best that it be done in the first session. If I don't get it the first session. I try the second session, but I do not stop trying to solve the issue of the operational diagnosis until I have an answer.

3. Create a therapeutic contract. Initially, psychologists at Biodyne get 130 hours of training before they are allowed to see a client, and then they get a year of in-service training after that. So I'm only going

to discuss this concept in their training very briefly. Every patient makes a therapeutic contract with every therapist in the first session, every time. But in 99% of the cases, the therapist misses it. A therapist must have not only a third ear but also fourth, fifth, sixth, and seventh ears to hear that therapeutic contract.

As Paul Watzlawick (personal communication, May 1979) has pointed out to us, if the patient gives the therapeutic contract and the therapist doesn't hear it, then because the patient wants to be a good patient, he or she goes along with what the therapist says the contract is. And then a wrestling match occurs between patient and therapist that the therapist, as a psychologist, erroneously labels resistance. Now there is such a thing as resistance. But I find that 80% of what most therapists term resistance is nothing more than a therapist's failure to recognize a patient's goals in treatment. For example, if a patient comes into the office and says, "Doctor, I'm glad you have this comfortable chair because I'm going to be here awhile," and the therapist doesn't respond to that, the therapist has just made a contract for long-term therapy. If the patient says, "I want to come in here and save my marriage, but whatever I do, I'm going to end up getting divorced," the therapist has just made a contract for that patient to divorce. And if the therapist breaks his or her neck over the next two years trying to save that marriage, the therapist is going to wonder, "Why? What's happening?" I could give you hundreds of examples. Listen for the therapeutic contract. After you discern the patient's therapeutic contract, talk about it. Then say, "Now that our goals are clarified, I would like to add the following to that contract: I will never abandon you as long as you need me. In return for that, I want you to join me in a partnership to make me obsolete as soon as possible." Don't just allow perfunctory answers. Discuss it, and eventually the patient will agree to this amended contract. Demonstrate that you, as the therapist, mean what you say.

4. Do something novel the first session. This isn't easy, but find something novel, something unexpected, to do the first session. This will cut through the expectations of the "trained" patient and will create instead an expectation that problems are to be immediately addressed.

5. Give homework in the first session and every therapy session thereafter. It isn't possible to have some cookbook full of homework that you just arbitrarily assign. Tailor the homework to be meaningful for that patient's goals and the therapeutic contract. The patient will realize, "Hey, this guy isn't kidding. I'm responsible for my own therapy."

6. If you take steps 1 through 5, you'll find that there is no such thing as a therapeutic dropout. Patients know when to terminate better than we, as therapists, do.

I was trained in analysis, and I did long-term therapy. In my career, I remember when I had so honed my craft as a psychotherapist that by the appropriate interpretation I could prevent any patient from terminating. And then I went through six weeks of some of the most soul-wrenching self-examinations I've ever gone through because I asked myself, "Am I doing this for the benefit of my patients or for the benefit of Nick Cummings?" I finally concluded that I was doing that for the benefit of Nick Cummings, and I cut it out.

Now the interesting thing about this model is that it is not necessary to have session limits. Biodyne has the only mental health package in the United States that has no top dollar amounts, no session limits, no co-insurance, no first dollar amounts, no deductibles: the patient gets what the patient requires. We find 10% of our patients require and get long-term therapy. And you say, "Well Nick, that doesn't add up. If 85% prefer brief therapy on the Intermittent Life Cycle Model and 10% need long-term therapy, what happened to the other 5%?" That 5% includes those patients who are interminable. Those are the people who never quit once they get into psychotherapy. They are the people we all rely on in private practice because they constitute our annuity. And they're the people that scare the insurance carrier that has to foot the bill. Now, if 5% of all patients that you see never quit, in 20 years you'll be the Veterans Administration; you'll still be seeing patients from the Spanish-American War. So we've developed special programs not only to treat the interminable patient but also to identify the potentially interminable patient before they become interminable.

And let me offer one last piece of advice. Acquaint yourself with the medical offset literature. There are now 58 replications of my original work. They all have the same results. Psychological services reduce medical costs because 60% of all doctor visits are made by patients who have no physical illness and who are somaticizing emotional problems. At the Bethesda Consensus Conferences three years ago, the federal government concluded that psychological intervention does indeed reduce medical overutilization. The problem is that it reduces it from as little as 5% to as much as 79%. Psychotherapists begin to break even when medical overutilization is reduced by 15% or more. The greatest reduction, 79%, occurs with the Biodyne model. Why do we get so much more medical offset than anyone else? Because we use targeted psychotherapy in our brief intermittent psychotherapy throughout the life cycle model. I'm persuaded of that because when I looked at all the medical offset studies and found out what kinds of services were performed for the clients, the closer the method of treatment is to a traditional model, the less the medical offset.

I think the future for psychology is bright for those psychologists who are prepared for it. Don't worry about the fact that you've had rigorous training. I will not hire anyone at Biodyne who has not had rigorous training. But I also have to hire people who not only have had rigorous training, but also who have the flexibility to get out of their "psycho religion." So don't worry about the fact that you've been doing what you've been doing for many years. You can still go back to school. You can still learn the parameters of brief therapy. You can learn how to market yourself, get help, and form a PPO.

I want to give you one caveat. A lot of you are going to join independent practitioner associations (IPA models). You will be told. "Sign up with us and you will stay in your office, and we will send you patients." You will agree to see these patients under their peer review and to see them for certain reduced fees. Many of them start out with very little or no reduction in fee. Now, the caveat I want to give you is that the IPA model cannot compete with the HMO staff model, under which everyone goes to a center where therapists work together with different skills and utilization is monitored, not by artificial peer review or by computers, but by practitioners enthusiastically working together and consulting and helping each other. The HMO model is more centralized and, therefore, less expensive to run than an IPA. So the IPA cannot compete with the HMO. And, when the money crunch comes, the IPA will make up the difference by reducing your fee. And after they reduce it the first time, the year after they they're going to reduce it again, and the year after that they may reduce it again. And you will have no alternatives because now your practice is dried up and you're married to the IPA occupationally. With that caveat in mind, think about forming your own groups. I don't want psychological care to suffer in quality because we're owned by huge corporations. I want us, as psychologists, to be in control of our own mental health delivery so that we can have the most effective, efficient, highest quality delivery system that the United States has known.

{ 12 }

CORPORATIONS, NETWORKS, AND SERVICE PLANS: ECONOMICALLY SOUND MODELS FOR PRACTICE*

TWO MEN WERE on a mountain trek through the high Sierra Nevada of California when they were confronted by a ferocious grizzly bear. Neither man was armed. As one stood frozen in fear, the other quickly removed his hiking boots and began to put on his running shoes. "You don't really believe you can outrun that bear," jeered his companion, somewhat out of contempt but mostly out of fear. "I don't have to," replied the first. "All I have to do is outrun you."

Psychologists are ill prepared for the competition that is heating up and will soon permeate all of health care delivery. This chapter offers some examples of successful practice models that can guide psychologists who are willing to change from traditional approaches to survive the new competition. But first it may be well to sketch briefly how the new climate of competition came about and some of its characteristics.

*With Herbert Dörken, Ph.D.

Note: The Biodyne model and part of this chapter were presented by Cummings in his award address. "The Dismantling of Our Health Care System: Strategies for the Survival of Psychological Practice," at the annual meeting of the American Psychological Association, Los Angeles, August 25, 1985. The descriptions of the Delaware Valley Psychological Clinics and the California Psychological Health Plan were presented in part at the Panel on Future Markets under the egis of the APA Committee on Professional Practice during the August 1983 annual meeting in Los Angeles by Janice Kenny and Donald D. Marsh, respectively.

During the Great Society era of the Lyndon Johnson presidency, the government began to fuel our health economy, first through the Hill-Burton legislation and then through Medicare and Medicaid. The important fact is that the government was fueling a *noncompetitive* health economy, because the medical profession had the clout to prevent a more competitive model of funding. The rest is history. Health care costs escalated at several times the inflation rate of the rest of the economy and currently account for 11 percent of our gross national product.

For several years government struggled in vain to slow down the rate of inflation in our health economy. Finally, in the early 1980s those who pay the bills for our health care, the employers, decided they had had enough. Overnight the industrial might of our nation formed health consortia in all our major cities, and these organizations included not only our largest corporations but also unions, farmers, consumers, and senior citizens. These consortia are effecting the changes in rapid succession that the government alone was powerless to bring about, and the American Medical Association is coming to realize it is unable to slow down the momentum for change. This climate is stimulating the mushrooming of health maintenance organizations (HMOs) and preferred provider organizations (PPOs), and large health corporations are applying their efficient management techniques and staking out increasingly larger market shares of our patient population. Meanwhile the employer is turning from payer to buyer and is doing so with data on use, cost, and benefits. It is industrial corporation to health corporation, industry to health dealing through negotiated contracts. As these health corporations, through consumer choice (selection and use) and employer contract (negotiated rates and services), capture more of the market, independent practitioners find their practice and their influence dwindling. Such circumstances are forcing more and more physicians to make arrangements with these health corporations.

Psychology is particularly vulnerable in this new health care delivery climate. Third-party payers do not understand the nature of mental health care and are wary of the seemingly endless quality of psychotherapy. Many segments of psychiatry are abandoning psychotherapy to the psychologist and are forming hospital-based PPOs that promise mental health delivery on a medical model of drugs and hospitalization. For now this evades the competition of the nonphysician providers and captures the typically higher inpatient benefits of group health insurance policies. This "adjustment," although it will be costly, is at least understood by the accountants' mentality, whereas psychotherapy seems ethereal and unmanageable to those who must pay the reimbursement bills. For the services that psychotherapy HMOs must provide for various reasons, there is a trend to hire social workers, who are paid less, or even mental health counselors with lesser training, who are cheaper still.

Health care is not just entering a period of change but is in the throes of a revolution. It is our prediction that during the transition period quality will suffer in the interest of cost containment. Eventually, however, those HMOs and PPOs that do not maintain quality will go out of business, yielding in favor of providers that are both efficient and effective. This time competition has been deliberately built into the system. For psychologists, it is important to note that, for those predicting the extinction of the private practice of psychotherapy as we now know it (Duhl & Cummings, 1985; Dörken, 1983), it is not a question of whether but when, simply because it cannot be delivered at competitive cost. There will be psychologists who will insist that the profession should fight against the formation of HMOs and PPOs. We would remind them that the might of the California Medical Association, in its 1983 attempt to undo the legislation that authorized PPOs, suffered its greatest legislative humiliation and defeat. The health revolution is here and will continue, because those who pay the bills have decided that health costs must be contained. Major changes are in the offing.

GROUP PRACTICE

The solo practice of psychotherapy is clearly on the defensive. Psychoanalysis, the most cost-intensive of all the psychotherapies, is fighting a battle for survival in the face of the cost containment efforts of third-party payers. As more and more of the patient market goes into HMOs and PPOs, in an attempt to preserve their private practices many psychologists will sign up with independent practice associations (IPAs). These organizations typically limit the reimbursement to the providers and also monitor their performance in an effort to reduce utilization. The IPA increases efficiency and cuts costs, but it cannot compete with the HMO or PPO that operates on a capitation basis and provides centers where all services are delivered, as opposed to the cost-intensive, solo practitioner's private office. When the squeeze comes, the IPA will attempt to compete with the HMO and PPO by giving the provider less and less fee-for-service reimbursement. The psychologist may be an independent contractor but at that point will have become the captive of the IPA and must either accept the reduced compensation, close the office, or find other practice markets. One alternative is for psychologists to form group practices and market themselves as a psychological PPO to general PPOs and full-range HMOs that may well wish to contract out their mental health care at an efficient cost rather than struggle with something they do not fully comprehend.

It is important from the outset to stress that group practice does not mean the usual mode of several independent solo practitioners operating under one roof, sharing overhead and participating in a pooled referral system. Rather, we have in mind a small, intensive group practice wherein all the psychologists are trained in intensive, targeted brief psychotherapy and provide a range of modalities that would not be possible in the traditional "group" of solo practitioners all essentially doing the same thing. It is a well-known fact that psychologists form groups with like-minded colleagues, thus making a truly multimodal group practice unlikely (Cummings & VandenBos, 1979). The participants in a group practice as newly conceptualized here hold common goals and agree to efficient management and aggressive marketing of their product.

Certainly the large health corporations will move swiftly to capture a large market share, but these giants have one major flaw: the loss of personal care or the human touch. There will be room in the future for psychologists who would form group service delivery models that can cut costs and still maintain the quality and personal caring that are essential to the real psychological model. Unfortunately, most psychologists eschew anything that smacks of business, almost as if in their aloofness they disdain the business reality of practice in the fantasy that the public is dependent on them. But quality care is not incompatible with efficiency, and we submit that the psychotherapists who survive the 1980s will be the individuals who have mastered what has been termed "social entrepreneurship," or a melding of humanism and efficiency (Cummings & Fernandez, 1985).

MARKETING

The word *marketing* seems almost obscene to many otherwise enlightened psychologists. In 1985 the Board of Professional Affairs (BPA) of the American Psychological Association instructed its innovative Subcommittee on Future Markets that the word *marketing* has an ominous quality and that another term should be used. (More than twenty years earlier the BPA had instructed the predecessor of its Committee on Health Insurance that the word *insurance* was not respectable.) The Subcommittee on Future Markets replied that it was its intention to alert the profession to the importance of marketing, and to do so, the word itself must be used. (This response was similar to the response given BPA more than twenty years earlier that the word *insurance* was not only respectable but vital to the survival of psychology as an autonomous profession.)

Even the best program will fail without proper marketing, and "Marketing or morbidity" will be the practitioner's version of the academician's slogan "Publish or perish." It will be strictly a buyer's market, in which the practitioner will have to demonstrate that better mental health care can be delivered more efficiently and at less cost (Cummings & Fernandez, 1985).

Psychologists must learn to market themselves if they are to succeed, and market research is essential to a successful marketing program. Psychologists do not possess the expertise to mount their own marketing campaign and should seek appropriate professional help. Consultant fees range from $2,500 to $5,000 per month, and research and advertising can add to the bill (Bean, 1985). The social entrepreneur who will survive the 1980s must be prepared to invest not only time but also money in his or her own future success. Even though the burden is shared in the group practice, there is little room for the timid.

TARGETED INTERVENTION

It has been said that a peculiarity of psychotherapy is that the patient receives what the practitioner has to offer rather than what may specifically be required. For example, whether one has a marital, occupational, or alcohol problem, if one goes to an orthodox Freudian, one will be put on the couch. If the patient goes to a Jungian psychologist, pictures will be painted and archetypes will be discussed. If one goes to a behavioral therapist, desensitization will be applied. This is tantamount to a physician's giving penicillin whether the patient has pneumonia or a broken leg. Such a state of affairs existed in medicine at the turn of the century. Each physician had five or six favorite medications, and if one did not work, another was tried, and so on until the physician's limited repertoire was exhausted. Since that time medicine has matured so that there are scores of *specifics*: specific treatments for specific conditions.

The remarkable thing about the state of affairs in psychotherapy is that even though the patient receives whatever the therapist has to offer regardless of the presenting condition, it does work to an extent. The problem is that it works inefficiently, and many more sessions are required to bring about amelioration than are really necessary. The number of sessions required to accomplish remediation can be drastically reduced by using targeted interventions directed to specific conditions (Cummings & VandenBos, 1979). Psychology has more "specifics" than practitioners generally acknowledge, and Cummings (1984) uses over fifty targeted interventions applied to specific conditions. The maturity of a profession is measured by the number of specifics at its disposal, and psychology must begin using these targeted modalities, for research has shown that it is not the number of persons seen in treatment that creates the inordinate cost of mental health services but the number of sessions each is seen in order to bring about the desired effect.

Magaro (1985), advocating the use of performance contracts as the most cost-effective model for securing therapist involvement in changing patient behavior, would emphasize the skills an individual needs to function in society and would direct treatment to those deficits. With reimbursement tied to outcome, rather than to time on the job or rank, this private sector orientation would focus on brief interventions and the modification of a specific behavior as the treatment product.

THE CONCEPT OF CURE

It is more timely than ever that psychologists reexamine their professional conceptions of the outcome of psychological intervention. Our conception of treatment outcome might well be termed the "ultimate cure." Any contact with a former mental health patient is labeled a "relapse" and is viewed as evidence that the earlier intervention was either unsuccessful or incomplete (Cummings & VandenBos, 1979). No other field of health care holds this view of treatment outcome. Moreover, the objections that the patient had a flight into health and now has a substitution of symptoms are not warranted by research (Cummings & Follette, 1976).

Psychologists also need to reconsider the problem of "diagnosis." Brief psychotherapy is not facilitated by accepting a vague description of the patient's problem or by giving a simplistic DSM-III diagnosis, which characterizes the nature of the dysfunction rather than its impact on the person. We believe that central to the initial interview is the establishment of what Cummings and VandenBos (1979) called the "operational diagnosis." It stems directly from the question "What brings the individual here today?" (rather than last week, last year, or next month).

The operational diagnosis formulates the problem(s) that the brief intervention must address, and the abandonment of the concept of cure permits the patient and therapist to interrupt the treatment as soon as the problem is solved. The patient is free to come in again if another problem arises, personally or with others. Again, the operational diagnosis defines the problem to be addressed, and treatment once again is interrupted rather than terminated. This approach to the psychologist's functioning as a general psychological family practitioner, which Cummings has termed "brief, intermittent psychotherapy throughout the life cycle," is the essence of his Biodyne model (Cummings & VandenBos, 1979; Cummings & Fernandez, 1985). The salient features are that the concept of cure is abandoned, diagnosis is redefined operationally, therepy is specific and brief, and the concept of termination of treatment is eliminated. Research has shown that brief, intermittent psychotherapy throughout the life cycle involves far less treatment than is required by traditional long-term therapy and is considerably more cost-effective.

BRIEF PSYCHOTHERAPY

Most private practitioners in independent practice today will require additional training in brief psychotherapy regardless of their previous orientation or training. Brief psychotherapy is not merely a compressed version of long-term therapy but has its own parameters and techniques. Most effective brief therapies involve a melding of dynamic, behavioral, and systems approaches, in spite of the insistence of the adherents of these "schools" of therapy that they cannot be fused into one approach. Budman and Gurman (1983) describe the integration of various approaches so that therapy will be beneficial within a well-planned, limited amount of time.

Malan (1963, 1976), working in Great Britain under socialized medicine, discovered that brief therapy works with therapists who believe in brief therapy. Cummings (1977, 1979), working for a quarter of a century at Kaiser Permanente in San Francisco, found that therapists who believe in brief therapy are those who are trained in brief therapy, regardless of their original orientation or previous adherence to long-term practice. In fact, reporting eighteen years of research, Cummings found that when a workable brief therapy model is offered, and without any prior screening for suitability, 85 percent of the patients will select brief therapy and will improve significantly with short-term treatment. Only 10 percent will self-select long-term therapy and will need that more protracted intervention. The implication is obvious: with 85 percent of patients profiting from brief therapy, the 10 percent who require long-term therapy and should receive it can be financed. There remains the 5 percent of the total therapy population reported by Cummings who prove to be interminable. This is the psychotherapy group that terrifies every third-party payer and provides virtually an annuity for some private practitioners. Every provider seeking to survive in the competitive health climate must develop effective techniques for dealing with the interminable patient. Otherwise, the mental health package will not be cost-effective. But even more important, the psychologist of the future must address the fact that most long-term therapy may well be, as P. Watzlawick (personal communication, 1979) has suggested, iatrogenic (provider-caused). What, then, can psychology do to survive these changes? Following are several highly viable options.

A COMMUNITY MODEL IN MINNESOTA

Many, especially the federally qualified, community mental health centers, are, to quote Albee, "old wine in new bottles." Many lessons were learned, however, in the development of the Minnesota Community Mental Health Services network (Dörken, 1962a, 1962b). Though twenty-five years old, some of those lessons are pertinent today. Minnesota was the second state to enact a community mental health services act. At the time it had four state mental hygiene clinics. The state was very largely without any mental health services over vast regions. How to develop cost-effective outpatient mental health services statewide was the foremost question.

The act, authored in part by input from the U.S. Public Health Service, in part by the mental health association and reflecting the social conscience of this Midwestern state, established some basic principles and encoded them in law (Dörken, 1960). The program was developed center by center and was in effect an ongoing laboratory. There were no indigenous professionals to recruit, but each community was unique and had specialized needs. With funding limited, the decision was made to recruit nationally, employ the best, and pay competitively. That yielded skills, diversity, and minimal turnover. It was quickly apparent that county civil service had neither the flexibility nor the salary structure to accommodate the caliber of staff desired, and so most of the new centers were established as nonprofit corporations in the private sector outside civil service where salaries were negotiable, premiums could be paid for excellence, and conditions for national recruitment became feasible. To have a sufficient population base of 50,000 to 100,000 usually required two or three counties. They became participants, contracting jointly with the state for the center's services. Thus, marketing, contracting, local representation, and service matched to community need were key considerations.

As the program developed further, several other facts emerged. Originally, centers were staffed with a three-person team per each 50,000 of population, the basic "holy trinity" of those days: psychologist, psychiatrist, and clinical social worker. The basic unit of concern—treatment, if you will—was the community. How to resolve community problems was the prime objective rather than simply developing a caseload or treating individuals. The training of gatekeepers and other community resources became essential. Thus, the problem was not tackled one person at a time but through a community plan (Dörken, 1962a). The services addressed the contractees' problems, not so much the traditional concerns of most mental health professionals (Dörken, 1971).

A public health philosophy prevailed, with its focus on positive mental health in harmony with the American value system, wherein the capacity of the individual to achieve is fundamental. The objective was to optimize personal resources and functionality rather than to seek a "cure" for psychopathology.

In rural areas a very pertinent question was how far a center could stretch. By plotting distance and presenting clinical problems, it was discovered that beyond an hour's drive by car, about forty to sixty miles in Minnesota then, the character of the incoming patients changed dramatically from the full range of emotional, family, behavioral, and mental conditions to predominantly acute psychotic disorders (Hodges & Dörken, 1961). Of course, the latter could not be served effectively by a distant outpatient service. Consequently, a geographical limit was set.

Three full-time equivalent (FTE) staff members per 50,000 population did not leave much idle time. It was intended that they be faced with a just manageable level of work. The traditional mental hygiene clinic model of social work intake, psychological evaluation, and psychiatric diagnosis followed by a team meeting to determine a course of action—that is, no intervention until the seventh professional time unit $(1 + 1 + 1 + 3 \rightarrow 7)$—was quickly shut down as an unworkable extravagance. Rather, the private-practice model was implemented. Patients were assigned on triage by the receptionist, matching problem to professional skills. The therapist would refer or seek consultation only when needed. As the private-practice model was implemented, it became obvious that the cost per unit of patient care in this model, the higher salaries of these corporate staff members notwithstanding, was much less than in the mental hygiene clinic model. The many hours not spent in staff meetings, multiple-staff treatment decisions, and so on substantially increased the hours directed to patient care or community service. Thus, when salaries were divided by effective program hours (as distinct from overhead), it became apparent that the higher-paid private-practice model yielded a lower cost per unit of service than the traditional mental hygiene clinic. Three state mental hygiene clinics were accordingly converted to community centers under local administration, and one was terminated, this change effected one year ahead of the legislative schedule.

In the process of this development, another major lesson was learned. None of the mental health professionals were trained as administrators, and yet competent local leadership was essential. There had to be one responsible contact for the state administrator. Competence, not profession, was then adopted as the criterion for appointment of program directors, with an administrative increment added to salary. The adoption of this competency principle for program direction statewide in 1960 was a first among the states and is as valid today as then. Interestingly, in those days the three professions always became program directors in about equal numbers.

To acquire an optimum mix of skills, it was often necessary to have close to or somewhat more than a double "team," five to eight FTE professionals. Further cost studies showed that the cost per unit of service dropped as staff size increased from one to five and bottomed through eight (one and two-thirds to two and two-thirds teams) and then began to climb again, rapidly. By ten to eleven the cost exceeded that of a solo professional. Reasons included the higher cost of psychiatrist salaries, exceeding the optimum ratio in economy of scale of support staff, increased housekeeping, elimination of many smaller and less costly site options, and the necessary substitution of formal administrative staff exchanges instead of the knowledge transfer by osmosis possible in a small, tight-knit organization. When an organization grows, its growth is not linear—its surface is squared and its volume is cubed. Individuality soon becomes lost. Considering necessary diversity of skills, cost, efficiency, and geographical coverage, an FTE staff of five to eight was adopted as the most effective: small enough so that everyone knew what was going on, small enough that the workload was at a just manageable level of difficulty without idle time, but substantial enough to have the diverse skills to serve the target area. Where there was a demand for growth, adjacent counties were encouraged to form a new center. Sixteen centers were developed over a three-year span (1959–1962), with a network of twenty-six projected. The full network was implemented several years later and has been operative since.

Thus, the lessons in developing new cost-effective mental health services in Minnesota community mental health have many features in common with the Biodyne model to be discussed later: highly qualified professional staff, diversity of skills pertinent to the community served, accessible location and businesslike appearance, small and close-knit staffing organization with minimal overhead, above-par competitive remuneration with realistic fringes, time commitment sufficient to assure close identity, and progressive innovation and zeal to outreach and effect change. We will not argue that Biodyne is the only model, however, space does not permit more than a mention of several other interesting models, each of which is viable in its own right.

DELAWARE VALLEY PSYCHOLOGICAL CLINICS

As the community mental health centers were just beginning to emerge across the country to bring ambulatory mental health care to reachable catchment areas, a totally private-sector network was founded in Philadelphia in 1958 by Janice Kenny and Aaron Smith. Beginning in rented basement offices, it moved into its own building in 1963.

It was the first private clinic in the area owned by psychologists and employing psychiatrists. In 1975 Smith moved to Nevada, and Kenny, with the plan of a major expansion, chose a new associate, Jan Grossman. Although the idea of expansion was appealing to Grossman, the idea was new, seemed unworkable, and therefore did not take shape until 1978. However, by 1983 they had established thirteen clinics and eight branch offices throughout the greater Philadelphia area of five counties in a ten-mile radius. The Delaware Valley Psychological Clinics (DVPC) is a privately owned partnership and is the largest group of private mental health professionals in the area. It is 100 percent supported by client fees and related third-party reimbursement and by policy accepts no government funds. Responsibility for coverage of over 39,000 patients through an affiliation with the Health Maintenance Organization of Pennsylvania has led to expansion of the clinic's network into Allentown, Bethlehem, and Easton, Pennsylvania, some fifty miles from Philadelphia. Plans are presently in the offing for expansion into the Williamsport and Lewisburg area.

No one joins the staff without passing a series of rigorous interviews and background checks. All professionals are required to have a strong background in general mental health care (psychotherapy, psychodiagnostics, and consultation) as well as at least one specialty that adds a unique coverage in service available for the clinic's clientele. Any client seeing one of the clinic's professionals has ready access to the entire specialty system, and on any given day there are numerous cross-consultations taking place among staff members. There is staffing for home visitation and shut-in services, and multilingual therapists are available who speak Spanish, French, Hebrew, Yiddish, Polish, and German.

In addition to licensed psychologists and psychiatrists, the clinics have fourteen Pennsylvania-certified school psychologists geographically distributed across the Delaware Valley. Only certified school psychologists can by state law prescribe special educational programs for learning-disabled or socially or emotionally disturbed children. DVPC is a teaching clinic with working agreements for training and teaching at Hahnemann Medical College, Fielding Institute, Bryn Mawr College, and Temple University. Internship programs in adult, child, and forensic psychology saw twenty-one young professionals in training in 1985–86. DVPC also has hospitalization privileges at six area health facilities.

Within the DVPC is a forensic division with over twenty psychologists, psychiatrists, and social workers and three sections: domestic, civil, and criminal. The domestic section is involved in over 100 divorce and custody situations each year, while the civil section handles over 200 referrals for such services as Social Security disability evaluation, worker's compensation litigation, and rehabilitation agencies. In a typical year, 50 to 100 patients are evaluated and treated in the criminal section. All services are rendered with the expectation that court testimony will be required, so that there is solid documentation, and as a result DVPC has earned considerable confidence within the legal community.

The clinics advertise, maintain a twenty-four-hour phone service, provide a computer testing service, and use computerized billing and computer-ready forms. Thus, although each of the clinics and branch offices is a small, efficient unit, the network gains economies of scale through centralized support services. As DVPC's size, coverage, and reputation grew, so did its ability to attract clients. Thus, quite apart from the professional attraction of working with competent peers, there is a distinct economic advantage to the professional affiliation.

Still another advantage to organization is in-service training provided at low cost to the staff members. Last year a two-day seminar was presented by out-of-state experts at a cost of only $50 per clinic member, compared with a customary seminar fee of $300.

The other side of the symbiotic relationship between clinic and practitioner is that the organization retains a portion of the practitioner fee. For new therapists, 100 percent of their first-session fee is retained by DVPC and 50 percent of subsequent fees. However, when the new therapist attracts or transfers in a new referral, his or her share rises to 55 percent, to 60 percent with the sixth referral, and to

65 percent with the eleventh, and after twenty referrals the therapist retains 70 percent of fee. Senior staff members who then serve a clientele of $600 or more a week for at least twenty-six weeks retain 75 percent. The financial incentive for involvement and productivity is clear. A bonus of 5 percent is given to those who arrange to see patients from home offices, thereby cutting clinic overhead. All members of the staff have an equal opportunity to reach the senior staff level.

The DVPC comprehensive psychological service network sees about 1,500 patients a week, and therapists may vary their time and therefore their income. They may also trade referrals for ones they prefer. The clinics share referrals, so that if a service is needed, a determination is made about who can deliver it. When a new client calls, he or she is connected as soon as possible with a psychologist who performs an immediate assessment of the client's problem and determines when it is convenient for the client to come in and which office is closest to the client's home or business. An appointment is then set up with the appropriate specialist within days—within hours if it is an emergency. There are no waiting lists and no awkward intake procedures. The objective is to provide the finest-quality private mental health care available in the community, promptly, appropriately, and effectively. No single (solo) practitioner or even a small group can match the in-depth professional resources of DVPC, its twenty-four-hour access, and its linkages to numerous community agencies and hospitals.

CALIFORNIA PSYCHOLOGICAL HEALTH PLAN

The California Psychological Health Plan (CPHP) is the product of a year-long study by a task force of the Division of Clinical and Professional Psychology of the California State Psychological Association (CSPA) in the early seventies. Following the recommendations of that task force in 1972, CPHP was incorporated in 1973, registered with the attorney general in 1974, and became independent of CSPA in 1975. In 1975 CPHP became the first statewide, prepaid mental health care plan licensed by the state Department of Corporations. Under California law, CPHP is a Knox-Keene licensed specialized health care service plan and, as such, must meet rigorous state standards of solvency, reserves to meet obligations, evidence of sufficient numbers of providers, and quality-of-care assurance. A nonprofit corporation, it is essentially a closed-panel program in which the contracting providers, licensed psychologists, and psychiatrists have been screened and agree to deliver services in accord with the CPHP service plan. Services are provided in the provider's own office. Donald D. Marsh, a member of the original CSPA task force, is director of professional services.

CPHP client organizations today number more than fifty, among which are fourteen municipalities, six school districts, and various corporations including, recently, Hughes Aircraft Company. Enrollment is only for organized groups of employees, and typically CPHP is marketed as the outpatient mental health arm of a comprehensive health care plan. It operates mainly on a capitation model and currently serves about 200,000 individuals. The organization is at risk to provide and pay for all required services and administration from its capitation revenue (per person per month, prepaid), although this risk is significantly reduced where employers underwrite direct treatment costs.

A geographical directory of contracting providers is distributed to all subscribers—the eligible employees of the client organization. Utilization is encouraged, and there are orienting health education sessions with members. A reverse copayment is used whereby the first five visits are without cost to the patient. There is a 15 percent copayment for the next five, 30 percent for a subsequent five, and 50 percent from the sixteenth visit. There is no deductible and no arbitrary limit on visits. Complete confidentiality from the employer is assured, and there is easy direct access to the CPHP provider of choice. There are no claim forms.

Initial capitalization of the plan was achieved through provider member contributions ranging from $300 to $1,300. Today there is a nominal annual membership fee of $25. Provider members agree by contract that their services are subject to review and that before the sixth visit, if further services are considered necessary, a written treatment plan of the case will be formulated for discussion with a district professional standards management committee (PSMC) chair. Treatment planning and review conferences are arranged at this point and usually every fifteen visits thereafter. The purpose is not peer review in the usual sense but a collaborative, educational system to assure more effective and definitive help for covered subscribers.

The current fee allowance (adopted in August 1984 and effective through 1985) for contracting providers is $60 for a forty-five- to fifty-minute sessions, which is less than UCR in most areas of the state and certainly in Southern California, where CPHP has the majority of its members. The copayments beyond the fifth visit are paid by the patient to the provider on the basis of the current ($60) rate. These are then "alternative," or negotiated discounted, rates under California law and are agreed to as payment in full. To ensure that CPHP can maintain the reserves required by the Department of Corporations, provider members also agree to defer 20 percent of their fee on each case to be withheld in reserve, until that treatment is concluded. The reserve has been paid to providers each year. Except for any copayment, the fee then is paid not by the patient but by CPHP to the provider.

It should be noted that CPHP is not an exclusive provider organization. A subscriber may go to a noncontracting provider, but that provider is paid only 50 percent of the CPHP rate (progressively less after five visits), and the subscriber is obligated to the provider for the difference from the provider's usual charge. There is also a limit per family per year on payment to noncontracting providers, ranging from $500 to $1,000 according to the contractual arrangements with the employer group. Thus, there is a substantial financial incentive for subscribers to use CPHP providers, as in a preferred provider organization. However, CPHP is more accurately described as an IPA-type HMO (individual practice association).

CPHP has been in the business long enough and with enough clients now to have accumulated some very positive outcome data. First its concept and then its results have attracted the attention of the insurance industry. In 1975 Crown Life and Massachusetts Mutual added the CPHP benefit at no cost to the policyholder in two plans, one a multiemployer trust. In the first year, the paid/loss ratio dropped from 92 to 67 percent, and despite rapid inflation in health care costs, there was no rate change under the policy until after the fourth year (Mercer, 1980). Other positive experiences are briefly referred to in "Psychological Health Plan Nips Insurance Premium Increases" (1981). More definitive is the report from the city of Redondo Beach (Casey & Siegel, 1982). The city's interest was in part sparked by the high incidence of family problems among safety employees and three successive disability retirements for psychological reasons. Instead of annually rising health insurance premiums, Redondo Beach saw its premiums remain constant from 1979 to 1981 while the group health insurance plan generated $160,000 in dividend reserves. Only one public safety employee was granted a valid psychologically based disability retirement during this period, and there were no further applicants. Moreover, the rate of absenteeism due to sickness dropped from 3.2 to 1.6 percent—all very positive outcomes and clear evidence of the impact of psychological intervention in reducing total health care costs.

CPHP serves only its subscriber members—the employees of organizations with whom it has a contractual relationship and their dependents. Its provider members, of course, serve not only CPHP subscribers but their other clients as well. As CPHP has gained major new client organization contracts, several providers are known to have moved their offices so as to be more optimally located. Of course, over time, the greater the percentage of an area population that is under contract to CPHP—or to a local HMO or other plan with a lock-in or use-incentive feature—the smaller will be the number of those inclined to use noncontracting providers. Independent practitioners will face a progressive dwindling of available clients as organized entities contract into and take over the market.

THE BIODYNE MODEL

American Biodyne Centers, based in San Francisco, offers a mental health maintenance organization (MHMO) type of PPO to HMOs, PPOs, insurance indemnity plans, medical service associations (Blue Cross/Blue Shield), and large employer groups that may wish to contract for a low-cost, effective, and comprehensive outpatient mental health benefit. The Biodyne model implements the concepts described above. It is psychology's first nationwide MHMO and can serve as a model or a point of departure for future psychological PPOs. Biodyne has already contracted to establish three centers in Arizona (in Phoenix and Tucson) and another in Florida on a for-profit basis. The Arizona centers are a joint venture with Blue Cross/Blue Shield in which the Blues will market Biodyne as an exclusive. Other centers are under negotiation in a number of states. The model might best be understood through a description of its prototype center in Honolulu. Biodyne/Honolulu, established as a subcontractor in a cooperative agreement (No. 11-C-98344/9, 10/83-9/88) between the state of Hawaii and the federal Health Care Financing Administration, is a nonprofit clinical center conducting offset research and, in the process, providing unlimited outpatient mental health care for 68,000 eligibles, 34,000 of whom are Medicaid beneficiaries and 34,000 of whom are employed or retired federal workers and their dependents.* Thus, there are two contracts for two types of enrollees: the state of Hawaii for the Medicaid population and Hawaii Medical Service Association (a Blue Shield affiliate) for the employed group.

All practitioners are indigenous and are selected for their clinical expertise, knowledge of area problems, and adaptability to the Biodyne model. For example, of the ten current professional Honolulu staff members, three are Caucasion. All are independent contractors who received 130 hours of training in the Biodyne model at the outset. This includes an extensive training manual with programs for over fifty targeted interventions for specific conditions, and participants are given the opportunity to view the hands-on application of these interventions by the clinical director and his assistant. Thereafter, there are weekly clinical case conferences that serve not only as continual on-the-job training but also as "peer review" aimed at maintaining the integrity of the model.

No investment is required of the participating practitioners. In the for-profit centers, the practitioners, at the end of the year, have the opportunity to share in the divisible surplus resulting from having performed efficiently enough to create such a surplus from the capitated dollars to Biodyne from the contractees. The practitioners work in a well-appointed center that is limited to ten or eleven practitioners. When Biodyne increases its enrollees, it forms additional centers and staffs them similarly. In this manner each center is maintained as a small, intensive, and efficient group practice.

In addition to providing an unlimited outpatient benefit with its targeted programs, house calls when appropriate, and other services not usually seen as part of a benefit package, Biodyne also provides an outreach program for the 10 percent highest utilizers of health care. Periodically, the contractee provides Biodyne with a computer printout of the utilization record of these 10 percent highest utilizers by incidence rather than dollar amount. A printout according to dollar amount would merely produce the organ transplants, the kidney dial-

*N. Cummings and H. Dörken are principal and co-principal investigators for the Impact of Psychological Intervention on Health Care Utilization and Costs. 11-C-98344/9 awarded by the Health Care Financing Administration to the Hawaii Department of Social Services and Housing (state Medicaid agency) under contract with the Biodyne Institute. Any opinions expressed here regarding Biodyne are those of the authors and should in no way be attributed to either the Health Care Financing Administration or the state of Hawaii.

yses, and other users of costly service rather than the somaticizer. To the 10 percent highest utilizers. Biodyne applies its program and elicits the 5.5 percent who are overloading medical resources without there being any physical basis for it. An outreach nurse or medical social worker contacts these patients and, without threatening their belief that their problems are physical, helps them to make an appointment with a Biodyne psychotherapist. About half of a center's resources are expended in providing a comprehensive, efficient, and effective mental health package, the other half in the outreach program. In this way Biodyne renders for its contractees/clients both a comprehensive, unlimited outpatient mental health package at competitive cost and an outreach to the somaticizers that results in considerable cost containment in the provision of overall health care.

Biodyne is able to maintain a low operating overhead at each center by having each of the centers connected by computer and voice lines to a streamlined corporate headquarters in San Francisco. The integrity of the Biodyne model is maintained by scheduled visits from the clinical director and the assistant clinical directors, who, during these visits, conduct clinical case conferences and further training sessions as well as arrange for the center providers to view them in hands-on therapy through one-way screens. Finally, the American Biodyne Centers are committed to providing annual research funds to the Biodyne Institute, a nonprofit research corporation, for ongoing research designed to perpetually refine the model and keep Biodyne on the cutting edge of the profession.

Biodyne operates as an HMO-type PPO; that is, a center is maintained centrally where all the providers see their contracted patients. It has been found that not only is this more efficient and cost-effective than the IPA model, where the practitioners function out of their own individual offices, but also it fosters a stronger identification with the Biodyne model. There is a tendency for practitioners to do in their own offices what they have traditionally done there. However, Biodyne is flexible enough to adapt the model in situations that warrant modification. Two examples are illustrative.

Biodyne/Honolulu serves all of the island of Oahu from its central, convenient location adjacent to the Ala Moana Shopping Center, where the island's extensive bus system converges. This location has proved satisfactory for most Biodyne enrollees. However, the residents of Waianae, a Polynesian "ghetto" northeast of Honolulu, will not come into the city. Furthermore, about one-third of the island's Medicaid population resides in Waianae. A satellite center was established that is staffed part-time by practitioners from the Honolulu center, and this has significantly increased the impact on that segment of enrollees. Similarly, a satellite has been opened in the Pearl Ridge area, where there is a high concentration of federal enrollees.

In Brevard County, Florida, it was apparent from the outset that a modification would be necessary. Brevard County, where NASA's satellite launching station is located, is a narrow county almost 100 miles long. Because of this length, the population divides itself into northern, central, and southern county areas, and the residents of the respective areas will not usually travel the distance to another area. For this reason, Biodyne in Florida is planning for a center in the central county, with satellites in the north and south counties as part of its start-up planning and costs. In the beginning, the satellites would be the private offices of two of the participating providers in the north and south sections of the county. It would be clear from the outset, however, that all practitioners would relate to the one centrally located center for clinical case conferences, meetings, the outreach program, and the other activities of the Biodyne model. This departure from the usual Biodyne Centers model is applicable not only to a 100-mile-long county such as Brevard where there are not yet enough enrollees to form three centers but also to rural settings where there will never be a sufficient cluster of enrollees to maintain one central location serving 30,000 to 80,000 enrollees.

The organizational model of the Biodyne Centers contributes to the efficiency and effectiveness of the delivery system. But to an even greater degree, this efficiency and effectiveness is attributable to the over fifty therapeutic interventions targeted for specific conditions. Empirically tested by Cummings and his colleagues over a twenty-five-year period and known collectively as the "Biodyne model," these techniques dramatically reduce the number of sessions required to achieve patient stability as they enhance the therapeutic outcomes. The literature on select interventions is scant. This specificity of treatment is a distinctive Biodyne feature.

These techniques range from necessarily tightly drawn approaches to the several types of suicidal behavior to a more open technique for dealing with midlife crises, so differentiated because the first is life-threatening and the latter requires more latitude for self-actualization. The Biodyne training manual includes a technique for getting house-bound and even bedridden agoraphobics out of bed and out of the

house with mostly one but sometimes two house calls. It further includes specific interventions for each of a series of addictive behaviors, which include not only alcohol and chemical abuse but also
compulsive eating and gambling, anorexia and bulimia, love and sex
addictions, and even therapy addiction. Because Biodyne is a capitated
delivery system, it can include a number of interventions that would
not normally be reimbursed in a fee-for-service practice but are,
nonetheless, important to both recovery from stress and prevention of
stress. These include stop-smoking programs, stress management programs, mind-body groups, group biofeedback training, and programs
designed to help the chronically unemployed find and keep a job.

The Biodyne model has melded techniques from dynamic therapy,
behavioral models, and systems approaches into cohesive interventions that belie the often-stated dogma from adherents that these approaches cannot be mixed with one another. Empirical research has
shown that insight is very useful in some conditions and relatively
worthless in others, and the same holds true for desensitization or
family systems approaches. The important consideration is that these
amalgams have been empirically tested over two and a half decades
and tested with Cummings' cost/therapeutic–effectiveness ratio,
which requires parsimoniously that the techniques used will render
the greatest benefit in the least number of sessions.

The Biodyne model employs a substantial number of group therapy
techniques, not because these cost less to deliver, but because empirical research has shown that clients with certain conditions (addiction
and agoraphobia, as two of many examples) recover faster and sustain
the recovery longer with group therapy. Biodyne has developed a
group for crisis intervention: patients needing to be seen that very day
are seen in a group with other such patients. The discovery that crises
are best met in crisis groups, even for an initial session, was startling
indeed, but the twenty-five years of empirical research that developed
the Biodyne model yielded a number of surprises that challenge several therapeutic sacred cows.

For those contracting with American Biodyne Centers there are distinct financial advantages. The Blue Cross/Blue Shield contract in Arizona is illustrative and led to the opening of three centers on
September 4, 1985, two in Phoenix and one in Tucson. With Biodyne
paid on a capitated basis, the "Blues" have a provider that is sharing the
risk. By being able to market Biodyne as an "exclusive," the Blues gain
a clear marketing advantage and one likely to increase their market

penetration. With capitation, there are no claims to review or reimburse and no individual providers to be qualified, all saving administrative costs. In addition, using a provider that outreaches the many high users of health care whose utilization is the result of somaticizing psychological problems produces a substantial offset of medical care costs.

Even if the joint venture between the Blue Cross/Blue Shield of Arizona and Biodyne Centers of America corporations had no direct financial advantages, it would still have distinct quality-of-care advantages. Biodyne holds quality of care paramount. All the professional staff members are licensed/certified by the state—no paraprofessionals are used. All were selected with care for clinical competence and diversity of skills. All have received intensive training in the Biodyne model. All services provided receive regular in-house oversight for appropriateness and progress in achieving the treatment goals.

From the subscribers' perspective there are also distinct advantages. There is no deductible or copayment and no arbitrary limit on the number of visits. There are also services, when appropriate, atypical of the benefits in most health plans, such as home visits, outreach, phone consultation, biofeedback, and lifestyle management programs. And since no claim forms and no employer approval of services are involved, the confidentiality of the practitioner/patient relationship is strengthened.

There are also distinct advantages for the members of Biodyne's professional staff. They work in new, modern offices with state-of-the-art equipment. They work with colleagues whom they can respect for their training and competence. And they practice without direction by or dependence on referral from another profession. Further, as self-employed contractors, they receive a highly competitive contract income. They are also partners in the "Biodyne family" and thereby eligible to participate in each year end's divisible surplus. As a longer-term incentive, practitioners continuing to contract with Biodyne for three or more years have the option of buying a specified number of corporation shares at nominal cost.

The above describes the many four-way advantages to the participants in the joint venture: the Blues, its subscribers, Biodyne, and its practitioners. They are incentive-oriented realities that promote the enterprise while forming the catalyst that will shape the endeavor and its success.

In reflecting on all the details, reflect also on the ultimate potential.

Here is a health care corporation under psychological direction in which services are delivered predominantly by psychologists. Its focus is not services to the mentally disordered but psychological intervention in the total spectrum of health care. The federal Health Care Financing Administration (HCFA) has funded a major five-year cost-offset research project with Biodyne through the Hawaii State Medicaid program. To the extent that the Biodyne psychological intervention succeeds in reducing total Medicaid health care costs, it will have major implications for psychological services in all state Medicaid programs and the operative federal law and regulations. Blue Cross/Blue Shield of Arizona has also entered into a multimillion-dollar contract with Biodyne to develop three centers to serve the subscribers of a number of its plans in two cities. The Arizona Blues are, of course, a member of the national Blue Cross/Blue Shield Association, headquartered in Chicago. To the extent that this Arizona contract proves a success, it has major implications not simply for future Biodyne contracts but also for the inclusion of clinical psychology nationally by the country's largest underwriter of health care. Thus, as a result of demonstrating the effectiveness of psychological services in the full spectrum of health care, the ultimate and not too distant potential is to gain for clinical psychology a collegial standing, recognition, and participation throughout the health care systems of the nation.

HOSPITALS

Hospitalization is heavily favored over outpatient care in most health insurance plans, is often without deductibles, often has a copayment of 20 percent rather than the more common 50 percent for ambulatory mental health care, and usually has a higher ceiling on days of care than outpatient visits allowed. It is therefore not surprising, even though the large majority of clients receive their care as office or clinic outpatients, that hospitalization accounts for more than half of the mental health dollar—indeed, 70 percent of the Medicaid mental health dollar, so that Medicaid is now the largest mental health program in the country. Big money usually attracts big business. The only wonder, really, is that the involvement of large corporations in psychiatric hospitals is so recent.

Levenson (1983) summarizes the recent rapidly growing ownership of private psychiatric hospitals by investor-owned hospital chains. In

1982 there were 198 nongovernmental (private) free-standing psychiatric hospitals in the country, of which 86, or 43 percent, were affiliated with for-profit (investor-owned) hospital chains. In 1980 only 41 (or 25 percent at the time) were so affiliated, and before the late sixties, the chains did not exist. The four major chains alone in 1982 owned 71 of the psychiatric hospitals affiliated with the National Association of Private Psychiatric Hospitals. The Hospital Corporation of America owned 22 psychiatric hospitals in 1982 and has since gone on to form a psychiatric division. Obviously "big business" is attracted to a major market and one it senses to be growing. Kiesler (1982b) has clearly documented that while public attention has been focused on the deinstitutionalization of the state mental hospitals, there has been since 1962 a linear increase in "psychiatric" hospitalizations into general hospitals without psychiatric units. In effect, hospitalization for mental disease has not decreased at all—quite the opposite. The locus of care has, however, changed dramatically. With third-party reimbursement, acute care in general hospitals has become feasible, while much of the chronic care at public expense is now situated in intermediate-care nursing facilities, which have lower operating costs than state hospitals. Kiesler (1982a) also found that in all controlled studies of alternatives to hospitalization none was less effective (the majority were more effective) and all were less costly. If there is to be any substantial direct reduction in the cost of mental health care (as distinct from mental health services offsetting total health care costs), it will likely be achieved by residential alternatives to hospitalization that emphasize effective and intensive treatment.

The California legislature wrestled with this issue in 1978 and established a new class of health facility, the psychiatric health facility, or PHF (pronounced "puff"), in S.B. 1496-Gregorio, chapter 1234. This law recognized a twenty-four-hour acute residential care nonhospital in which it was intended that the per diem costs would not exceed 60 percent of the average of similar services in an area general hospital. Of particular interest to psychology, the mandated basic services included "clinical psychology." Within thirty days of the effective date of the legislation (January 1979) the Department of Health Services appointed an ad hoc committee to assist in the formulation of regulations. Seven years later, in January 1986, the draft regulations were finally given public hearing. County mental health programs had established eighteen PHFs on waivers under guidelines of the Department of Mental Health, but private facilities could not be operated

without a license. Without a Certificate of Need (CON) it was not possible to grant a license. Without regulations there were no licensing
criteria that could be met. And, of course, third parties would reimburse only for services in a licensed facility. Double catch-22.

Legislation in 1984 (S.B. 2160, chapter 1367) resolved much of the
impasse when it required that if the health insurance included coverage for services in a general acute care hospital or an acute psychiatric
hospital, then the coverage must extend to a PHF operating under either state guidelines or licensure. Finally, in the spring of 1985, the
new state administration, seeking to encourage private-sector development, sent word to its Office of Statewide Health Planning that applications should be granted a waiver of the otherwise required CON.
Frustrated with the years of bureaucratic delay, Senator Paul Carpenter
introduced S.B. 1414 in 1985 to waive the CON requirement when the
Department of Mental Health determines that the applicant either will
not create excess beds in the area or will deliver services in an innovative and more competitive way or at a lower cost than services at
other area facilities. The state administration then moved to incorporate these provisions into the draft regulations and the bill was then
converted to another purpose. Thus, finally, the stage is set for the flexible development of cost- and program-competitive acute care mental
health services in twenty-four-hour residential facilities. Hospitals, psychiatric and general, will experience the competition.

The first private-sector PHF waiver was granted to Treatment Centers of America (TCA) in the spring of 1985 to open a facility in
Panorama City (San Fernando Valley), California. Of its 146 beds, half
will function as a PHF with acute intensive treatment. The other half
are licensed by the Department of Social Services for residential treatment, much like a halfway house but with active treatment programs.
Thus, TCA-Valley can offer two levels of care in a quality professional
environment at rates at least 40 percent less than psychiatric hospital
care in the area.

TCA also has a thirty-four-bed behavioral health treatment center for
psychological conditions and chemical dependency in adults at Scotts-
dale, Arizona. This operation is licensed as a behavioral health specialty unit within a skilled nursing facility. Plans are underway for the
development within the year of other PHF facilities in Southern California. Samuel Mayhugh, president of TCA and a psychologist, is convinced that this model not only enables the development of residential
facilities accessible to psychological practice but holds the potential

for behavioral health centers to emerge as the more effective alternative to psychiatric hospitalization as measured both by cost and by multilevel treatment effectiveness. Moreover, such facilities can serve as the hub for a range of psychological health services in their area.

IN RETROSPECT AND PROSPECT

There are, no doubt, other viable psychological organizations across the country engaged in the delivery of health care. We hope that the descriptions of community mental health centers as nonprofit corporations, a Philadelphia metropolitan area partnership network of twenty-one offices, the California Psychological Health Plan, the Biodyne model, and Treatment Centers of America will prompt other psychologists to organize new and even more effective models for behavioral health practice. We are convinced that the viable mode of future practice will be within competitive organizations and systems.

The 12 Couches

When I first came to Kaiser in 1950, I had just come from analytic training at William Alanson White Institute in New York City, and psychoanalysis was considered to be the only true way to get people better in psychotherapy. The only indispensable piece of hardware was the psychoanalytic couch. Since I was hired as a Chief of Mental Health at Kaiser, what was the one thing I needed for everyone? You got it! Everyone should have a couch!

New psychoanalytic couches were not purchased in department stores. They had to be custom-made, particularly if you were on the West Coast. So, as a good psychoanalyst, I had 12 couches custom-made for my staff shortly after I got to Kaiser. After all, this was the way you do REAL psychotherapy. Now, an analytic couch is not much good for anything but analysis. You can't sit comfortably on it, and you can't sleep on it. And having it custom-made is quite expensive.

Many of the patients we saw at Kaiser were blue-collar workers, laborers, longshoreman, and often non–high-school graduates. The idea of having them lie down on psychoanalytic couches was not going to work. We also had to have a more accessible kind of psychotherapy.

I called my staff together and said, "We are going to have to change the way we do therapy."

They said, "How is that?"

I said, "I have no idea. But we have got to get rid of those couches."

I called Goodwill, and a man came up and looked at me oddly. He said, "You can't sleep on them, you can't turn them into beds." "We don't want them," he said, and he walked away. He wouldn't take my couches!

I then called the Salvation Army. "Oh yes," the person who answered the phone said, "we'd love to have 12 couches."

I said, "And they're only a couple months old. Hardly been used."

So two men from the organization parked their truck in front of the hospital and came upstairs with their dollies. One said, "What do you do with them? You can't sleep on them. You can't lie on them." And they walked away, too.

This time I said, "Well, let me not make this mistake again." I called St. Vincent DePaul and said, "I've got 12 couches, brand-new, two months old, hardly been used."

"Oh, we want them," was the response. My staff and I carried them to the elevator, took them downstairs, and stacked them up on the street. And we stood there, and when the St. Vincent DePaul truck pulled up, I said, "Look, they're yours. I got them to the street. You agreed on the telephone to take them and if you don't, I'll report you to the city for littering the sidewalk in front of the hospital." They took them.

{ 13 }

THE FUTURE OF PSYCHOTHERAPY: ONE PSYCHOLOGIST'S PERSPECTIVE

The inefficient manner in which psychotherapy is delivered renders mental-health practitioners vulnerable to the new emphasis in health-cost containment. It is estimated that in 1995 most health-care delivery will be controlled by five or six giant health corporations. Fifty percent of the mental-health practitioners in independent practice today are unlikely to survive. Those who do survive will either have learned the new delivery system, or they will be employees of corporate health. As frightening as these predictions may seem, there is also a window of opportunity for psychotherapists to get their house in order and to meet the challenge.

FIRST, I MUST confess I am not a futurist. I have no idea how psychotherapy will be practiced in the year 2025. So I should like to bring us back to the 20th century, which is rapidly expiring, and talk about what we can expect in the next ten years. That is about as far as I can see, which closely approximates the length of my nose.

We are in the process of dismantling the largest and most successful health-care system ever devised on the face of this earth (Cummings, 1986), and we are dismantling it very rapidly. How is this going to affect us as mental-health practitioners? There is no doubt but that it will affect us drastically, but even more drastically, it is going to impact on the American people. I believe we are about to enter an era of chaos, where the American consumers, our patients, are going to experience a sharp decline in the quality of care they will receive. This period will persist until we emerge from the turbulence that will affect not only them, but you as providers.

How did we get into this mess? It is important to talk about that, because without understanding how we got here, it is difficult to comprehend what will occur in the next decade. And since most of you who have been in independent practice for at least several years are doing so well, you will not wish to hear that over half of private practitioners in the mental-health field will be out of practice by the middle of the next decade. If you believe that is too drastic a prediction, consider the forecast of the American Medical Association which holds that only 5 percent of physicians practicing in 1995 will be in independent solo practice. Only 5 percent! This means that 95 percent of physicians will be with HMOs and PPOs in less than ten years.

THE PARADOX: RATIONING OUR SURPLUS OF HEALTH-CARE RESOURCES

There is a paradox facing us. The year 1986 found us with the highest number of hospital beds per capita anywhere in the world. The excess of hospital beds is so serious that hospitals are resorting to marketing programs to fill beds by converting to substance-abuse, psychiatry, and adolescent care. At the same time, we have entered the doctor glut. Health-care providers of of all kinds are mushrooming far ahead of need. And during this era of surplus, what are health economists talking about? It is the rationing of our surplus! You ask, and properly so, how can we have a surplus and a need to ration at the same time? It is because the cost of health care in the United States now accounts for 11 percent of the Gross National Product (GNP), and those who pay the bills are determined that inflation of health care at two or three times the general inflation rate must stop. To understand how this determination evolved, and how rationing can be brought about in spite of a surplus, we must trace the two health-care eras immediately preceding the present one, and then look to economics.

THE THREE MODERN HEALTH-CARE ERAS

Immediately following World War II the United States entered the *Era of Health-Care-Resources Expansion*. This era can roughly be identified by the years 1945 through 1970. During this period the government especially, but the private sector as well, pushed for a major increase in our health-resource capacity. The Hill-Burton legislation was fueling in a noncompetitive fashion the building of new hospitals and the expansion of existing facilities. The federal government was funding seemingly endless stipends for the training of health-care providers, and psychiatry, psychology, and social work all benefited. In my own profession of psychology, graduate departments built their laboratories and academic programs on government monies earmarked for the stimulation of clinical training. Also during this era we launched the paraprofessional movement, having concluded there would never be enough mental-health-care professionals to fill the demand. Now we have so many professionals that the paraprofessionals are merely regarded, by those who hire providers, as a cheap form of labor.

In 1970 we entered the second major period in health care since World War II, the *Era of Social Reform in Health Care*. Following the era of expansion, we awakened to the fact that in spite of all of the growth in resources, there were still segments of our society that were not receiving adequate care: the poor and the minorities, our rural areas, and the elderly. Clearly, social reform was needed, and the nation responded with Medicare and Medicaid, and with incentives for practitioners to settle in rural areas. We also began to train practitioners to address the needs of ethnic minorities. This new emphasis in health care was a significant part of what came to be known as the Great Society.

Then, after only ten short years, we ushered in the *Era of Health-Care-Cost Reform* in roughly the year 1980. By that year, most of health care in the United States was reimbursable through a third-party payor, which was either the federal government in Medicare and Medicaid, or insurers in the private sector. Ultimately, however, either through employee benefits or Social Security, much of the burden for the health-care bill fell on the employer. In 1980 the industrial might of the nation began to organize health-planning consortia in our major cities, and it was the avowed purpose of these business interests to bring down health-care costs. These consortia were joined by government, which for years, through a series of initiatives, had failed to halt the escalating spiral of health-care costs. Then industry and government were joined by the unions, farmers, and eventually consumer-action groups. The driving force in this third modern era of health care is cost containment! Lip service is paid to maintaining quality, but cost containment is clearly the real mission. In this relentless drive for cost containment, you, the provider, will be one of the casualties.

As I travel about the country speaking to provider groups, it is not difficult to ascertain if the impact of the current era has yet hit the provider community. The give-away is the size of the audience. Two years ago I lectured in one state that had not a single HMO to an audience of eleven practitioners. A little over a year later there were 28 HMOs in that state and the private practices of many mental-health practitioners dried up almost overnight. I was asked to return with my "survival kit" for mental-health practitioners, and where two years earlier there had been an audience of eleven, there were now fourteen hundred.

GUCCI LOAFERS AND HEALTH CARE: A LESSON IN ECONOMICS

Most health-care practitioners do not like the field of economics, and I must confess that I regard economics to be an occult science. Economists have pet theories, such as deregulation will bring competition which will reduce prices. Once stating their bias, they massage their theories. And when one goes awry, such as the breaking up of the Bell System raising rather than lowering prices to the consumer, they are quick to find rationalizations. Yet there are health economists who have had a remarkable record in predicting the course of the health-care marketplace. Two of these are Eli Ginsberg of Columbia and Uwe Rhinehardt of Princeton, who gave most illuminating addresses to the Western Conference of Prepaid Medical Service Plans, held in Tucson, Arizona, in November 1986.

Professor Rhinehardt rather whimsically, yet in all seriousness, compares health care to Gucci loafers. Anyone who has been in New York City is impressed that there is seemingly an endless supply of Gucci loafers, yet the price does not come down. Rhinehardt states there is a simple social contract. There are Gucci loafers on one side, and Yuppies on the other. The Yuppies ask, "How much are the Gucci loafers?" "Four hundred dollars," comes the reply. The Yuppies respond, "Go to hell!" Then, "How about a hundred and fifty?" "You've got a deal." The Yuppie has a stake in keeping the cost of Gucci loafers somewhat high, for if everyone could afford them, how could the Gucci loafer remain the badge of the Yuppie? I said, "Don't tell me that is how health care is negotiated." And Rhinehardt's response is, after thousands of hours of debate, that health care is no different than Gucci loafers, except for the social contract. Whereas no one insists that the Yuppie and the hobo are equally entitled to Gucci loafers, the social contract in health care in the United States is that the hobo and the millionaire should get the same health care. This has never been accomplished successfully anywhere in the world, but this ethic remains the basis of the social contract in health care and tends to overly fuel health-care costs. In the Soviet Union, where I lectured during a recent summer, there is a two-tiered health system. One system is for the privileged, defined as the four million members of the Communist Party, and the second is for everyone else. The poor are not even allowed to peek into the front door of the other system.

Rhinehardt goes on to propose a three-tiered health system. The first tier would be for the unemployed which would be HMO medicine paid for by the government. The second would be for the employed, and would be Kaiser Permanente type HMOs, which are a cut above the usual HMO. This would be provided by the employer. Finally, there would be Yuppie care at 100 percent copayment (that is, out of pocket), and would include such non-essentials of modern medicine as breast and thigh reduction, cosmetic surgery on a vanity basis, and hair transplants. No one would seriously propose Rhinehardt's three-tiered system, yet, interestingly, it may just come about by default.

Probably my favorite health economist is Professor Ginsberg. In 1980 he startled the assembly in New York of health-care experts who were heralding the *Era of Cost Reform in Health Care*. Ginsberg was the sole dissenting voice to the notion that health-care costs would come down. He predicted that costs would continue to rise. And now, six years later, although the rate of inflation of health care has slowed, total costs continue to rise. Ginsberg predicts that even though productivity is down and expenditures are up, capitated* health care will continue to grow. This will include capitated mental-health care, which is currently only a small share of the market.

---

*A *capitated* health-delivery system is one in which a group of providers is given a monthly payment per enrollee to provide all of the contracted health benefits to those enrollees. Thus capitation differs markedly from fee-for-service. In the former, the providers are prospectively reimbursed and are responsible in advance for providing whatever care may occur in the future while in fee-for-service the provider is reimbursed only aftr the service has been rendered.

Schwartz (1987), a health economist at the Tufts University School of Medicine, asserts that the recent slowing in health-care cost is misleading, and that costs will skyrocket after 1990 unless there is a "painful" health-care rationing. He goes on to state that nothing short of wiping out the hospital system will prevent increases in health costs unless access to expensive high-technology medicine is severely limited.

OUR SUPPLY-DRIVEN MENTAL-HEALTH SYSTEM

The paradox is that although generally health costs are demonstrating a slowing in the rise of expenditures, mental-health costs are escalating at the phenomenal rate of 30 to 40 percent per year. Psychiatric hospital chains increased their bed capacity by 37 percent in the year ending July 1, 1985, and general hospitals, while divesting their acute-medical-care facilities, are opening lucrative 28- to 45-day substance-abuse centers and adolescent units eagerly prepared to keep teenagers hospitalized for six months and even one year. The national average of 40 percent mental-health-cost increases per annum was shattered last year in Los Angeles where psychiatric hospitalization rose 88 percent. Clearly, we are a supply-driven industry: if we have a bed, we'll fill it. This is shown to be true on the outpatient side as well, although the figures are not as clear and dramatic. There is a glut of mental-health practitioners, with ever-increasing competition for the patients available. The incentives are decidedly in the wrong direction for cost containment. Psychiatrists are joining hospital-based practices and colluding to fill the new psychiatric, substance-abuse, and adolescent beds that are heart-renderingly advertised on nightly television. Those who remain mostly in outpatient practice are given the incentive, once you find a patient, to keep him or her as long as possible. This does not mean that mental-health practitioners are dishonest or cynical. Yet as students of the unconscious, we know that people behave in their own best interest. We can always rationalize another few months of psychotherapy in the interest of the patient's growth, or choose a 28-day detoxification program even though research (Miller & Hester, 1986) reveals this is no more effective than intensive outpatient treatment.

The result is a boomerang effect on the part of those who must pay the bills: the third-party payor. Through benefit-design mental health is being severely limited and cut back in policy after policy. Undaunted, the mental-health community is responding by seeking laws that mandate mental-health coverage such as have been enacted in Massachusetts and Maryland. Texas recently enacted what is virtually a mandated, unlimited substance-abuse benefit. So mental-health practitioners continue, in most instances, to do well in 1987. They have been lulled into complacency. If third-party payors lose the right to limit mental-health benefits by virtue of state legislation mandating mental-health coverage, this will only hasten the advent of managed mental-health care through HMOs and PPOs. All indicators point to the fact that this is beginning to happen. It is only common sense that third-party payors and employers will not allow mental-health expenditures to grow at their current phenomenal rate while all other health-care costs are slowing down. When most mental-health professionals realize what is happening, their practices will already have substantially dried up.

No More Gucci Loafers

The reader may well ask, "Nick, what is the problem? You were with Kaiser Permanente for 25 years. So perhaps we will all go to work for HMOs and PPOs, what's the big deal?" I would point out that Kaiser Permanente was a provider-driven system, and remains the only such national capitated program that is owned and operated by the professional providers. The giant health corporations are business driven. Kaiser Permanente, during the quarter of a century I was with them, put quality care and the dignity of the practitioner as its highest priorities. Businessmen do not and would not place these priorities in the same perspective as would a practitioner.

Economists like to pick on how much you and I make for a living. When one is a college professor, the income of a physician or a surgeon must seem like a great deal of money. The giant health corporations, with their economist advisers, are going after the paycheck of the physician. There is no question that under managed health care physicians' incomes will shrink, and so will those of mental-health professionals. In fact, a story circulating among economists today is revealing. The question is asked, what will be the difference in 1990 between a pigeon and a physician? The answer is that a pigeon will still be able to make a deposit on a Mercedes-Benz.

Ginsberg argues that reducing practitioners' salaries will not reduce costs. The only thing that will reduce costs is the limitation in the number of practitioners we train and graduate. In 1959 when the nation was troubled by the shortage of physicians, Ginsberg had stated there should be no worry. There were so many physicians in the pipeline that in 20 to 25 years there would be a glut of doctors. Ginsberg's prediction was even more accurate for mental-health providers. In the 1950s we launched the paraprofessional movement because we sincerely believed there would never be enough professionals to meet patient demand. Now the paraprofessional is seen as a cheap form of labor preferred by many HMOs to the more expensive psychiatrists, psychologists, and even psychiatric social workers. In one HMO I visited, a quarter of a million enrollees were receiving all of their mental-health needs by a staff of one psychiatrist, two psychologists, and 26 paraprofessionals who were doing all of the so-called mental-health intervention.

Prepare for capitated mental-health care. Buy your Gucci loafers now while you can still afford them.

A SURVIVAL KIT FOR MENTAL-HEALTH PRACTITIONERS

What alternatives do mental-health practitioners have to becoming the employees of the dozen or so health-industry giants that will dominate and control health-care delivery in the 1990s? The relatively small market share of the health-delivery system previously held by HMOs will grow to the point where traditional fee-for-service will constitute only a small part of the industry. In other words, most health-care delivery (including mental-health-care delivery) will be managed care. Mental-health practitioners will either have learned how to form their own provider-controlled HMOs and PPOs, or they will have become employees of business-driven health corporations. These changing financing mechanisms will promote dramatic cost reduction and lower-cost health-delivery substitutes while maintaining acceptable levels of quality (Fig. 1).

In 1985 we formed American Biodyne, Inc., the first national Psychological HMO (PHMO). It was founded under the dedicated principle that it would become the standard of the industry in quality, efficiency, and comprehensiveness. In meeting this objective, we soon learned that we must challenge some of the most cherished notions in mental health. I should like to share these with you.

Figure 1. Trends in Payment Mechanisms.

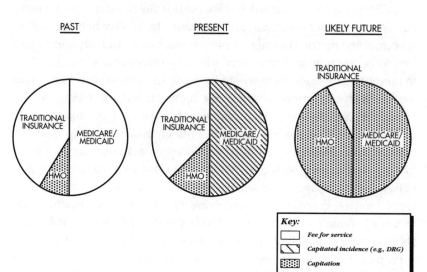

1. There is no such thing as the ideal therapist. The psychotherapy of the future will see a blurring of the distinctions among the various schools, with a melding of dynamic, behavioral, and systems approaches into techniques that will not be identifiable as Freudian, Jungian, Adlerian, behavioral, and so forth. There will be an array of therapeutic skills, some of which will be negatively correlated. Therefore, no one provider will be equally adept at all of these techniques, and the group practice will be the only viable response. Traditionally, psychotherapists who formed group practices joined several colleagues who practiced exactly the same way, obtained common office space, and shared a secretary and other expenses. This is not a group practice. Rather, it is several individual practitioners practicing under one roof, and will not meet the challenge of providing an array of skills among practitioners. It is difficult for mental-health providers, being fiercely individualistic, to give up the notion of independent solo practice. The most fiercely independent members of our society have been psychological professionals and gas-station owners. I would like to point out as a warning what happened to gas-station owners: they are all now working for the company store.

2. Mental-health-provider groups are going to have to learn to market themselves. To many of us, the term marketing borders on the unethi-

cal. It is almost as if the psychological practitioners went into our profession so as to eschew anything that smacked of business or entrepreneurship. Consequently, we are ill-prepared to face the competitive market that lies ahead and has already begun. Yet "marketing or morbidity" will become the practitioner's equivalent to the researcher's "publish or perish" (Cummings & Duhl, 1987). As part of your survival kit you must learn Social Entrepreneurship, or a melding of humanism and efficiency.

3. Abandon the concept of cure. This is part of the medical model that has no basis in psychotherapy. It is the one concept above all others that has held psychotherapy back from developing more effective and efficient parameters. Of all of the treatments in health, psychotherapy is the only one where the doctor and patient get only one chance. The goal has been to so analyze every possible unconscious conflict that the patient will never again experience anxiety. A physician who treats a patient for pneumonia does not feel the treatment was a failure should the patient return a year later with a broken leg. Yet in psychotherapy, should a terminated patient once again experience depression or anxiety, the statement is made that "something was missed," or the person was not "fully analyzed." This has led to psychotherapy becoming more and more protracted, for when can it be stated that every problem has been addressed, or self-actualization realized? Both a therapist and a client can always rationalize a few more sessions, or more often, a few more months of therapy. In fact, anxiety will be gone when the person is dead, because anxiety is a condition of living.

At Biodyne we have developed "brief, intermittent therapy throughout the life cycle." It is problem-oriented therapy, which is interrupted (not terminated) when the problem is solved. The client returns in the future when there is another problem of living that requires attention. And the psychotherapist functions similar to the old-fashioned family doctor, who treats on the psychological side not only the problems of the individual client, but those of the spouse and children. Another term for it is "the general practice of psychology" (Cummings & VandenBos, 1978).

4. Psychotherapy must be integrated into the entire field of health. With most health plans, and in the minds of most physicians, psychotherapy is a necessary nuisance. The consumer demands it, or it would not be a covered benefit. Nonmedical practitioners envy the psychiatrist, believing erroneously that psychiatry is an accepted part of medicine. It remains a fact that the majority of physicians do not

fully accept their psychiatric colleagues as truly physicians, and the remedicalization of psychiatry that is currently in vogue will not better the situation.

At Biodyne we have integrated the entire process into health psychology, addressing the 60 percent of all physician visits that do not deal with physical disease, but rather with somaticized stress. The discovery in the 1950s (Follette & Cummings, 1967) that psychotherapy directed at the high utilizer of medical resources can reduce medical utilization significantly (the so-called medical-offset phenomenon) has been summarized by the federal government along with over two dozen replications of the original research in a variety of settings. (Jones & Vischi, 1979). At Biodyne we outreach the 10 percent of the highest utilizers of medicine routinely from a periodic list provided by our client health plan. The savings to the client organization are something that the health plan and its physicians understand and appreciate, and result in the Biodyne Model being a totally integrated health resource. In addition to its core services of group and individual psychotherapy, Biodyne also provides what we term soft services: smoking-cessation programs, stress-management training, biofeedback, parenting programs, individual lifestyle and health appraisals, and a host of other protocols intended to direct the consumer to healthier lifestyles. Even the word Biodyne, coming from two Greek words, means "life change."

5. Targeted interventions are the essence of brief therapy. It is the embarrassing characteristic of mental-health practice that, with a few minor variations, all patients are treated alike and by whatever predominant therapeutic orientation is held by the practitioner, be it a substance-abuse problem, an occupational problem or a marital problem. Regardless of the presenting complaint, should one go to an orthodox Freudian, he or she will receive long-term psychoanalytic therapy. Should the practitioner be a Jungian, pictures will be painted. The behaviorist will provide desensitization. Our professions have traditionally lacked what are known as specifics: specific techniques targeted for specific conditions. The maturity of a health profession can be measured by the number of specifics at its disposal. Fifty years ago medicine had few specifics; now it has thousands. Without these specifics, it is a wonder that psychotherapy works at all. It does work, albeit very inefficiently. It often requires years of treatment. By targeting specific interventions designed to treat specific mental-health conditions, the length of psychotherapy is remarkably reduced.

At Biodyne, where in a quarter of a century we empirically researched over 60 targeted interventions, our average case requires about 6 sessions. Thus, at Biodyne, we can provide unlimited psychotherapy without restriction because 85 percent of our patients respond well to brief therapy, permitting us to provide longer-term therapy for those who need it and should receive it. Most health plans attempt to limit abuse by "benefit design": limiting sessions, requiring copayments or first-dollar amounts.

When psychotherapy is effective and efficient, artificial limiting structures, which deprive worthy patients of receiving all the treatment they need, are not necessary and are counterproductive. And, not to be overlooked, the client health plan enjoys a competitive edge by being able to market a mental-health benefit that is truly comprehensive and without limitations. The targeted interventions employed at Biodyne are not only effective, but aggressive in making most psychiatric hospitalization unnecessary. Since most patients can be treated effectively on an ambulatory basis, they and the family are spared the ultimate intrusion into their lives which psychiatric hospitalization represents. Our rate of hospitalization is under 3.5 days per enrollee per year, the lowest of any full mental-health benefit plan in the nation. This effective outpatient treatment efficiently saves millions in psychiatric hospitalization.

6. You will need training in effective brief therapy. Brief therapy is not a "dehydrated" version of long-term treatment. It has its own concepts, parameters, and techniques. Most brief therapy performed in the United States is done by the seat-of-the-pants. It is called eclectic, and the therapist is essentially doing whatever seems appropriate without a fully organized and well-trained approach. At Biodyne we extensively train our providers in brief therapy and our targeted interventions, and the training and monitoring never stop as it is a peculiar propensity of our mental-health practitioners to drift back to whatever they learned in their analytic training, graduate programs, or practical placements.

While other areas of health care are being brought under control, mental-health expenditures rose a whopping 40 percent last year. The glut of mental-health providers makes us vulnerable as the health-care industry tackles the job of curtailing mental-health costs. So far we have been left somewhat alone. The tendency in the health arena to ignore mental health in favor of addressing what are regarded as more essential problems has given us some breathing space. But the planners are about to descend upon us. There is much fat in the system, yet there are many who require mental-health services who do not have them available. As mental health becomes more rationed or more efficient (both approaches will proceed side by side), we shall need fewer providers. My prediction is that 50 percent of the practitioners flourishing today will not be needed and will be out of practice.

It is my hope that those who survive will be the ones who are innovative and resourceful enough to develop quality practitioner-owned delivery systems. The alternative is that the majority of practitioners who survive will be working for business-driven health corporations. If the latter occurs, I predict that the quality of mental-health delivery will decline and the American consumer will be the primary loser.

SUMMARY

There has never been a time when more health-care resources were available to the American people. There is a surplus of hospital beds as well as a glut of providers, yet the nation has embarked on a decade of health-care rationing in an attempt to contain skyrocketing costs. A period of chaos is predicted as we dismantle America's health-care system. There will be a period of severe transition during which quality of services will deteriorate markedly. Psychotherapeutic practice is particularly vulnerable to disruption for two reasons: third-party payors do not regard mental-health coverage as an essential, and the glut of provider-psychotherapists is greater than that of any other health profession. In spite of these facts, we continue to spawn new mental-health professions to add to the surplus. This paper deals with the necessary strategies for the survival of psychotherapy during the next ten to twenty years.

{ 14 }

Triaging the "Somaticizer" Out of the Medical System Into a Psychological System*

SUMMARY. *An effective system for triaging somaticizing patients out of the medical system and into a psychological system is proposed. The system is based on over 25 years of research performed in a Health Maintenance Organization setting. It is suggested that by involving "somaticizers" in a psychological system, therapeutic relief of pain, anxiety, and depression can be accomplished, as well as the realization of significant decreases in inappropriate medical utilization and reduction of psychiatric costs.*

THE USE OF the word or description of a condition as "psychosomatic" has earned the dubious distinction of taking its place in the psychological literature in a similar way to that of historical figures such as Lizzie Borden. However, in the last 20 years it has become increasingly apparent that psychosomatic conditions are not only real, but are, as a group, one of the major presenting problems seen in the psychotherapist's office. In an investigation at the Kaiser Health Plan in San Francisco, Follette and Cummings (1967) found that patients in emotional distress were significantly higher users of both inpatient

* With Jeffrey I. Bragman, Ph.D.

and outpatient medical services. In fact, as much as 60% of visits to physicians were made by patients with no diagnosable physical illness but who were experiencing somatic symptoms related to their emotional problems. We have now come to call these patients somaticizers.

In testimony before the United States Senate (Cummings, 1985), it was reported that these patients who are experiencing emotional stress generally find "an unsympathetic or uncomprehending ear" when they attempt to discuss their distress with their physician, and quickly begin to translate their problems into physical symptoms for which they receive a great deal of attention in the form of x-rays, laboratory tests, prescriptions, and return visits to the physician. The Follette and Cummings study (1967) indicated that there were significant declines in medical utilization in those emotionally distressed individuals who received psychotherapy. In fact, further research by Cummings and Follette (1976) demonstrated that one session of psychotherapy, with no additional visits, could reduce medical utilization by 60% over the following 5 years and that there was a 75% reduction in medical utilization over a 5-year period for those patients receiving two to eight psychotherapy sessions.

It was on the basis of the above research that American Biodyne, Inc., was founded in 1985. American Biodyne, Inc., is a for-profit, Psychological Health Maintenance Organization (PHMO). The focus of Biodyne is twofold: (1) to provide the highest quality, comprehensive mental health care available, and (2) to treat the somaticizing patients by triaging them out of the medical system and into the psychological system.

We would like to focus on the latter goal, that of the effective treatment of the somaticizing patient. At Biodyne, the first step in accomplishing this task is through an active outreach procedure aimed at these "somaticizing" patients. The outreach is integral to the entire operation of a center. As noted earlier, a major focus at Biodyne is to triage the somaticizing patient out of the medical system into a psychological system and eventually into physical and emotional well-being. Each center, as part of its contract with a third-party payer, receives a monthly print-out of the 10% highest utilizers of medical facilities and resources. Of these patients, more than half will be either somaticizers or persons suffering from physical illness whose treatment is enhanced by psychological intervention. The outreach system is directed toward getting that 5 to 6% of the patients into psychological treatment.

Because of their extensive knowledge of physical illness and their ability to be conversant with such conditions, coupled with their psychotherapeutic skills, psychiatric nurses are usually employed by Biodyne to conduct the telephone outreach. A medical social worker possessing similar knowledge and skills is an acceptable substitute for the psychiatric nurse. As a new center is being implemented, our procedure is to utilize, however, the initial free time of psychologists at least until the therapeutic load builds to the level as to preclude such time being available. Therefore, it is necessary for each therapist on staff to learn the outreach procedure.

The nurse, social worker or psychologist is responsible for calling a predetermined number of these high utilizer patients. From the outset, it is important that the patient's belief in the somatic nature of his or her complaints not be challenged, even to the slightest degree. The patient's interest can usually be aroused by the statement, "Someone who has had as much illness as you have had certainly must be upset about it." This statement usually elicits an immediate reaction, ranging from an exposition of symptoms to the complaint that physicians don't seem to understand or to be sympathetic to the patient's plight. After hearing the patient out sufficiently to permit the development of some initial trust, the patient is invited to come in to explore how Biodyne might be of help. The service is free and perhaps Biodyne can investigate the possibilities of alternatives to the treatments that have not worked, or perhaps the patient, once the difficulty is better appraised, may be put in touch with a more sympathetic physician. Then, an initial appointment for psychotherapy is made. If the psychologist is doing the outreach, there is the immediate advantage that an appointment can be made with that therapist.

The telephone outreach is but one method used in an attempt to bring the somaticizing patients into therapy. At Biodyne, there are periodic mailings of brochures or newsletters to remind these high medical utilizers of the services offered. In addition, the monthly newsletter features an article about a specific somatic complaint in each issue. The condition is discussed and suggestions for change are made, along with the suggestion that an appointment at Biodyne may be appropriate. Psychologists and outreach personnel are also encouraged to take part in community presentations and presentations to local industries in an attempt to further identify the high utilizers and encourage their participation in psychotherapy.

Once the patient comes to Biodyne, it is vital that the therapist continue meticulously not to challenge the somaticization. The therapist's interviewing skills are marshaled to detect the problem that is being somaticized. Once this problem or set of problems is determined, the therapist treats these without ever relating these to the physical symptoms. In fact, most patients conclude rather brief therapy with a relief of somatic symptoms without ever consciously relating psychological discoveries to the previous physical complaints.

It is important to note that the Biodyne Model of training somaticizers out of the medical system and into a psychological system was not developed as a cost-containment procedure. Rather, it was developed first to bring therapeutic effectiveness and relief of pain, anxiety, and depression to the patient in psychological distress. It became an integral part of a therapeutically effective, comprehensive mental health treatment system, and only then was it discovered that it was also cost-effective.

In cases of actual physical illness, the psychologist accepts the illness as a given. At that point, the therapist concentrates on the patient's reaction to the condition (depression, rage, despair), and also to any neurotic conflicts that may be impeding or slowing recovery. These issues are then addressed in the course of psychotherapy with the patient.

It's Hard to Do Psychoanalysis Face Down

Shortly after I was hired at Kaiser, I ordered a dozen psychoanalytic couches—custom-made in leather. We had our couches in place, and were ready to do our psychological treatment. One of my first patients was a man in his mid-30s who complained of low back pain. He had had two back surgeries, the physicians had done everything possible for him, and he had exhausted the roster of orthopedists in the Kaiser system. He was not getting better, and there was no physical reason for his back problem. The referring doctor thought it might have a strong psychological component.

The man came into my office, and I introduced myself and shook his hand. Then I asked him to lie down on the couch—my new psychoanalytic couch. So he did—face down!

I said, "No, you should be lying face up." And he asked, "But then how are you going to examine my back?"

I looked at him and said, "I want you to turn over and lie on your back." Like most blue-collar patients, he was very compliant, "Sure, Doc!" He turned over onto his back, remarking, "How are you going to examine my back if I'm lying on it?"

I said, "Very simple. I'm not going to examine your back. We're going to talk."

"Oh, OK." He sat up, grabbed a chair, put it opposite me, and sat on it. "Well," he asked, "what are we gonna talk about?"

He was a blue-collar worker, as were most of the Kaiser enrollees. The idea of doing psychoanalytic treatment made no sense to them—that is, lying on one of these couches. It also occurs to me that all human beings know that when you talk, you sit across from each other—everyone, that is, except psychoanalysts.

{ 15 }

MENTAL HOSPITALIZATION:
DANIEL ENTERS THE LION'S DEN*

THE KIESLER AND Sibulkin volume is a unique and intriguing research monograph analyzing national trends in mental hospitalization. The volume provides a comprehensive review of national mental health policy that serves as a model for those of us interested in policy analysis and policy research.

The authors examine various sources of national data in a low-key, empirical style that is an asset to the reader in synthesizing the implications of a set of complex data. The picture of national practice that emerges is altogether different from that which the public and the policy/professional community seem to believe. The reality of national trends toward increased hospitalization for mental disorder is a disturbing and largely unacknowledged consequence of national policy. As a result, we think that the volume also provides the empirical base from which to evolve a more effective, and cost-effective, national mental health policy.

The context for the volume is an implicit set of beliefs ("myths") about mental health and mental hospitalization held by both public

*A review with Michael S. Pallak, Ph.D., of the book of the same title by Charles A. Kiesler and Amy E. Sibulkin of Vanderbilt University, Nashville, Tenn.

and professional communities. Most of us probably believe that hospitalization for mental disorder has declined, that the length of stay during a hospital episode has shortened, that hospitalization is more effective for "serious disorders," and that the lion's share of mental health dollars nationally goes for outpatient psychotherapy. Whether one does or does not hold these beliefs personally is not the point. Such beliefs are held uncritically in policy circles, remain unexamined empirically, and thereby forestall effective national discussion of alternative approaches to mental health issues.

The authors examine trends in all institutional sites where mental hospitalization takes place: state hospitals, private psychiatric hospitals, Veterans'Administration (VA) hospitals, Community Mental Health Centers (CMHCs), Residential Treatment Centers (RTCs) for emotionally disturbed children, hospitals administered by the Indian Health Service (IHS), military hospitals, general hospitals with psychiatric units, and general hospitals without psychiatric units. In separate sections, the authors consider data regarding nursing homes, readmissions, and the homeless. In light of some of the "beliefs" noted above, we summarize major trends but refer the reader to the volume for greater detail.

The total number of inpatient episodes for mental hospitalization per year (1980) was just under 3 million nationally, excluding nursing homes—a figure much greater than the 1.8 million episodes widely accepted based on NIMH reports. The difference in estimates revolves around the fact that NIMH surveys have never included general hospitals without psychiatric units. Thus NIMH has included hospitalizations only in the specialty mental sector (i.e., state hospitals, psychiatric hospitals, general hospitals with psychiatric units, etc.).

Just under 500,000 episodes took place in state and county mental hospitals, down from 819,000 in 1955 (however, during the 1965-1975 period the number of admissions increased while the number of residents declined—a more complex picture). VA hospitals had 198,000 episodes, representing a modest decline from 214,000 in 1976. Private psychiatric hospitals increased from about 98,000 in 1971 to about 177,000 in 1981 (representing an increase in both residents and admissions). CMHCs in 1980 accounted for 254,000 episodes in contrast to 27,000 in 1967 (recall that CMHCs grew from 100 centers in 1967 to 700 in 1981). RTCs accounted for 34,000 episodes, up from 21,000 in 1969. About 4,000 episodes occurred in IHS hospitals and 34,000 took place in military hospitals.

As the authors point out, episodes of hospitalization have dropped but only in state and county hospitals and in VA hospitals. Note, however, that average length of stay in state hospitals still remains about 143 days (4.5 months). For psychotics in the VA system, length of stay was 160 days and 53 days for other diagnoses. In all other sites, episodes of mental hospitalization have increased.

The most striking data, however, concern hospitalization for mental disorder in general hospitals. About 60% of all mental hospitalizations in this country take place in general hospitals, only 20% of which have a psychiatric unit. Kiesler and Sibulkin estimate that 1.1 million episodes of mental hospitalization (out of the national total of 3 million) take place in general hospitals without psychiatric units—a sixfold increase from 184,000 episodes in 1965. In contrast, episodes of mental hospitalization in general hospitals with psychiatric units have remained stable from 1965-1980 at 520,000-578,000 per year. In other words, almost as many mental hospitalizations take place in general hospitals without psychiatric units as in state and county mental hospitals, VA hospitals, and general hospitals with psychiatic units combined.

The authors assess a number of explanations for the sharp increase. For example, the rate of hospitalization (i.e., the number of hospital episodes per 100,000 population—an important index because the absolute number of episodes may increase solely because of general population increases) was reported previously by NIMH as 800 per 100,000 and stable since 1955. In contrast, by including mental hospitalization data from general hospitals without units, the rate of hospital episodes jumps from 950 per 100,000 in 1965 to about 1,250 per 100,000 in 1981—a 32% increase nationally.

The length of stay per episode of mental hospitalization in general hospitals without psychiatric units is 8-9 days (about the national average for all general hospital health care episodes). Based on the authors' review of available data, the mental health treatment rendered is not trivial, does not consist of merely holding patients for transfer or discharge to another facility, is not accounted for by declines in episodes at state hospitals, or by the often hypothesized "revolving door" (i.e., a shift from long-stay residents to shorter stays and more frequent readmissions).

Consider two other points examined by the authors in rounding out the national picture: (a) Kiesler and Sibulkin derive conservative estimates of just under $13 billion in annual direct public expenditures for mental hospitalization (excluding nursing homes). In short, 70–75% of every public mental health care dollar is spent on mental hospitalization. (b) A review of the experimental research literature, that is, with random assignment of patient to traditional hospital treatment versus some form of alternative care (e.g., outpatient, nonhospitalization) demonstrates that mental hospitalization is no more effective, and often much less effective, than alternative outpatient care. Taken together, these data bring the reader to the conclusion that the effect of national policy has been to increase mental health hospitalization (and dollars spent on hospitalization), a form of treatment that is probably the least effective and least cost-effective national alternative for mental health care.

The authors note that de jure mental health policy (i.e., law, regulation, appropriations dealing with mental health such as CMHCs) emphasizes deinstitutionalization and outpatient, community-based, treatment. However, de facto national mental health practice is driven by an emphasis on mental hospitalization in order to receive treatment through the Medicare, Medicaid, and private health insurance systems. The insurance mentality reimburses for "medically necessary" treatment when rendered in an inpatient facility and erects major barriers to reimbursement for outpatient or nonhospital mental health treatment (e.g., large deductibles, substantial copayment requirements, and annual dollar expenditure limits).

Thus national reimbursement practice forces people to seek, or to acquiesce to, mental hospitalization in order to receive help or treatment. Keeping a family member in outpatient treatment, and at home, may involve substantial out-of-pocket expense under typical insurance coverage. However, if the family member is hospitalized, then out-of-pocket expense for mental health treatment is minimal and covered by insurance.

In essence, the typical insurance configuration embodied in Medicare, Medicaid, and private health insurance plans drives the system of national practice toward inpatient hospitalization for treatment—thereby setting the stage for unnecessary and expensive overutilization of mental hospitalization. Kiesler and Sibulkin estimate that Medicare pays $995 million for inpatient hospitalization and that Medicaid pays $4.09 billion for inpatient mental hospitalization in contrast to federal expenditures of $240 million (last available figures) for

CMHCs. About 25% of all days spent in hospitals for all diagnoses are for mental health treatment.

Without consistent national policy, mental health treatment has fallen, de facto, under the umbrella of traditional health insurance mechanisms geared toward hospitalization. The myth that reimbursement for outpatient treatment leads to frivolous use of the benefit dominates the insurance mentality in spite of the fact that only 2–4% of an insured population will use the benefit (even in a system with no barriers) and that 80% of treatment is completed in 6–10 outpatient visits.

The authors' analyses delineate the consequences of beliefs and national practice in terms of an increasing rate of mental hospitalization. Mental hospitalization may well be the least effective treatment since the vast array of those treated could be handled by alternative, non-hospitalized care. Ironically, arguments have raged for years about the effectiveness of psychotherapy, while implicitly accepting the practice of hospitalization for mental disorder.

At the time of this writing, recent Medicare legislation introduced in the House points toward greater support for outpatient treatment. The latter initiative suggests that the Kiesler and Sibulkin analyses have begun to have national impact—impact that we applaud. We note, however, along with the authors, that these policy issues and the critical examination of policy alternatives in mental health remain as yet largely ignored nationally.

The volume clearly fulfills the authors' intention of presenting "the most thorough and integrated analysis of data on hospitalization for mental disorders yet attempted."

{ 16 }

ARGUMENTS FOR THE FINANCIAL EFFICACY
OF PSYCHOLOGICAL SERVICES
IN HEALTH CARE SETTINGS

INTRODUCTION

By the beginning of the 1980s, it was generally conceded that psychologists had won their hard-fought struggle to be included in third-party payment for mental health services. The notable exception was in Medicare and Medicaid, where the inclusion of psychological services was, at best, sparse and spotty and indicated a job yet to be concluded. The history of this movement, which began in the late 1950s, was detailed by Cummings (1979) in an article that fell just short of signaling victory.

The effort to achieve parity with psychiatry in the recognition of psychology by the insurance industry and the government is a case history in the struggle for the autonomy of the psychological profession, most often bitter, sometimes comical, but always colorful. Professional psychologists had to overcome the resistance not only of the insurance industry, which was reluctant to add another class of practitioners, but also of their own American Psychological Association (APA), which was then academically dominated and was indifferent to the professional psychologists' struggle for survival. This phase of the struggle concluded with psychology's being recognized along with psychiatry as one of the dominant practitioner forces in the field of mental health. It also concluded with a thoroughly professionalized APA, which, in contrast to the prior era, now spends a very significant portion of its resources on professional issues.

Now all of this is rapidly changing. Those who would plead for the financial efficacy of psychological services in health care settings are once again on the defensive. This threat has been brought about by what has been termed the *health care revolution* (Kiesler & Morton, 1988; Kramon, 1989), which has created an array of new health and mental health delivery systems to which psychology must adapt in its effort to be included. In the original struggle for the inclusion of psychologists in third-party reimbursement in private practice, failure to be included would have spelled economic extinction. Again, in the present situation, failure to be included in the new delivery systems may result in the demise of professional psychology. The arguments for the financial efficacy of psychological services in health settings have never been more crucial.

The original arguments for the inclusion of psychology in third-party payment are delineated here, for they are as valid now as they were then. Second, the health care revolution, with its implied threat to professional psychology as it is now constituted, is described. Finally, how the arguments for the financial efficacy of the inclusion of psychologists in health care must be modified in the face of the health care revolution is addressed.

THE HISTORICAL PERSPECTIVE

Immediately following World War II, the Kaiser Permanente Health Plan on the West Coast began offering total health benefits to millions of enrollees without the usual limitations, copayments, first-dollar deductibles, and other such restrictions that were customary in all other health plans at that time. In that era, mental health and substance abuse benefits were totally excluded, as they were also at Kaiser Permanente. The research that led Kaiser Permanente to include mental health and substance abuse as covered services became the basis of over two dozen research replications and constituted the arguments for the inclusion of psychologists in health care. The 20-year experience at Kaiser Permanente, which demonstrated the financial efficacy of psychological services and the public policy implications in favor of the inclusion of psychologists, was summarized by Cummings and VandenBos (1981).

The Beginning of the Kaiser Permanente Mental Health Benefit

Kaiser Permanente soon found, to its dismay, that, once a health system makes it easy and free to see a physician, there occurs an alarming inundation of medical utilization by seemingly physically healthy persons. In private practice, the physician's fee has served as a partial deterrent to overutilization, until the recent growth of third-party payment for health care services. The financial base at Kaiser Permanente is one of capitation, and neither the physician nor the health plan derives an additional fee for seeing the patient. Rather than becoming wealthy from imagined physical ills, the system could have been bankrupted by what was regarded as abuse by the hypochondriac.

Early in its history, Kaiser Permanente added psychotherapy to its list of services, first on a courtesy reduced fee of five dollars per visit and eventually as a prepaid benefit. This addition was initially motivated not by a belief in the efficacy of psychotherapy, but by the urgent need to get the so-called hypochondriac out of the physician's office. From this initial perception of mental health as a dumping ground for bothersome patients, 25 years of research has led to the conclusion that no comprehensive prepaid health system can survive if it does not provide a psychotherapy benefit.

The Patient with "No Significant Abnormality"

Early investigations (Follette & Cummings, 1967) confirmed physicians' fears they were being inundated, for it was found that 60% of all visits were by patients who had nothing physically wrong with them. Add to this the medical visits by patients whose physical illnesses were stress-related (e.g., peptic ulcer, ulcerative colitis, and hypertension), and the total approached a staggering 80%–90% of all physician visits. Surprising as these findings were 30 years ago, nationally accepted estimates today of stress-related visits range from 50% to 80% (Shapiro, 1971). Interestingly, over 2,000 years ago, Galen pointed out that 60% of all persons visiting a doctor suffered from symptoms that were caused emotionally, rather than physically (Shapiro, 1971).

The experience at Kaiser Permanente subsequently demonstrated that it is not merely the removal of all access barriers to physicians that fosters somatization. The customary manner in which health care is delivered inadvertently promotes somatization (Cummings & Vanden-Bos, 1979). When a patient who has not been feeling up to par attempts to discuss a problem in living (e.g., job stress or marital difficulty) during the course of a consultation with a physician, that patient is usually either politely dismissed by an overworked physician or given a tranquilizer. This reaction unintentionally implies criticism of the patient, which, when repeated on subsequent visits, fosters the translation of this emotional problem into something toward which the physician will respond. For example, in a purely psychogenic pain patient, the complaint that "My boss is on my back" may become at some point a lower back pain, and neither the patient nor the physician may associate the symptom with the original complaint. Suddenly, the patient is "rewarded" with X rays, laboratory tests, return visits, referrals to specialists, and finally, even temporary disability, which removes the patient from the original job stress and tends to reinforce protraction and even permanence of the disability.

Estimates of stress-related physical illness are subjectively determined, whereas the number of physician visits by persons demonstrating no physical illness can be objectively verified through random samplings of all visits to the doctor. After more-or-less exhaustive examination, the physician arrives at a diagnosis of "no significant abnormality," noted by the simple entry of *NSA* in the patient's medical chart. Repeated tabulations of the NSA entries, along with such straightforward notations as "tension syndrome" and similar designations, consistently yielded the average figure of 60%. This figure is now generally recognized in the medical profession, which refers to these patients as *somaticizers*, and in behavioral health, which has named them the *worried well*.

During the early years of Kaiser Permanente, there was considerable resistance to accepting such estimates because it was reasoned that if 60%–90% of physician visits reflected emotional distress, 60%–90% of the doctors should be psychotherapists! This concern, as will be demonstrated below, was unfounded because subsequent research indicated that a relatively small number of psychotherapists can effectively treat these patients.

In an effort to help the physician recognize and cope with the distress-somatization cycle, Follette and Cummings (1967) developed a scale of 38 Criteria of Distress. These criteria do not use psychological jargon; rather, they are derived from typical physicians' entries in the medical charts of their patients. The researchers worked back from patients seen in psychotherapy to their medical charts, on which the diagnosis NSA had been made. They gathered extensive samplings of typical entries that connoted distress and validated these into the 38 criteria shown in Table 1. Physicians were urged to refer patients for psychotherapy who scored 3 points or more on this scale as attested by the physician's own medical chart entries.

After expending considerable effort and time validating this scale, it was discovered that emotional distress could be just as effectively predicted by weighing the patient's medical chart. The reason is that patients with chronic illness (or those involved in prenatal care) tend to see a physician at more-or-less scheduled appointments, whereas a patient suffering from emotional distress tends to use drop-in services, night visits, and the emergency room. In the instance of the chronically ill patient, the physician makes each entry in the chart immediately under the one bearing the date of the previous visit; thus, several visits are recorded on one sheet, front and back, in the medical chart. By comparison, when emotionally distressed persons make nonscheduled visits, the medical chart is not available, and the physician makes the entry on a new and separate sheet, which is later filed in the chart by medical records librarians. Repeating this practice through months and years builds up enormous medical charts, sometimes into the second and third volume.

Once the patient enters the somatization cycle, there is an ever-burgeoning symptomatology because the original stress problem still exists in spite of all the physician's good efforts to treat the physical complaints. The patient's investment in his or her own symptom is only temporarily threatened by the physician's eventual exasperation, often accompanied by that unfortunate phrase, "It's all in your head." A new physician within the care system is found, one whose sympathy and eagerness to determine the physical basis for the symptom have not been worn down by this particular patient. The inadvertent reward system continues, as does the growth of the medical chart. In a similar fashion, stress can impact on an existing physical illness, exacerbating its symptomatology and increasing its duration. The baffled and frustrated physician uses such terminology as "failure to respond" to account for the ineffectiveness of the treatment and often silently suspects noncompliance or malingering.

Table 1. *Criteria of Psychological Distress with Assigned Weights*

One Point	Two Points	Three Points
1. Tranquilizer or sedative requested.	23. Fear of cancer, brain tumor, venereal disease, heart disease, leukemia, diabetes, etc.	34. Unsubstantiated complaint there is something wrong with genitals.
2. Doctor's statement pt. is tense, chronically tired, was reassured, etc.	*24. Health Questionnaire: yes on 3 or more psych. questions.	35. Psychiatric referral made or requested.
3. Patient's statement as in no. 2.	25. Two or more accidents (bone fractures, etc.) within 1 yr. Pt. may be alcoholic.	36. Suicidal attempt, threat, or preoccupation.
4. Lump in throat.		37. Fear of homosexuals or of homosexuality.
*5. Health Questionnaire: yes on 1 or 2 psych. questions.	26. Alcoholism or its complications: delirium tremens, peripheral neuropathy, cirrhosis.	38. Non-organic delusions and/or hallucinations; paranoid ideation; psychotic thinking or psychotic behavior.
6. Alopecia areata.		
7. Vague, unsubstantiated pain.	27. Spouse is angry at doctor and demands different treatment for patient.	
8. Tranquilizer or sedative given.		
9. Vitamin B$_{12}$ shots (except for pernicious anemia).	28. Seen by hypnotist or seeks referral to hypnotist.	
10. Negative EEG.	29. Requests surgery which is refused.	
11. Migraine or psychogenic headache.	30. Vasectomy: requested or performed.	
12. More than 4 upper respiratory infections per year.	31. Hyperventilation syndrome.	
13. Menstrual or premenstrual tension; menopausal sx.	32. Repetitive movements noted by doctor: tics, grimaces, mannerisms, torticollis, hysterical seizures.	
14. Consults doctor about difficulty in child rearing.		
15. Chronic allergic state.	33. Weight-lifting and/or health faddism.	
16. Compulsive eating (or overeating).		
17. Chronic gastrointestinal upset; aereophagia.		
18. Chronic skin disease.		
19. Anal pruritus.		
20. Excessive scratching.		
21. Use of emergency room: 2 or more per year.		
22. Brings written list of symptoms or complaints to doctor.		

* Refers to the last 4 questions (relating to emotional distress) on a Modified Cornell Medical Index—a general medical questionnaire given to patients undergoing the Multiphasic Health Check in the years concerned (1959–62).

THE EFFECT OF PSYCHOTHERAPY ON MEDICAL UTILIZATION

In the first of a series of investigations into the relationship between psychological services and medical utilization in a prepaid health plan setting, Follette and Cummings (1967) compared the number and type of medical services sought before and after the intervention of psychotherapy for a large group of randomly selected patients. The outpatient and inpatient medical utilization by these patients for the year immediately before their initial interview in the Kaiser Permanente Department of Psychotherapy, as well as for the five years following that intervention, was studied for three groups of psychotherapy patients (one interview only, brief therapy with a mean of 6.2 interviews, and long-term therapy with a mean of 33.9 interviews) and a "control" group of matched patients who demonstrated similar criteria of distress but who were not, in the six years under study, seen in psychotherapy.

The findings indicated that (1) persons in emotional distress were significantly higher users of both inpatient facilities (hospitalization) and outpatient medical facilities than the health plan average; (2) there were significant declines in medical utilization by those emotionally distressed individuals who received psychotherapy, compared with that of the "control" group of matched patients; (3) these declines remained constant during the five years following the termination of psychotherapy; (4) the most significant declines occurred in the second year after the initial interview, and those patients receiving one session only or brief psychotherapy (two to eight sessions) did not require additional psychotherapy to maintain the lower level of medical utilization for five years; and (5) patients seen two years or more in continuous psychotherapy demonstrated no overall decline in total outpatient utilization (inasmuch as psychotherapy visits tended to supplant medical visits). However, even for this group of long-term therapy patients, there was a significant decline in inpatient utilization (hospitalization), from an initial rate several times that of the health plan average to a level comparable to that of the general adult health plan population. Thus, even long-term therapy is cost-effective in reducing medical utilization if it is applied only to those patients that need and should receive long-term therapy.

In a subsequent study, Cummings and Follette (1968) found that intensive efforts to increase the number of referrals to psychotherapy by computerizing psychological screening with early detection and alerting the attending physicians did not significantly increase the number of patients seeking psychotherapy. The authors concluded that, in a pre-paid health plan that already maximally uses educative techniques for both patients and physicians, and that provides a range of psychological services, the number of subscribers seeking psychotherapy at any given time reaches an optimal level and remains constant thereafter.

In another study, Cummings and Follette (1976) sought to answer, in an eighth-year telephone follow-up, whether the results described previously were a therapeutic effect, were the consequences of ex-traneous factors, or were a deleterious effect. It was hypothesized that, if better understanding of the problem had occurred in the psy-chotherapeutic sessions, the patient would recall the actual problem rather than the presenting symptom and would have lost the pre-senting symptom and coped more effectively with the real problem. The results suggest that the reduction in medical utilization was the consequence of resolving the emotional distress that was being re-flected in the symptoms and in the doctor's visits. The modal patient in this eighth-year follow-up may be described as follows: She or he denied ever having consulted a physician for the symptoms for which the referral was originally made. Rather, the actual problem discussed with the psychotherapist was recalled as the reason for the psy-chotherapy visit, and although the problem had been resolved, this resolution was attributed to the patient's own efforts, and no credit was given the psychotherapist. These results confirm that the re-duction in medical utilization reflected a diminution in the emotional distress that had been expressed in symptoms presented to the physi-cian.

Although they demonstrated in this study, as they did in their earlier work, that savings in medical services do offset the cost of providing psychotherapy, Cummings and Follette insisted that the services pro-vided must also be therapeutic in that they reduce the patient's emo-tional distress. Both the cost savings and the therapeutic effectiveness demonstrated in the Kaiser Permanente studies were attributed by the authors to the therapists' expectations that emotional distress could be alleviated by brief, active psychotherapy. Such therapy, as Malan (1976) pointed out, involves the analysis of transference and resistance and the uncovering of unconscious conflicts and has all the characteristics of long-term therapy, except length. Given this orientation, it was found over a five-year period that 84.6% of the patients seen in psychotherapy chose to come for 15 sessions or fewer (with a mean of 8.6). Rather than regarding these patients as "dropouts" from treatment, it was found on follow-up that they had achieved a satisfactory state of emotional well-being that had continued into the eighth year after the termination of therapy. Another 10.1% of the patients were in moderate-term therapy with a mean of 19.2 sessions, a figure that would probably be regarded as short-term in many traditional clinics. Finally, 5.3% of the patients were found to be "interminable," in that, once they had begun psychotherapy, they had continued, seemingly with no indication of termination.

In another study, Cummings (1977) addressed the problem of the "interminable" patient, for whom treatment is neither cost-effective nor therapeutically effective. The concept that some persons are so emotionally crippled that they may have to be maintained for many years or for life was not satisfactory, for if 5% of all patients entering psychotherapy are "interminable," within a few years a program will be hampered by a monolithic caseload, a possibility that has become a fact in many public clinics where psychotherapy is offered at nominal or no cost. It was originally hypothesized that these patients required more intensive intervention, and the frequency of psychotherapy visits was doubled for one experimental group, tripled for another experimental group, and held constant for the control group. Surprisingly, the cost–therapeutic-effectiveness ratios deteriorated in direct proportion to the increased intensity; that is, medical utilization increased, and the patients manifested greater emotional distress. It was only by reversing the process and seeing these patients at spaced intervals of once every two or three months that the desired cost–therapeutic-effect was obtained. These results are surprising in that they are contrary to traditionally held notions that more therapy is better, but they demonstrate the need for ongoing research, program evaluation, and innovation if psychotherapy is going to be made available to everyone as needed.

The Kaiser Permanente findings regarding the offsetting of medical-cost savings by providing psychological services have been replicated by others (Goldberg, Krantz, & Locke, 1970; Rosen & Wiens, 1979). In fact, such findings have been replicated in over 20 widely varied health care delivery systems (Jones & Vischi, 1978). Even in the most methodologically rigorous review of the literature on the relationship between the provision of psychotherapy and medical utilization (Mumford, Schlesinger, & Glass, 1978), the "best estimate" of cost savings is seen to range between 0% and 24%, with the cost savings increasing as the interventions are tailored to the effective treatment of stress.

The Effects of Behavioral Medicine on Medical Utilization

The foregoing addresses interventions with the patients who comprise 60% of all physician visits: somaticizers who have no physical disease but are replicating physical symptoms as a result of stress, and who are commonly referred to as the *worried well.* There is also the worried sick patient whose physical illness is a source of stress (secondary stress attendant on physical illness, e.g., fear of death following a myocardial infarct), or whose stress has contributed to succumbing to a physical illness or complicates a physical illness (e.g., tension-induced peptic ulcers or ulcerative colitis, failure-to-thrive syndrome). Finally, there is the asymptomatically sick patient who experiences no discomfort and for whom a medical evaluation is necessary to establish the existence of the disease (e.g., essential hypertension). Mechanic (1966) estimated that, if one looks at all three of the preceding categories, 95% of all medical–surgical patients could profit from psychotherapy or behavioral medicine interventions. Even with many supposedly biologically based physical health disorders, psychotherapy and behavioral medicine work and are cost-effective in that they reduce medical utilization (VandenBos & DeLeon, 1988; Yates, 1984).

Although physicians are becoming increasingly cognizant of the somaticizer, there still is resistance to referring to a mental health professional in cases of actual illness. This resistance prompted an editorial in *Newsweek* by a journalist with breast cancer (Kaufman, 1989):

> Curiously, while I was advised to see an internist, a surgeon, cosmetic surgeon, an oncologist and radiation therapist, at no point did anyone in the medical fraternity recommend that I see a mental health professional to help me cope with the emotional impact of breast cancer. Perhaps they didn't realize that breast cancer had an emotional impact. But I did. So, I went to see a psychologist, ironically the one specialist not covered by my insurance. It was worth the cash out of pocket. (p. 32)

Patients like this journalist report beneficial effects from counseling and behavioral medicine. That this benefit translates into a medical offset for the physically ill is demonstrated by a growing body of research, a few studies of which will serve as examples.

Schlesinger, Mumford, and Glass (1980) found that the greatest medical offset was obtained in the chronic diseases of diabetes, ischemic heart disease, airways diseases (e.g., emphysema), and hypertension. This finding was corroborated by Shellenberger, Turner, Green, and Cooney (1986), who reported a 70% reduction in physician visits in a chronically ill population following a 10-week biofeedback and stress management program. Fahrion, Norris, Green, and Schnar (1987) were able to alter dramatically, through behavioral medicine interventions, including biofeedback, a group of hypertensives' reliance on medication. A 33-month follow-up revealed that 51% had been well controlled off medication, an additional 41% had been partially controlled, and only 8% had been unsuccessful in lowering their blood pressure without medication. Assuming a five-year medication cost of $1,338, the authors demonstrated significant cost savings.

Olbrisch (1981) found a savings of 1.2 hospital days on average in surgical patients who received preoperative interventions. Similarly, Jacobs (1988), using biofeedback training before surgery, reduced hospital days by 72% and postoperative outpatient visits by 63%. Friedman, Ury, Klatsky, and Siegelaub (1974) found that they could predict through an automated screening the recovery rate following myocardial infarct and could influence that recovery rate through behavioral medicine interventions. This recovery period varied more than six months, which reflects high potential savings through behavioral medicine. Flor, Haag, Turk, and Koehler (1983) reported a significant reduction in physician visits and medication rates in rheumatological back pain patients after EMG biofeedback.

Impressive as the savings to the medical system can be through behavioral medicine, the potential savings in workers' compensation costs can even be greater. Steig and Williams (1983) calculated, for both treatment costs and disability payments, the estimated lifetime medical savings per patient as a result of a behavioral outpatient pain treatment program. Gonick, Farrow, Meier, Ostmand, and Frolick (1981) studied hospital costs five years pre- and posttreatment for 235 consecutive patients referred to behavioral medicine. The cost of providing the behavioral interventions, related to the savings in medical offset, yielded a cost–benefit ratio of $5 to $1.

Cummings and VandenBos (1981) described in detail the public policy implications that resulted in the eventual inclusion of psychologists as mental health providers in health care settings, as did DeLeon, VandenBos, and Cummings (1983). These conclusions indicated that any comprehensive health system that did not include a mental health or behavioral health benefit would pay for that lack of benefit in its medical–surgical benefit. Also, that cost would amount to far more than the cost of providing a psychological benefit. Insurers became convinced. Then came a whole new ballgame (Duhl & Cummings, 1987).

THE HEALTH CARE REVOLUTION

Actually, the health care revolution has been occurring since the early 1980s (Bevan, 1982), but it did not impact on the field of mental health until a few years ago because the initial cost containment efforts focused largely on reducing medical and surgical costs. An early alert was sounded by Cummings and Fernandez (1985) and three years later by Cummings (1986). By the time Duhl and Cummings (1987b) described it extensively and Kiesler and Morton (1988) sought to inform all of psychology, the mental health part of the health care revolution was well under way, with over 31 million Americans covered under *managed* mental health rather than traditional fee-for-service. The figure is growing at 25% a year, and it is predicted that, by 1995, at least half of all Americans will receive their mental health benefits under managed mental health care and that 50% of all present fee-for-service mental health practitioners will be out of business (Cummings, 1986; Cummings & Duhl, 1985, 1987). At the same time, psychiatry is undergoing what it terms *remedicalization*, a euphemism for the position that only the *medical* aspects of mental health should be covered, and is fiercely opposing the extension of hospital privileges to psychologists ("Supreme Court to Review," 1988). In the absence of such privileges, psychiatry would have no competitors, as it is the only mental health profession licensed to perform medical services. Because federally chartered health maintenance organizations (HMOs; to be described further below) are largely exempt from state statutes, they are under no duress to recognize and employ psychologists. Many are seduced into "going on the cheap" in mental health and employing less expensive providers, not only social workers who are qualified, but also mental health "counselors" with as little as one or two years of community college psychology training (Cummings & Duhl, 1987). This is a crisis for psychology of enormous proportions.

The fuel for the health care revolution came from spiraling health care costs, which were exceeding twice the rate of inflation for the rest of the economy, and the thrust came from the entry into the health care arena of the new heavy hitters: American corporations. Where, in the previous struggle, professional psychologists had to persuade the insurance industry and their own APA, now they are confronted by those who pay the bills and who have cried, "Enough!" The new drive for health care cost containment not only has produced such unlikely bedfellows as industry and labor but has been joined by farmers and consumers as well. In 1965, health care accounted for 6% of the gross national product (GNP). The projections made from the accelerating costs in 1979 predicted a doubling to 12% of the GNP. The beginning of 1989 saw it at just over 11% of the GNP, attesting to the success of cost containment efforts to slow it down. The exception has been the cost of mental health, which is running away.

Whereas the current inflation in the health care field is about 9% a year, in 1988 mental health care was increasing at almost twice that rate, at 16.5% per year (Mullen, 1988). Aside from the fact that the health care industry was not confronting mental health care costs because of the overriding priority of medical and surgical costs, how did this happen? The efforts to control health care costs caused mental health care to balloon like an aneurism in a blocked artery. Primary among these efforts was the introduction of diagnosis-related groups (DRGs) by Medicare and Medicaid. DRGs imposed on hospitals lengths of stay limited by the diagnosis for each patient (or category of patients, over 300 in all). This limitation resulted in thousands of empty hospital beds throughout the nation, threatening the financial stability of the American hospital system. Hospitals were quick to note that DRGs did not apply to psychiatry and substance abuse, and they began a rapid conversion of their excess beds to adult psychiatry, substance abuse, and the new phenomenon of adolescent psychiatric hospitalization. They embraced huckstering, and marketed these beds in slick television commercials that were guaranteed to frighten any spouse or parent into hospitalizing a husband, wife, or child. General hospitals, which never had psychiatric beds, soon had 50% of their beds converted to mental health and substance abuse. Something that was never predicted became commonplace. Psychiatrists were lured into lucrative hospital-based practices and began to fill these beds. In 1986, the last year for which statistics are now available, psychiatric hospital beds increased by 37%, and expenditures for psychiatric hospitalization increased by 44% in the United States (Mullen, 1988). Preliminary data for 1988 and 1989 suggest similar increases for each of those years (Mullen, 1989). There is now a saying in the psychiatric units of private hospitals: "A built bed is a billed bed."

Outpatient psychotherapy still accounts for a relatively small portion of the increase in mental health costs, and hospitalization is responsible for the runaway costs. Nonetheless, the health care industry is turning its attention to aggressively reducing the cost of mental health. Some insurers, regarding mental health services as unimportant, are severely reducing this benefit. Others are aggressively turning to managed mental health. This reaction has created an industry where none existed before, with companies such as American Biodyne, American PsychManagement, Metropolitan Clinics of Counseling (MCC), Preferred Healthcare, Plymouth, United Clinics of Counseling (UCC), and U.S. Behavioral Health, to name only a few, suddenly having an impact on the manner in which mental health care is dispensed.

NECESSARY MODIFICATIONS

Any health system that does not include a comprehensive mental health service will pay for stress-related conditions through the overutilization of its medical services. This fact was learned by the insurance industry in the 1980s, and resulted in the inclusion of mental health services (and the subsequent inclusion of psychologists as providers). Now there is an entirely new set of players that have to be persuaded: the giant health corporations that are rapidly gaining control of our health system and instituting managed care. The foregoing arguments are all still valid, but they will have to be reiterated.

There is an array of new delivery systems, sometimes called the alphabet soup of health care, which psychologists and other mental health practitioners must learn (Cummings & Duhl, 1987). These managed-care systems include the HMO (health maintenance organization, which is capitated and closed-panel), the PPO (the preferred-provider organization, the purpose of which is to compete with existing providers), the EPO (the exclusive provider organization, in which all health enrollees must seek the benefit services), and the IPA (the independent provider association, where capitated providers practice in their own office), to name only the dominant few. Psychologists will have to adapt to and be willing to assume the risk for mental health services, which means that, if a prospective reimbursement is not sufficient because of provider inefficiencies, the provider sustains the financial loss. Psychologists will need a great deal of training, as well as encouragement from the APA and the leadership of the profession. Unfortunately, most of our resources at the present time are expended in attempting to preserve the status quo and to stave off the rapid emergence of managed care.

Psychologists are in an excellent position to innovate delivery systems. Psychiatry has all but abandoned psychotherapy, and because the psychologist can not prescribe medication, our profession has developed an impressive number of targeted, brief interventions. These targeted interventions, focused on specific psychological conditions, can bring rapid relief from pain, anxiety, and depression that is a change of behavior, rather than the masking of behavior that is accomplished by most chemotherapies (Cummings, 1985a, 1988b). The managed health care industry must be made aware of our expertise in this regard.

We must abandon the concept of cure (Cummings & VandenBos, 1979). This concept has held back psychotherapy more than any other. First of all, we are dealing with psychological conditions, not an illness. Furthermore, behavioral health has shown that stress derives from the way we live: what we eat or do not eat; how we eschew exercise; how we smoke, drink, and pollute; and an array of other lifestyle variables. Psychologists have developed wellness programs and need to demonstrate their importance in any comprehensive health system. We are on the defensive here, because many in the health industry remember psychologists as those ethereal beings who were committed, for all their patients, to the nirvana of self-actualization and human potential, the so-called happiness variables that no one has ever been able to measure adequately in psychotherapy outcome studies. Psychology has innovated brief, intermittent therapy throughout the life cycle, which is focused, problem-solving therapy at stress points in a person's life (Cummings, 1986, 1988b; Cummings & VandenBos, 1979). The ultimate cure of anxiety is never the focus, as anxiety is a normal accompaniment of life. Rather, the person is encouraged to seek brief therapy at various stress points throughout the life cycle.

Because most increases in mental health expenditures in the past several years have resulted from unnecessary psychiatric hospitalization, psychology is in an excellent position to demonstrate that it has proven outpatient alternatives to the overhospitalization of emotionally disturbed adults and adolescents, as well as of substance abusers. The average for nonmanaged mental health plans currently exceeds 100 hospital days per year per 1,000 enrollees, and we have seen it approach 300. Contrast these numbers with those for a well-run HMO, which average between 40 and 50 hospital days per year per 1,000 enrollees. American Biodyne, a psychology-driven mental health maintenance organization (MHMO) using a wide array of aggressive psychotherapy protocols, has achieved what is regarded as the lowest psychiatric and substance abuse hospitalization in the nation. On its entering one market, the 178,000 enrollees averaged 114 days of hospitalization per year per 1,000 enrollees. Within 60 days, Biodyne reduced the yearly hospital days to 4 per 1,000 enrollees per year and demonstrated what can be accomplished with the appropriate application of current psychological services.

Psychology is now engaged in a national struggle to obtain hospital privileges for psychologists. It will one day succeed, but at that time, it would be a tragedy if psychologists were to succumb to the temptation of the temporary, lucrative, hospital-filling practices that have attracted many psychiatrists. Rather, psychologists need to continue to demonstrate that outpatient psychotherapy can reduce unnecessary psychiatric hospitalization. Care outside the mental hospital is likely to be the wave of the future because it is more effective and can be less expensive (Kiesler, 1982a, 1982b; Kiesler & Sibulkin, 1987).

Finally, psychologists are uniquely prepared to render program evaluation and outcome measures of the effectiveness of all of health care, not just mental health care. In an era of health care rationing, public policy concerns center on the adequate distribution of our health care resources, the elimination of waste and duplication, the quality assurance, and the strengthening of our limited resources through efficacy of treatment and efficiency of delivery (Reinhardt, 1987). The profession of psychology, with its scientific base, is integral to the design, delivery, and outcome evaluation of *all* health care (Cummings, 1987).

OUTREACH: PHYSICIAN COOPERATION AND CONSUMER EDUCATION

It has been demonstrated that physician referral is the most effective way to triage a patient into a behavioral health system (Friedman et al.,

1974). Patients respect their physicians and will generally accept such a referral. Unfortunately, in the case of the somaticizer, the exasperated physician often refers in a manner not conducive to compliance: "It's all in your head." Various methods have been used to help the physician identify and refer the somaticizer early in the cycle, by far the most frequent of which has been screening through computer-based test instruments (CBTI). Cummings (1985a) issued a note of caution. In a study of the practice patterns over a two-year period of 34 primary-care physicians who received regular CBTI printouts identifying somaticizing patients, it was found that the rate of missed diagnoses of actual physical illness increased dramatically. The physicians began to rely overly on the results of CBTI screening and did not look further into the symptomatology of patients identified as somaticizers, thus failing to heed the age-old adage, "Hypochondriacs can get sick, too."

The economics of practice influence whether a physician will refer a somaticizing patient. Capitated physicians readily refer such patients, as there is no economic incentive to hang on to them, whereas fee-for-service physicians regard the high utilizing patients as a source of revenue (Rand Corporation, 1987). It becomes useful, in such a setting, to access the somaticizer directly through outreach and consumer education.

One of the most successful triaging methods to directly address the overutilizer has been in operation for several years at American Biodyne and was reported on by Cummings and Bragman (1988). Founded in 1985, American Biodyne is a for-profit behavioral health maintenance organization (BHMO) that services the mental health and behavioral health needs of 2.1 million enrollees of several health insurers (e.g., Blue Cross and Blue Shield, CIGNA, Humana, and SelectCare) in eight states. Where its triage is in operation, Biodyne receives a monthly computer printout of the highest of 10% utilizers of medical facilities and resources as identified by frequency of service, not cost. The somaticizer is characterized by excessive visits to a physician, whereas high dollar amounts identify supercostly interventions such as open-heart surgery, organ transplants, and other medical heroics. Of these 10%, more than half are either somaticizers or persons suffering from physical illness whose treatment may be enhanced by behavioral health intervention. The outreach program is directed toward getting that 5%–6% of the patients into mental health or behavioral health treatment.

Because of their extensive knowledge of physical illness, and their ability to be conversant with patients about physical illness, coupled with their psychotherapeutic skills, psychiatric nurses are usually employed by Biodyne to conduct the telephone outreach. A medical so-cial worker having similar knowledge and skills is an acceptable sub-stitute for the psychiatric nurse. However, as a new center is being implemented, our procedure is to use the initial free time of psychol-ogists, at least until the therapeutic load builds to the level where their time is not available. Therefore, it is necessary for each therapist on the staff to learn the outreach procedure.

The nurse, the social worker, or the psychologist is responsible for calling a predetermined number of these high utilizers. From the out-set, it is important that the patient's belief in the somatic nature of his or her complaints not be challenged, even to the slightest degree. The patient's interest can usually be aroused by the statement, "Someone who has had as much illness as you have had certainly must be upset about it." This statement usually elicits an immediate reaction, ranging from an exposition of symptoms to the complaint that physicians don't seem to understand or to be sympathetic to the patient's plight. After the patient has been heard out sufficiently to permit the devel-opment of some initial trust, the patient is invited to come in to ex-plore how Biodyne can investigate the possibilities of an alternative to the treatments that have not worked, or perhaps, the patient, once the difficulty is better appraised, may be put in touch with a more sympa-thetic physician. Then, an initial appointment for psychotherapy is made. If the psychologist is doing the outreach, there is the immedi-ate advantage that an appointment can be made with that therapist.

The telephone outreach is only one method used in an attempt to bring somaticizing patients into therapy. At Biodyne, there are peri-odic mailings of brochures or newsletters to remind these high med-ical utilizers of the services offered. In addition, each issue of the monthly newsletter features an article about a specific somatic com-plaint. The condition is discussed, and suggestions for change are made, along with the suggestion that an appointment at Biodyne may be appropriate. Psychologists and outreach personnel are also en-couraged to take part in community presentations and presentations to local industries, in an attempt to further identify the high utilizers and to encourage their participation in psychotherapy.

Once the patient comes to Biodyne, it is vital that the therapist con-tinue meticulously not to challenge the somaticization. The therapist's interviewing skills are marshaled to detect the problem that is being somaticized. Once this problem or set of problems is determined, the therapist treats these without ever relating them to the physical symptoms. In fact, most patients conclude rather brief therapy with a relief of somatic symptoms without ever consciously relating psychological discoveries to the previous physical complaints.

It is important to note that the Biodyne model of triaging somaticizers out of the medical system and into a psychological system was not developed as a cost containment procedure. Rather, it was developed first to bring therapeutic effectiveness and relief of pain, anxiety, and depression to the patient in psychological distress. The model became an integral part of a therapeutically effective, comprehensive mental health treatment system, and only then was it discovered that it was also cost-effective.

In cases of actual physical illness, the psychologist accepts the illness as a given. At that point, the therapist concentrates on the patient's reaction to the condition (e.g., depression, rage, or despair), and also to any neurotic conflicts that may be impeding or slowing recovery. These issues are then addressed in the course of the psychotherapy or the behavioral health intervention with the patient.

Perhaps one of the most effective methods developed for triaging the worried well into a behavioral health system and the asymptomatic sick into the medical system has been automated multiphasic health screening, which includes psychological screening (Friedman et al., 1974). In the early 1980s, it was by far the approach of choice in most comprehensive prepaid health plans, and some had as many as 30 to 35 laboratory and other health checks by computer on-line and all within a two-hour period. Eventually, such elaborate automated systems proved too costly, and they have given way to smaller, less ambitious health-screening systems, most of which can be quite effective when there is an awareness of physicians' propensity to miss physical diagnoses (as noted above).

SUMMARY

Like all health care disciplines, clinical psychology is increasingly confronted with the need to prove not only its clinical effectiveness, but also its *cost*-effectiveness. Numerous powerful forces, whether in the form of DRGs or HMOs or some new form that has yet to appear on the health care scene, will continue to require accountability and justification for the expenditure of health care dollars. In part because of the scientific motivation of clinical psychologists to study what they do, data relevant to the clinical *and* the financial efficacy of services in health care settings are available to address these issues. The evidence thus far suggests that psychological services can reduce the inappropriate utilization of expensive medical care among the "worried well" and can improve medical management and behavioral outcomes among the chronically ill.

The Mobilization of Rage in the Service of Health

We did a follow-up on the 1967 and 1968 papers, and found that, indeed, the patients had altered the behavior that had brought them into the original session. And this was, in some cases, a single session. Generalization had occurred, and even after eight years, they no longer had the problem. They were amnesic about the physiological problem that had brought them to psychotherapy, but they remembered the psychological issue. Many did not remember, for example, that they had had a lower back problem, but they remembered the stress. "I never had a back problem. But I remember that the boss had been giving me a hard time for six months," they would say.

As they remembered it, the physician didn't help them, but neither did the psychotherapist. They denied that they had ever had a headache or a back problem.

Remember what we were discovering here: It is the mobilization of rage in the service of health. They got mad and told the doctor that he or she was wrong. "The doctor says I have these headaches because I don't know how to handle my boss. That is nonsense! I walked in and I told my boss off!" All of a sudden, the headaches were gone. So the patient asks, "What headaches?"

"And the fact that I told the boss off proves that the psychologist didn't know what he was talking about."

L. T.: What did they think the psychologist was talking about?

N. C.: The psychologist was insulting them by questioning their symptoms.

L. T.: But this isn't very good public relations for psychologists.

J. C.: Well, it is, because they will report these positive results in an outcome study. Plus, they will send us all their friends. It works, but in an indirect way.

N. C.: As it says in the article, they'll refer all their friends.

J. C.: I found that this would happen at Biodyne, too. Thus, a really key question in outcomes research is not, "Did you like the doctor?" but, "Would you go back to the doctor?" Another key question would be, "If you had a friend who was having difficulties, would you send the friend to that doctor?" It is likely that the answer would be "Yes."

N. C.: This is the point. When we build our system of integrating psychotherapy into medical care, we need to look at the outcomes that really count. Remember, these are people who attend only one or two sessions. Patients in long-term therapy remember their doctors.

J. C.: These people forget about the psychotherapist because there is not enough time to establish a relationship. After one or two sessions, they go out and get well.

N. C.: But remember, not all of our patients had only one session. That's why when Moshe Talmon came out with a book on one-session therapy and quoted my work as proof of its effectiveness, I thought it was not a correct characterization. Those who had only one or two sessions decided to quit on their own initiative. We used to call these patients therapeutic failures—until we did the follow-up study. They were not failures at all!

L. T.: Of course, this has been replicated, hasn't it? After a single session, and being considered "dropouts," these people would report that they got a lot out of therapy.

N. C.: Yes. Budman and Gurman (1988) also found that. In fact, Budman and Gurman, without ever talking to me, stumbled onto this phenomenon, and we both, simultaneously, dropped the term "therapeutic failure" with regard to those who had had only one session.

L. T.: But Budman knew you before the two of you wrote your articles.

N. C.: Of course, he knew me. I helped him set up the Harvard Community Health Plan. We go way back, historically.

I worked with Budman around 1975 or 1976. Historically, Congress, under Nixon, passed the HMO Act, which encouraged the formation of HMOs. Funding was provided for the first three years. Edgar Kaiser, son of Henry Kaiser, decided we were going to give the technology away. We were each assigned to advise and help build three HMOs. Seven out of eight start-up HMOs founded under the Nixon plan went bankrupt when the federal start-up money was exhausted. I was given the Harvard Community Health Plan and the Group Health Cooperative of Puget Sound. Both are raging successes even today. That was where I got to know Simon Budman, George Vaillant, Michael Bennett, and Michael Quirk, among others.

{ 17 }

INPATIENT VERSUS OUTPATIENT TREATMENT OF SUBSTANCE ABUSE: RECENT DEVELOPMENTS IN THE CONTROVERSY

ABSTRACT: *There has been considerable controversy the past decade on which is more effective, inpatient or outpatient treatment of substance abuse. During this same decade substance abuse treatment grew into a $40 billion industry with for-profit hospital programs accounting for as much as one-half the total figure. Recently, controlled studies have replaced the previous research literature which was largely composed of uncontrolled studies. A research consensus is developing that states inpatient rehabilitation has no advantages over outpatient treatment and that even hospitalization for detoxification is unnecessary for 90% of patients. Implications for public policy are that we are over-spending in the treatment of substance abuse by misallocating resources to the most intrusive intervention.*

So MUCH CONTROVERSY has raged the past few years on the efficacy of inpatient versus outpatient treatment of substance abuse that three facts are often overlooked. First, inclusion of substance abuse treatment as a covered benefit in health insurance is a relatively recent phenomenon, primarily of the last 20 years. Second, the large-scale hospitalization of addicted persons is a very recent phenomenon, essentially of the past decade and in current numbers only in the past five years. Third, inpatient and outpatient treatment is not a difference of treatment modalities, but a difference in settings. In view of these considerations, it may be worthwhile to review the developments in substance abuse treatment over the past quarter of a century.

HISTORICAL PERSPECTIVE

Thirty years ago no major health plan in the United States reimbursed for the treatment of substance abuse. The medical consequences of alcoholism, such as cirrhosis of the liver, were covered, but the treatment of alcoholism itself was not. Even medical detoxification coverage was essentially absent. The wealthy went to plush private sanitoria where they paid out-of-pocket and their alcoholism was disguised by a medical diagnosis, such as pneumonia, while they were "dried-out." Poor alcoholics detoxified each other by use of what was termed a "hummer": The alcoholic detoxing the other alcoholic would ration small amounts of alcohol sufficient to prevent delirium tremens or other sequelae of withdrawal. In between was the middle class who could afford out-of-pocket expenses sufficient to dry-out in small motel or guest house settings operated by recovering alcoholics with little or no medical supervision. The technique was primarily that of the "hummer," with a strong helping of Alcoholics Anonymous philosophy thrown in during the few days the alcoholic was drying out.

The most conspicuous addicts were the chronic public inebriates who for the most part were remanded to the criminal justice system. A few of the more progressive states had provisions in their welfare and institutions codes for the involuntary commitment of chronic inebriates to the state hospitals in programs apart from those provided for the mentally ill. Most of these programs were on locked wards intended to enforce several weeks of abstinence. Treatment was mostly aversive conditioning: The patient was served cocktails in rapid succession in a simulated barroom setting, and after having been given Antabuse. Following what would be 48 hours of excessive vomiting and other unpleasant physical symptoms, the patient was given Antabuse and again ushered into the simulated barroom for drinks. This was repeated a prescribed number of times under the hypothesis that an aversive reaction to the consumption of alcohol would be created. Not surprisingly, the technique did not work and did not survive the state hospital era.

A unique program for heroin addicts was operated by the federal government at Lexington (KY) Barracks. With the guarantee of anonymity, the addict could enter the program for several weeks and under an assumed name while withdrawing from heroin. These heroin addicts seldom entered Lexington Barracks with the intent of going straight. Rather, they wanted to reduce the required daily quantity of heroin to which they had built up so as to make their addiction more affordable. This, of course, was impossible. Shortly after leaving the facility, the addict rapidly returned to the level of drug tolerance previously achieved. This pioneering program was regarded as a success by no one, and after several decades it was closed when the federal government began licensing experimental methadone programs.

In the 1960s health plans began to include mental health and chemical dependency treatment (MH/CD) benefits, and by the 1970s most plans were characterized by including such benefits. However, most hospitalization was for medical detoxification, not for rehabilitation, something that was to change drastically in the decade of the 1980s. For most of the health plans, it was simple to adopt the 30-day hospital benefit that had become standard in medicine and surgery, and reject recommendations for 60- and 90-day benefits. Some fewer health plans, however, did adopt 60- and 90-day benefits with others compromising at 45 days.

As a result of these insurance benefits the decade of the 1980s saw the emergence of a new industry: chains of private chemical dependency hospitals with formulated 28-day inpatient programs that dovetailed with the general indemnity benefit. There were also 45-, 60- and 90-day programs for those holding health policies with more liberal benefits, but the 28-day program which included both detoxification and rehabilitation in a hospital setting became standard.

In the beginning there was little concern on the part of the insurance industry because relatively few persons filed for this inpatient benefit. The emergence of employee assistance programs (EAPs) did much to accelerate the use of the CD hospital benefit as EAP counselors made certain the employee took full advantage of benefits available. In some industries, such as the auto workers, inpatient rehabilitation became the preferred mode, with health economists taking note of the "revolving door" nature of these programs as early as the 1970s (Gallant, Bishop, Mouledoux, Faulkner, Brisolara, & Swanson, 1973).

The giant leap in the use of inpatient CD rehabilitation programs occurred following the enactment by the United States Congress in 1985 of Diagnosis Related Groups (DRGs) in Medicare and Medicaid. Reimbursement to hospitals was no longer on a cost plus 15% basis, but on a schedule of a set number of days for each of over 300 DRGs. Seemingly overnight the occupancy rate of medical and surgical beds dropped drastically. Hospitals were in financial trouble until it was noticed that DRGs did not apply to MH/CD. By 1986 most hospitals converted empty beds to CD units and entered into aggressive multimedia advertising to market these newly proliferated programs. They were inordinately successful as the treatment of CD conditions in the United States increased in cost an average of over 40% for each of the succeeding four years. The treatment of substance abuse in the United States is an industry that now exceeds 40 billion dollars per year.

TREATMENT MODALITIES

As indicated above, the inpatient versus outpatient controversy is one of difference in settings, not treatment modalities. Treatment modalities cluster around four philosophies: medical, psychoanalytic, behavior modification, and 12-step. Any of these may be found in hospitals and outpatient programs.

Medical

The medical model of treating addiction potentially addicts a person to a stronger drug to get off the drug to which the person was previously addicted (Cummings, 1979). Just as in the 1910s heroin was introduced as a "cure" for morphine addiction, methadone is used to get addicts off heroin, Valium is used to get alcoholics off alcohol, and amphetamines are used to control calorie "addiction." This model sees addiction as a physical craving that must be interrupted by chemical means. Most psychiatrists, as well as physician addictionologists, and especially those who have hospital-based practices, subscribe to this model.

Psychoanalytic

The psychoanalytic model, which essentially strives to elicit insight into the underlying conflicts that lead to addiction, is out of favor in CD treatment circles. Until the recent era, however, it was the usual approach to treating addiction by independently practicing psychotherapists. It sees addiction as a set of unconscious emotional conflicts rooted in development that predispose the individual toward addictive behavior. As a unique application of insight therapy, Peele (1978) sees all addictions as "love addiction," with the understanding of the fear of commitment as the cornerstone to conquering one's addiction.

Behavioral Modification

This is the traditional psychological model. Based on behaviorism, and more recently cognitive behaviorism, it holds that addictive behavior can be controlled and that an addict can be restored to being a social user. The latter aspect became discredited with the allegedly fraudulent research of Mark and Linda Sobbell, but most psychologists are still trained in the behavioral model of treatment addiction. It holds that addiction is a constellation of learned behaviors that can be modified and is the direct opposite of the disease model (Cummings, 1979).

Twelve-Step Programs

In the 1930s Bill Wilson founded Alcoholics Anonymous with its disease model of addiction which holds that abstinence is the only response to addiction and that there are 12 steps to recovery. Originally AA was a self-help movement, but as more and more recovering alcoholics became alcoholism counselors, the 12-step philosophy has become the dominant modality in drug rehabilitation programs. Within the last two decades the AA philosophy has been expanded to include Narcotics Anonymous (NA), Cocaine-Abusers Anonymous (CA), Gamblers Anonymous (GA) and Overeaters Anonymous (OA). Even more recently the 12-step modality has been stretched to include conditions upon which there is disagreement as to whether they are really addictions (e.g., sex and love addictions, compulsive spending, and compulsive shoplifting).

There are other minor modalities, most of which are mixtures of these four main philosophies that dominate or have dominated the CD treatment sector. Within these, there are also two divergent points of view as to whether one needs to be a recovering addict to be effective, or whether being a recovering addict reduces effectiveness as a therapist or counselor. In delineating the 12th step as maintaining abstinence by helping others achieve abstinence, the founder of AA saw this as a volunteer endeavor, and he worried that the trend for recovering alcoholics to become *paid* counselors had the potential of corrupting the 12-step philosophy (B. Wilson, personal communication, May 1978).

THE OTA REPORT

In 1983 the Congressional Office of Technology Assessment (Saxe, Dougherty, Esty, & Fine, 1983) released a report on the effectiveness of outpatient versus inpatient treatment of alcoholism and unleashed a storm of controversy. This review of the extant research revealed that although high-cost treatments such as hospitalization were probably justified by cost-benefit analysis, there was a substantial body of evidence that indicated less costly outpatient care was equally effective. Several years earlier Cummings (1979) published the results of a seven-year Kaiser Permanente study which showed that 95% of addicts could be effectively treated outside an inpatient setting. These findings generated not a ripple of protest inasmuch as the for-profit sector of substance abuse treatment was still in its infancy and had not yet become a part of the giant mental health complex (Duhl & Cummings, 1987a), which was to be the case just a few years later.

The OTA report admitted that most of the studies upon which the conclusions were based were uncontrolled and that the conclusions could be regarded as only tentative. It argued, however, that there was sufficient evidence, even if not adequately controlled, to at least call into question the ultimate cost-effectiveness of inpatient care. Three years later Miller and Hester (1986) reviewed both the original uncontrolled studies and the more recent controlled studies and announced some startling conclusions. Whereas a host of confounding factors in the uncontrolled studies render their data inconclusive, the 26 controlled studies consistently reported no statistically significant differences between treatment settings or differences in intensity of treatment. They point out that these findings are consistent with the overall literature on inpatient psychiatric care (Kiesler, 1982b).

Five years after its initial report the OTA updated its findings (Saxe & Goodman, 1988), this time focusing on the controlled studies that had emerged. They reaffirmed their initial finding that both inpatient and outpatient treatment have demonstrable effectiveness, but that there is no evidence to suggest that inpatient treatment is better than outpatient treatment. They addressed public policy issues and flatly stated, " . . . the data strongly suggest that to the extent we have developed a system of providing care for alcoholism that rests on inpatient treatment, we are greatly overspending. Such overexpenditures have the result of inflating the necessary costs of alcoholism treatment and, perhaps, denying treatment to those who are unwilling or cannot afford inpatient programs" (pg. 3).

It may be worthwhile to consider in some detail the complexity of the question, and to review a number of these controlled studies.

Controlled Studies

Some of the problems inherent in studying the efficacy of inpatient versus outpatient treatment include the following. Length of hospital stay can be influenced by motivational variables, severity of the problem, coercion, and appropriateness of client-treatment match (Miller, 1985; Miller & Hester, 1987a, 1987b); clients judged as unmotivated may be terminated early by the staff (Holser, 1979) or even not referred for lengthy care (Sheehan, Wieman, & Bechtel, 1981). Studies controlling for confounding variables necessarily employ random assignment to control and experimental groups, such as those that follow.

In one of the most cited studies in substance abuse (Edwards, Orford, Egert, Guthrie, Hawker, Hensman, Mitcheson, Oppenheimer, & Taylor, 1977), 50 alcoholics seen in inpatient and outpatient care, and 50 alcoholics randomly assigned to receive only an evaluation and a single counseling session were followed-up one year and two years after treatment. No significant differences were found between groups on any measure of improvement. In another study (McCrady, Longabaugh, et al., 1986; McCrady, Noel, et al., 1986), no significant difference in improvement was found between patients randomly assigned to either inpatient or day care. Chapman and Huygens (1988) compared inpatient, outpatient and single confrontation interview situations and found no difference in outcome. The confrontation was in the presence of the patient's spouse, family member or close friend. As reported by the OTA (Saxe & Goodman, 1988), Newton and Bowman randomly assigned alcoholics following detoxification to aftercare alone, or 25 days' inpatient treatment plus aftercare. No significant differences were found at 2-, 4-, 7-, 10-, or 13-month follow-ups. In a similar study (Mosher, Davis, Mulligan, & Iber, 1975), 200 alcoholics were randomly assigned to receive or not receive 30 days of detoxification and inpatient treatment. No significant differences were found in abstinence, work status, drug use or anxiety on 3- and 6-month follow-ups.

The dangers of detoxification are often cited to justify hospitalization. Indeed, delirium tremens can be a severe form of alcohol withdrawal and withdrawal from several drugs can result in convulsions (e.g., alcohol, barbiturates, benzodiazpines). A number of controlled studies indicate that only a small number of addicts need to detoxify in the hospital (Feldman, Pattison, Sobell, Graham, & Sobell, 1975; O'Briant, Peterson, & Heacock, 1977; Hayashida, Alterman, McClellan, O'Brien, Purtill, Volpicelli, Raphaelson, & Hall, 1989). Annis (1987), in reviewing the literature, concludes that 90% of addicts can not only be detoxified outside of the hospital, they need no medication to do so. Annis further concludes that hospitalization should be reserved for those relatively few patients who need management of *medical* sequelae.

Neither length of hospital stay nor duration of outpatient treatment correlates with successful outcome. A number of studies (Mosher et al., 1975; Pittman & Tate, 1972; Page & Schaub, 1979; Walker, Donovan, Kivlahan, & O'Leary, 1983; Willems, Letemendia, & Arroyave, 1973) comparing hospital stays of from one to seven weeks found no advantages in longer over shorter stays. Similarly, length of outpatient care does not increase improvement (Robson, Paulus, & Clarke, 1965; Smart & Gray, 1978; Powell, Penick, Read, & Ludwig, 1985). Even more startling are studies that indicate 6 to 18 weeks of outpatient therapy was no more effective than self-help with minimal therapist contact (Miller, Gribskov, & Mortell, 1981; Miller & Baca, 1983; Buck & Miller, 1986).

Matching addicts to treatment on the basis of clinical dimensions has been the focus of several studies, and these yield the only demonstrable positive results for the variable of intensity. In general, more severe and less socially stable alcoholics do better in outpatient care, and even less intensive outpatient treatment (Annis, 1987; Kissin, Platz, & Su, 1970; McLachlan & Stein, 1982; McLellan, Luborsky, Woody, O'Brien, & Druley, 1983; Orford, Oppenheimer, & Edwards, 1976; Smart, 1978; Stinson, Smith, Amidjaya, & Kaplan, 1979; Willems,

et al., 1973). But as Miller and Hester (1987b) point out, when het-
erogeneous populations of alcoholics are averaged together, no significant advantage of inpatient over outpatient treatment emerges. They
conclude that brief hospitalization may be warranted for severe phar-
macologic dependence, suicidality, or homelessness, but for most patients outpatient treatment is as effective as inpatient.

Miller and Hester (1987a) reviewed five controlled studies evaluating partial hospitalization (day care or halfway house) and found no
advantage for inpatient versus partial residential treatment. They also
found only one study (Stinson, Smith, Amidjaya, & Kaplan, 1979) that
compared inpatient settings with a high density of staff to low density
of staff, with the surprising finding that the latter had a statistically significant advantage in measures of abstinence over the former. It was as
if the greater self-direction induced by the lower staff density carried
into the patient's life after release from the hospital.

Community Pressures

There is now a plethora of evidence indicating that inpatient care is
no more effective for most patients than outpatient treatment, and
when one compares the difference in cost, the advantage is decidedly
on the side of outpatient care. Yet the community continues to clamor
for inpatient care for a number of reasons. First, the addict is looking
for a magical "fix" of the problem in a setting where responsibility, self-
initiative, and pain will be minimized. The family also wants a vacation
from the addict who by the time of presentation for treatment has
been the source of familial disruption or chaos for weeks, months or
years. Similarly, the employer, who has felt the economic pinch of the
high cost of healthcare as well as the loss of productivity from addicted employees and those fellow employees they disrupt, wants the
addict out of the workplace until recovered. For all these, the inpatient setting is the obvious solution, for while the patient is away for
28 days all concerned can cherish the illusion that something is being
done to forever fix the problem.

Health plans, and especially managed health care plans that are sensitive to costs and are convinced that inpatient treatment is not better,
have begun restricting the unwarranted use of inpatient care (Cummings, 1986). Hospitals and psychiatrists with hospital-based practices, both of whom have a vested interest in filling the newly created
for-profit inpatient beds, find it relatively easy to incite patients, family,

and employers to protest that denial of inpatient admission is denial of benefits. The noise in the system intensifies as complaints mount. In response to this community pressure, there emerged in the 1990s two types of programs whose efficacy has yet to be tested, but whose immediate effect is to significantly lower the number of complaints from addicts, their families and their employers when the system deems that hospitalization is not warranted.

The first of these is the Intensive Outpatient Program (IOP) that in its ideal would combine the best of outpatient treatment with the intensity of partial residential care. The IOP is several hours of outpatient treatment daily for a specified number of weeks, or a number of weeks specifically tailored for each individual case. Patients are required to meet criteria of attendance, abstinence, and family involvement. A number of programs have suddenly emerged, seemingly overnight, in response to the perceived need. This author has investigated a number of these and would advise caution. Some are excellent programs and hold promise for increasing the continuity of care. Others are hastily organized by hospitals that have seen the impending reduction of hospitalization and want to enter a new, possibly lucrative outpatient market as inpatient revenues drop.

The second is what has been termed either an "Abstinence Training Group" or "Pre-addictive Group." In either case, they are psychoeducatinal programs that meet daily, with each series being five meetings. Their intent is to reduce the denial, coercion, or antagonism with which addicts present themselves. Devised by the author and his colleagues, they have been in effect in several Biodyne centers for more than a year. As shown in Table 1, preliminary results indicate a 50% increase in the number of addicts both entering a 20-week outpatient

Table 1. *Summary of the numbers of drug and alcohol patients presenting for treatment, actually entering treatment into a 5-month outpatient program, and completing that program, respectively, for the six months prior to the implementation of a 5-session psychoeducational program (before) and the six months following the implementation of that program (after).*

		Presenting for Tx	Entering Tx	Completing Tx
Before	N	232	59	29
	%		25.4	12.5
After	N	246	125	68
	%		50.9	27.6

addictive treatment program, and completing it. Further, it has subjectively greatly reduced the noise in the system.

CONCLUSIONS AND PUBLIC POLICY IMPLICATIONS

The research evidence indicating that inpatient treatment is not significantly more effective than outpatient treatment has increased to where the conclusion is inescapable. We are drastically over-spending to treat addiction because of a misallocation of resources. It is yet to be fully delineated which patients should be hospitalized for detoxification, but it is apparent that the percentage is much smaller than previously believed. The determination to hospitalize should largely be on the basis of medical, not psychological need. These findings as they are implemented are going to be painful for the relatively new for-profit multibillion dollar inpatient addictive treatment industry. Once society is aware of the facts, the re-allocation of resources will occur quickly. Those who doubt that addictive program hospital beds will be emptied need only to look at how rapidly society emptied the medical and surgical beds in the United States following the implementation of DRGs.

If only the public policy issue in substance abuse treatment were as simple as deciding between inpatient and outpatient settings! Those of us who work with addicts are aware that all of our programs are minimally effective. The finding that inpatient treatment does not increase this minimal effectiveness cannot rest there—we must increase the effectiveness of our outpatient programs, broaden the continuum of care, learn better to mobilize social support systems, and, above all, develop better clinical tools that will enable us to cut through the addict's denial that renders all help impotent until the addict is ready to give up that denial. Freed from a misallocation of resources, we should be prepared to expend more money and effort toward those techniques and modalities that would increase the patient's motivation to abstinence, rather than galvanize the patient's illusion that he or she can be a "successful addict," or as Peele (1978) has stated it, a "comfortable loser."

{ 18 }

FUTURE PRACTICE PATTERNS: INDEPENDENT PRACTICE AND MANAGED MENTAL HEALTH CARE*

MANAGED MENTAL HEALTH care is here to stay. This is the reality bitterly accepted by many of professional psychology's leadership which just two years ago was predicting the early demise of managed mental health care. There is hardly an independent practitioner who has not been impacted by the spectacular growth of managed care (Fox, 1992). Some have seen their practices "ravaged" or "devastated," to use two of Welch's (1992) favorite words in describing the effect. It is unfortunate that we missed the opportunity, but a few short years ago psychology could have owned managed care. This is because the American Psychiatric Association (ApA) took an early and vigorous opposition to it, and had our American Psychological Association (APA) heeded the warnings (Cummings & Fernandez, 1985; Cummings, 1986), psychology could have played a paramount role in the shaping of the future. Where psychiatry dug in its heels, psychology went into denial. Now psychiatry is accommodating managed care and is having a disproportionate impact on it, while psychology falls farther behind and is in danger of being shut out.

Six years ago I told the following simple story:

*Invited Distinguished Centennial Address to the American Psychological Association Convention, August 1992.

Two men were on a mountain trek across the high Sierra Nevada Mountains of California when they encountered a particularly ferocious grizzly bear. The first man froze in panic while the second man dropped to his knees and began to remove his hiking boots, replacing them with his running shoes. "You don't really think you can outrun that bear, do you?" sneered the first man. "I don't have to," replied his companion. "All I have to do is run faster than you."

This story is repeated because six years ago the grizzly of managed care could have been our dancing bear. Now we must survive by running faster than our colleagues. What happened in those six years while psychology was in denial?

HISTORICAL PERSPECTIVE

After two centuries as a cottage industry, health care in America began to industrialize, first in medicine and surgery, and finally in mental health and chemical dependency treatment. The characteristics of such an industrialization have been detailed elsewhere (Cummings & Wright, 1991), and suffice it to say here that the field of mental health is experiencing the painful evolution found in all industrialization: (1) Those who make the product (in our case, deliver psychological services) lose control over their own product; (2) the control shifts to business interests (in our case, the emerging giant managed mental health care industry); (3) the income of those who make (deliver) the product goes down as industrialization thrives on cheap labor; (4) there is standardization of the products (in our case, psychotherapy integration); and (5) industrialization results in efficiency and cost management, which makes the product (psychotherapy) available to more and more people.

In order to place this industrial revolution of health care in perspective, let us first look at the last several decades of psychological practice. Psychology is celebrating its first 100 years, but professional psychology is only 50 years old (Cummings, 1992). It emerged in World War II, and the Veterans' Administration was its first setting. Prior to that, there were a few psychologists in private practice, spread around the country, sometimes in improbable places. They were mostly women with masters' degrees, and they worked with children. They flourished because society was beginning to appreciate that children needed this kind of help, and the male-dominated psychiatry profession was not threatened by these apparently benign maternal figures.

These pioneers were replaced following World War II by first a trickle, and then a steady stream, of doctorally trained veterans who fled the psychiatric domination of our mental health institutions into independent practice. These new pioneers, of which I pride myself as being one, bootlegged their psychotherapy training and supervision off-campus from congenial psychiatrists who also referred their overflow of patients (VandenBos, Cummings, & DeLeon, 1992).

During the next several decades, psychology established itself as an autonomous profession, in spite of open warfare from the American Psychiatric Association and opposition, and sometimes even sabotage, from its own American Psychological Association. This history, sometimes tragic, sometimes comical, but always colorful, was first detailed by Cummings (1979). During those decades, professional psychology achieved statutory recognition in all states and jurisdictions, third-party payment status, and wide public acceptance. Psychotherapy became the undisputed province of professional psychology in the eyes of the American public.

It is the view of this paper that psychology flourished in spite of all odds and early resistances on the parts of both APAs because it met certain societal needs. In short, professional psychology succeeded because society, for many good reasons, wanted to make psychotherapy the province of psychology. Progress in psychotherapy and psychopharmacology occurred simultaneously. In society's eyes, psychology became identified with the former, psychiatry with the latter. Society wanted psychotherapy and elevated psychology against all odds. It is also our contention that the future of psychotherapy will be shaped less from within than by external forces. These are social and economic forces stemming from the extension of psychotherapy from the middle class to the blue-collar and laboring classes and to the ethnic minorities by (1) the community mental health movement, (2) the industrialization of health care (including mental health care) through managed care, and (3) finally by the eventual adoption of government-regulated universal health care. As these change points occur, the bandwagon effect of a profession abandoning its former resistance and opposition will make it appear that change is coming mostly from within, when in fact it is not.

In the 35 years following World War II, the APA was frighteningly out of touch with the needs of society for psychotherapy. This is understandable because during these years the APA was under the domination of the academicians who were attempting to impose their own view of what professional psychology should look like. But the past decade has seen the professionals in firm control of the APA, and we do not seem to be doing better. In fact, for the first time it is professional psychology *itself* that is asyntonic with the direction in which society is moving. As examples, the "mini-convention" on managed care that preceded the 1992 APA Convention did not have among its presenters a single recognized authority from managed care. The National College, designed to prepare psychologists for the marketplace, does not have a single board member from the managed care industry, which is rapidly becoming the dominant force in the marketplace. Each issue of *Advance-Plan* becomes more hysterical and is beginning to rival the American Medical Association's (AMA) polemics, which, during its most rabidly guild era, attacked the now commonplace programs of Medicare and Medicaid as "socialized medicine." The crescendo of recent issues of *Advance-Plan* makes even the historic rantings of the AMA appear to be scholarly treatises by comparison.

There are many flaws and failings in managed mental health care, which is not surprising in an industry still in its infancy and experiencing unprecedented growth. There needs to be a positive, corrective approach on the part of the profession to these shortcomings. An excruciating litany of horror stories is neither accurate nor productive. My own 9 years on the APA Insurance Trust taught me two things: colleagues who abuse and abandon patients, and who are incompetent and guilty of poor judgment, abound far more than we are comfortable admitting; and one cannot judge an entire profession by the bad apples among us. But my sense of humor, defined as the ability to survive adversity by laughing at oneself, compels me to share one case that was recently brought to my attention. A psychologist who was seeing a patient diagnosed as multiple personality, and whose insurance policy limited psychotherapy to 20 sessions, demanded 20 sessions for each of her 14 personalities, for a total of 280 sessions. When the insurance company sought a second opinion, the psychologist protested that this would violate the confidentiality of his patient, who was also a psychologist. Finally a second opinion was arranged in another state. My sense of humor compels me to believe that this psychologist was neither cynical nor incompetent, but was tweaking the noses of the bean-counters within the insurance company.

There are abuses on both sides, and clearly an accommodation must be reached in the interest of quality care. Managed care needs psychology, the premier psychotherapy profession, to maintain its clinical integrity. Psychology, which is falling farther and farther behind, cannot afford to be shut out of managed mental health care. It is the intent of this paper to be constructive, not polemic. Practitioners need help in this era of cost containment. But bear in mind that the current heated debate about managed mental health care is not just about money. It is also about "professional prerogatives, about power and about autonomy, things that most mental health professionals value highly but do not often admit" (Feldman, 1992, p. 5). Based on our 7 years' experience with a leading-edge managed care company, we wish to share with you a set of propositions that will be both predictions as to where mental health delivery is going and recommendations on not merely how to survive, but how to thrive in the new environment. In short, it will be everything your graduate program and the APA did not tell you.

Proposition 1: Managed Care Will Gravitate from Preferred Providers to Prime (Retained) Providers. (Excerpted from Cummings, 1992a, 1992c.)

Given the realities of the social, economic and market pressures on psychology, along with the lamentable missed window of opportunity, what can the profession do to meet the challenge of the future? An analysis of where managed mental health care is heading reveals another opportunity, which, although not as large as the one that got away, is nonetheless attractive in that it restores some of the autonomy and control that are important to the profession.

The First Generation of managed care, of which almost every reader is now aware, involves telephone utilization review and limited benefits. The Second Generation, which is not as frequent but is growing rapidly, continues telephone utilization review and limited benefits, but adds an unmanaged provider network administered through a negotiated, discounted fee-for-service. The Third Generation of managed care, which is just now beginning, is characterized by expansion of benefits made possible by networks trained in managed care and time-shortened therapy techniques, with clinical case management of outpatient services as well as on-site hospital review, a defined continuum of care, and the inclusion of lifestyle management programs. Within this Third Generation everyone has heard of networks of "preferred providers." There is emerging a new concept that goes beyond "preferred provider" to "prime provider," called "retained provider" in one progressive managed care company. Here is where the opportunity lies.

Retained providers are a group of practitioners who not only are able to deliver the wide range of services required, but have also demonstrated quality, efficiency and effectiveness. These groups of retained providers will contract with the managed care firm to be responsible for all the care to a specified enrolled population, and for a *prospective* reimbursement. Because it has proved its quality, effectiveness and efficiency, the managed care company no longer case manages the group, and only maintains an arm's-length monitoring to assure that services provided meet the contractual standards. Thus, the managed care company profits by saving the expense of case management, and the practitioners benefit by having their autonomy restored.

The group practices that achieve the status of retained providers will prosper in a climate of relative austerity. These groups will be multifaceted, able to perform the entire range of psychotherapy and lifestyle management services. They will be skilled in focused, targeted interventions and know how to practice brief, intermittent psychotherapy throughout the life cycle (Cummings, 1990). The group practice model, called "the general practice of psychology" and first proposed by Cummings and VandenBos (1979), is still relevant in this new arena, and farsighted psychologists are beginning to move rapidly in that direction and on their own initiative. These are the psychologists who will not only survive, but prosper, as they meet the needs of society during an industrial health care revolution.

The remaining 8 propositions are designated to aid the psychologist in thinking about, and preparing for, the new environment as a Prime (Retained) rather than Preferred Provider.

Proposition 2: Managed Care Will Become the Modal Delivery System in Universal Health Care in the United States.

This is inevitable. The price tag on universal health coverage will be staggering, and can only be made possible by the cost-efficiency of competing managed care companies, coupled with the savings realized through a government single claims/payor system. The Health Care Financing Administration (HCFA), after several successful demonstration projects, is putting more and more of Medicare and Medicaid under managed care contracts. This is only the precursor of what is coming.

Realizing this, some of the professional psychology leadership has embarked on a campaign to enact legislation in the states to restrict the growth of managed care. Curiously, some of these same leaders who a few years ago eschewed all government interference in the practice of psychology have suddenly, in their zeal to stop or restrict managed care, become born-again regulators! This is the path followed by the AMA, when in the 1960s it decided to stop the growth of HMOs by successfully passing a patchwork of inhibiting state laws. But society wanted HMOs, and after millions of dollars spent by the AMA, in the 1970s federal laws were enacted to enable HMO development, thus superseding the inhibiting state laws. There is little question but that the APA will succeed in passing a number of inhibiting laws. These will temporarily slow down the growth of managed mental health care as costs also increase. But society wants managed mental health care and these laws will, after millions in expenditures and much effort, be superseded. Further, universal health care can operate only when state laws are superseded by one national set of health care regulations.

Proposition 3: Managed Care Can Save the Independent Practice of Psychology.

Managed care will evolve in directions no one can adequately predict at this point in time. But whatever the eventual form, health care, once industrialized, will never return to the practitioners' halcyon days as a cottage industry based on fee-for-service. For all time to come health-care delivery will involve those who pay the bills, holding those who deliver the service accountable. If the practitioner can give up the nostalgia about the "good old days" when control was in the hands of the therapist, one might discern that managed care may save psychological practice, because it is an alternative to the current trend just to eliminate the psychotherapy benefit. In addition, it actually increases the amount of money diverted into the private practice of psychotherapy. It is the psychiatric hospital and hospital-based psychiatrists' practices that have been impacted by the appropriate level of care, which has seen an increase in psychotherapy as a valid clinical alternative to intrusive, disruptive and unnecessary hospitalization.

.Figure 1 demonstrates how, in a population of 100,000 enrollees, with 150 days per 1,000 hospitalization rate and a 4% outpatient penetration, the 95% reduction in the amount of unnecessary hospitalization to 20 days per 1,000 enrollees results in a 50% increase in outpatient psychotherapy. This is because outpatient psychotherapy becomes the appropriate treatment in lieu of inappropriate psychiatric hospitalization. The recipients of this increased volume in outpatient services are most often the psychologists participating in the network and working out of their own private offices (Cummings, 1992c).

Proposition 4: Mismanaged Mental Health Care Is Easy to Spot.

We are in the predicted period of consolidation in managed mental health care (Cummings, 1986) where the well-run companies are acquiring their less successful competitors. Managed care practices will continue to be highly variable, ranging from quality care to poor delivery of services. In the meantime, practitioners will be confronted with choices of networks to join. A review of the widely distributed "Ten Ways to Spot Mismanaged Mental Health" can spare the practitioner much grief. We can only refer to them here, and the reader desiring greater detail should consult the original publication (Cummings, 1991b). Briefly, if a managed care company fails three or more of the ten guidelines in Table 1, the psychologist had best beware.

Proposition 5: An Adversarial Relationship Is Neither Inevitable nor Desirable.

When confronted with a case manager, most psychotherapists will inadvertently fall into an adversarial role with the managed care company. Psychologists are highly individualistic and resent any intrusion into the doctor-patient relationship. Hence, they are likely to jump to the conclusion that the managed care company does not really care about the patient and just wants to save money. Unfortunately, there are enough marginal managed care firms from which an unwarranted generalization can be made, just as there are incompetent psychotherapists, from whom it would be unfair to damn the entire profession.

A well-run managed care company no more wants a suicide on its hands than you do. It knows as the so-called "deep pocket" that its legal exposure is financially even greater than yours. Therefore, it

Figure 1. Diversion of Inpatient Care to Outpatient Care

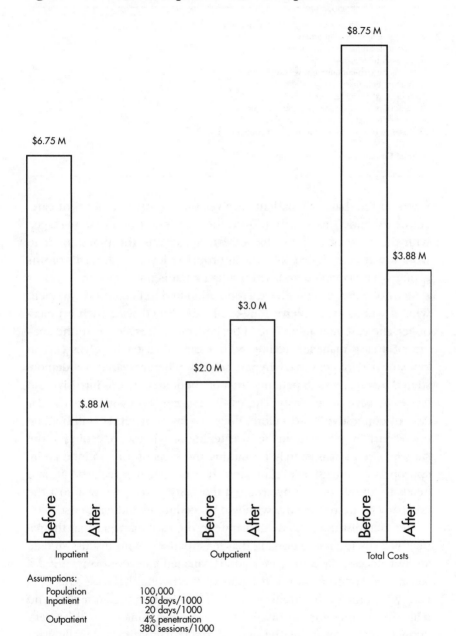

Assumptions:

Population	100,000
Inpatient	150 days/1000
	20 days/1000
Outpatient	4% penetration
	380 sessions/1000

Table 1. *Ten Ways to Spot Mismanaged Mental Health Care*

1. Signing up everyone who will join the network
2. Charging a fee to join a network
3. Nonprofessionals as case managers
4. Barriers to access of care
5. Focus on cost-containment versus clinical efficiency
6. Narrow benefits
7. Look hard at the leadership
8. Lack of professional development for providers
9. Lack of formal quality assurance measures
10. Absence of commitment to research (outcomes)

From Cummings, N.A. (1991b), pp. 79–83.

wants to see that your patient receives the *appropriate* level of care. Let us examine this situation from the standpoint of a case manager, with the view of helping that case manager and the practitioner to work toward the same goal—the appropriate level of care. This means giving what is needed and withholding what is unnecessary.

Many of our colleagues have a reputation for inefficiency. Any patient who is willing will receive long-term care. Faced with such a practitioner, the case manager is faced by a dilemma. It is similar to the analogy of a case manager dealing with a cardiologist who gives certain kinds of patients coronary bypass surgery when research has demonstrated that many such patients are more benefited by less intrusive and less expensive angioplasty. The case manager, discussing a particular case of congestive heart failure, does not know whether withholding open-heart surgery will be life threatening or whether acceding to the surgeon's request is merely permitting the surgeon to continue an inappropriately intrusive level of care. The case manager really wants and needs to know, for an unwarranted mortality potentially will cost the company far more than the withheld procedure would have cost.

The therapist needs to demonstrate to the case manager that the patient is a suicide risk, knowing that most patients who discuss suicide are not necessarily lethal. In a good managed care company, given a substantial concern on the the part of the psychotherapist, this concern will come to the attention of a clinician within the company who will call the therapist to discuss the case. This clinician will be very knowledgeable regarding the signs of true lethality and will really want to know the facts. If the therapist is equally knowledgeable, a collegial decision will be reached. If the therapist is not skilled in assessing and treating lethality, however, the company's clinician will still be left with the dilemma of whether or not the patient is potentially lethal to self or others. A second opinion from a more skilled psychotherapist is warranted, at which point the therapist may become more adversarial and complain that the doctor-patient relationship is being violated.

Limitations on patients' psychotherapy benefits are not new with the advent of managed care. For decades we have had fee-for-service indemnity insurance that limits psychotherapy to 5, 10, or 20 sessions. Psychotherapists long ago accommodated their practices to this reality. The current controversy stems from the fact that good managed care companies do not want to limit the number of sessions, preferring rather that the appropriate number of sessions be utilized. Such an "open benefit" means that the psychotherapist will be held accountable for his or her effectiveness and efficiency. Psychotherapists are not used to being held accountable. Frankly, most cannot provide adequate therapeutic rationale for their interventions, and I continue to be startled by the large number of psychotherapists who never formulate a treatment plan. The days are over when an insurance company will pay for what has been called "therapeutic drift." (Excerpted from Cummings, 1995.)

Proposition 6: Soon Managed Care Will Know More About Your Job Than You Do.

An organizational setting such as that provided by managed care makes possible extensive outcomes research (Pallak & Cummings, 1994). Insurers have long been mystified by what we do as psychotherapists. They had no basis upon which to question treatment decisions as to duration, intensity or outcome. This situation is about to change.

For decades, Budman (Budman & Gurman, 1983) and Cummings (Cummings & Follette, 1968; Follette & Cummings, 1967) have pointed to the growing irrelevance of schools of psychotherapy reporting research indicating that all schools have truth, but no one approach has all the truth. They called for specific treatments designed to ameliorate specific psychological conditions. Cummings was particularly scathing, pointing out that psychotherapy is the only field of health where the patient receives that which the therapist was trained to do, rather than that which the patient's condition requires (Cummings, 1987). In other words, whether one has a marital problem, a phobia or a job problem, one receives the couch, the painting of pictures, or desensitization, purely on the basis of whether the therapist is a Freudian, Jungian or Behaviorist. Cummings' criticism is admittedly overdrawn, but the point still remains that too often all patients, regardless of presenting complaints, receive essentially the same approach in treatment.

Working independently and on opposite coasts, Budman and Cummings reported research demonstrating that some conditions best respond to dynamic approaches, while others do well with behavioral or systems approaches, but most conditions do best with specific, empirically derived amalgams of all schools of psychotherapy. The admixture varies with the psychological condition. Budman predicted an eventual "blurring" of the boundaries dividing the various approaches, while Cummings foresaw the "melding" of all the schools of psychotherapy into admixtures. Cummings also predicted that instead of keeping a patient in therapy for protracted periods until all problems and potential problems were resolved; the psychotherapist of the future would practice "brief, intermittent psychotherapy throughout the life cycle," not unlike the practice of all the health fields, which treat specific problems as they arise, with continuity for chronic conditions (Cummings, 1990; Cummings, 1992a).

Now, in psychology's Centennial year, many of the leaders in psychotherapy who had been showing signs for several years of moving in that direction are flat-out predicting psychotherapy "integration." Diverse clinicians representing a wide range of approaches are predicting not only (1) an integration, but also (2) empirically derived, focused, targeted treatment of specific conditions, (3) emphasis on brief and time-limited interventions, (4) accountability, and even (5) treatment manuals (Austad & Hoyt, 1992; Beck & Haaqa, 1992; Coyne & Liddle, 1992; Goldfried & Gastonquay, 1992; Lazarus, Beutler & Norcross, 1992; Mahrer, 1992). In addition, some of the same authors predict (6) therapies specifically designed to address certain populations. This process will be evolving for years to come, but these predictions are inevitable, because they respond to social and economic forces. Primary will be managed care sponsored outcomes research that yields empirically derived targeted therapies for specific psychological conditions, resulting in more efficient and effective treatment.

Proposition 7: Successful Psychologists Will Reformulate Their Attitudes and Outlook.

An effective, clinically driven managed care system concentrates not on saving money, but on clinical effectiveness, which ultimately achieves this efficiency and cost-savings. This not only requires therapeutic skills that not all therapists possess, but as Friedman and Fanger (1991) have postulated, will require a "paradigm shift" on the part of the therapist.

What immediately comes to mind for the reader is forms of brief therapy. Effective, efficient psychotherapy is not necessarily brief therapy, although, if effective, it may be less time intensive. It is the appropriate level of therapy based on the patient's need to have the least intrusive intervention necessary to do the job. This may, for some patients, mean long-term therapy, but it is long term based on the patient's need, not the psychotherapist's ineffectiveness. In our own work we regard this as the Patients' Bill of Rights:

The patient is entitled to relief from pain, anxiety and depression in the shortest time possible and with the least intrusive intervention.

This presupposes that therapists will hone their skills to be able to fulfill this Patients' Bill of Rights. It follows from this and the foregoing that the therapy of the future will be pragmatic, eclectic psychotherapy. Efficiency is clinically driven rather than cost-containment driven. It allows for intermittent therapy throughout the life cycle of the patient, rather than one protracted episode intended to solve all problems for all time.

Proposition 8: The First Session Will Be Critical to Successful Pragmatic Therapy.

It is beyond the scope of this presentation to delineate completely the critical nature of the first session. Therapy can be made or lost in that first session, and a great deal of attention will be accorded to it in the outcome research and clinical literature. Budman's latest thrust (Budman, Hoyt, & Friedman, 1992) is typical.

In our own work we have formulated the work that needs to be accomplished in the ideal first session, as shown in Table 2. It must be emphasized that there are patients for whom this ideal first session is not possible, and the "first session" may require two or more sessions. It must be stressed, however, that until this work is accomplished, any treatment plan must be tentative and subject to modification.

The therapeutic contract, made before the treatment plan is augmented, is critical. It must embody the fact to the patient that we are here to serve as a catalyst, but the patient is the one who will do the

Table 2. *Cummings' General Psychotherapeutic Principles*

---

1. *Hit the ground running.* The first session must be therapeutic. The concept that you must devote the first session to taking a history. . .is nonsense.

2. *Perform an operational diagnosis.* The operational diagnosis asks one thing, "Why is the patient here today instead of last week or last month, last year, or next year?" And when you answer that, you know what the patient is here for. The operational diagnosis is absolutely necessary for you to set about your treatment plan, and it is best that it be done in the first session.

3. *Create a therapeutic contract.* Every patient makes a therapeutic contract with every therapist in the first session, every time. But in 99 percent of the cases, the therapist misses it.. . .If a patient comes into the office and says, "Doctor, I'm glad you have this comfortable chair because I'm going to be here a while," and the therapist doesn't respond to that, the therapist has just made a contract for long-term therapy.

4. *Do something novel the first session.* Find something novel, something unexpected, to do the first session. This will cut through the expectations of the "trained" patient and will create instead an expectation that problems are to be immediately addressed.

5. *Give hope in the first session.* This is not done by the usual "reassurance." Rather, have a small therapeutic gain in that first session. If this is not possible, give an example of a successful therapy of a patient with the same problem. But make certain the patient can identify with the example in terms of age, ethnicity, gender, and socioeconomic status.

6. *Give homework in the first session and every therapy session thereafter.* It isn't possible to have some cookbook full of homework that you just arbitrarily assign. Tailor the homework to be meaninful for that patient's goals and the therapeutic contract. The patient will realize, "Hey, this guy isn't kidding. I'm responsible for my own therapy."

Adapted and excerpted from Bloom (1991), p. 312.

---

growing. This contract, with variations to suit differences in education, intelligence and socioeconomic status, is stated:

> I will never abandon you as long as you need me, and I will never ask you to do anything until you are ready. In return for this I ask you to join me in a partnership to make me obsolete as soon as possible. (Cummings, 1983, pp. 312–313.)

Proposition 9: Less Than One-Third of Psychotherapy Will Be One-on-One.

This idea will be startling to most clinicians, and this will undoubtedly be the most controversial of our propositions. Individual psychotherapy, even when it is effective and efficient, is still labor-intensive. It drastically limits the number of patients a therapist can see in a given day. This would be acceptable if individual therapy were the best way to treat all patients. Recent outcome research, still in the preliminary stages, strongly suggests that what has been known for some time about alcoholics may be true for many, if not most, other patients: a group program format yields greater therapeutic outcomes.

Personality disorders, especially Axis II patients, do not generally respond therapeutically to the therapist (parental) transference. They defy authority, frustrate treatment by acting out between sessions, and are regarded as needing long-term treatment of as much as a decade or more. Whereas they defy parental (therapist) authority, these persons stuck in a perpetual mode of adolescent rage respond quite readily to the peer (group) transference. The peer pressure of the group can confront and control acting out in a manner that would not be accepted from the therapist. Because the number of persons presenting for treatment with these personality disorders is increasing, we predict that in the not too distant future, in effective delivery systems only 30% of psychotherapy will be one-on-one, while 70% will be group and targeted psychoeducational programs.

SUMMARY AND CONCLUSIONS

Although the wide-open window of opportunity to own managed care a few years ago is gone forever, there are still opportunities through which practitioners will not only survive, but thrive in the new environment. Managed care will gravitate from preferred providers to prime (retained) providers, and those practitioners who can hone their skills and competencies will prosper. A number of propositions designed to enable the psychologist to become a retained provider, which will restore the professional autonomy lost to the preferred provider, have been presented. Psychologists need to prepare for the fact that managed care in some form will be the modal delivery system in universal health care which is likely to be adopted this decade. Therapy will be pragmatic and eclectic, will favor the least intrusive and appropriate level of care (such as outpatient psychotherapy over unnecessary hospitalization), and will be focused and targeted therapy throughout the life cycle. Psychologists will not only have to hone their skills, but also re-examine their attitudes.

THE FUTURE OF PSYCHOTHERAPY: SOCIETY'S
CHARGE TO PROFESSIONAL PSYCHOLOGY

"Any body who visits a shrink should have his head examined."
Samuel Goldwyn, 1946.

THIS TONGUE-IN-check observation by the founder of MGM Studios was
not so much a remark concerning a social stigma, but an astute early
recognition of the ground-swell of interest in psychotherapy that was
beginning in the United States almost immediately following World
War II. Professional Psychology, having just survived its birth and infancy, rode this ground-swell and became a major profession.

As the American Psychological Association celebrates its Centennial
year, there seems to be a stampede of experts predicting that in the
future, psychotherapy will resemble a form that has been controversial and highly resisted by the profession itself for the past 30 years.
This bandwagon effect is not surprising, inasmuch as it has character-
istically occurred throughout the history of psychotherapy at each
point in which change has become obvious and inevitable. Even so,
the bandwagon is composed of the psychotherapy leadership, and the
effect takes considerable time to trickle to those in the trenches.

It is the point of view of this paper that psychology flourished in
spite of all odds and early resistances on the parts of *both* APAs, be-

cause it met certain societal needs. In short, professional psychology succeeded because society, for many good reasons, wanted to make psychotherapy the province of psychology. It is also our contention that the future of psychotherapy will be shaped less from within than by external forces. These are social and economic forces stemming from the extension of psychotherapy from the middle class to the blue-collar and laboring classes and to ethnic minorities (1) by the community mental health movement, (2) by the industrialization of health care (including mental health care) through managed care, and (3) finally by the eventual adoption of government-regulated universal health care. As these change points occur, the bandwagon effect of a profession abandoning its former resistance and opposition will make it appear that change is coming mostly from within, when in fact it is not.

We are now in such a change period with its accompanying bandwagon effect. But before we look at the pundits' rush for consensus, let us briefly review where we have been.

PROFESSIONAL PSYCHOLOGY'S FIFTY YEAR CENTENNIAL

Whereas psychology is celebrating its first 100 years, professional psychology as we know it today is only 50 years old (Cummings, 1992b). It was born in World War II, and the Veterans' Administration was its first home. Prior to that time, there was a handful of psychologists in private practice in widely scattered, and often improbable, places in the nation. Most were women, most had masters' degrees, and almost all worked with children. They flourished because society was beginning to develop a new perspective about children, and the male-dominated psychiatric profession, not feeling threatened by a seemingly maternal figure working exclusively with children, presented no opposition.

This author was privileged to have known several of these women, of whom Florence Mateer was characteristic. A pioneer and a thoroughgoing clinician, Mateer had an independent practice in Columbus, Ohio, where in 1928 she was called as an expert witness in court. This was decades before the first licensure, and long before psychology was recognized as a profession. The judge looked down at her from the bench and inquired, "What does it take to be a psychologist?" She fixed the judge with her formidable gaze and shouted back, "First of all, Your Honor, intelligence!" The judge was temporarily flustered, then recovered and brought down his gavel in declaration, "The court recognizes Florence Mateer as an expert witness."

These pioneers were replaced following World War II by first a trickle, and then a steady stream, of doctorally trained veterans who fled the psychiatric domination of our mental health institutions into independent practice. These new pioneers, of which I pride myself as being one, bootlegged their psychotherapy training and supervision off-campus from congenial psychiatrists who also referred their over-flow of patients (VandenBos, Cummings, & DeLeon, 1992).

During the next several decades, psychology established itself as an autonomous profession, in spite of open warfare from the American Psychiatric Association and opposition, and sometimes even sabotage, from its own American Psychological Association. This history, some-times tragic, sometimes comical, but always colorful, was first detailed by Cummings (1979). During those decades, professional psychology achieved statutory recognition in all states and jurisdictions, third-party payment status, and wide public acceptance. Psychotherapy be-came the undisputed province of professional psychology in the eyes of the American public.

So apparent is this fact that psychology came very close to ending its 50-year war with psychiatry. The latter was ready to acknowledge psychology's preeminence in psychotherapy, while it retained solely to psychiatry what it considered its medical prerogatives of medica-tion and hospitalization privileges. But professional psychology chose to expand into its natural frontiers to include prescription and hospi-talization privileges, thus assuring at least several more decades of warfare between psychiatry and psychology (Cummings, 1992c).

There are sound reasons why professional psychology became pre-eminent in psychotherapy. First, while psychology espoused psy-chotherapy and applied all of its clinical and research skills toward innovating and improving its parameters, psychiatry fell prey to the expedient and greater monetary reward of medication/ hospitalization practice. Psychotherapy and psychopharmacology advanced side-by-side, but psychology became identified with the first, and psychiatry with the second. Americans wanted psychotherapy, and elevated psy-chologists' status as psychotherapy providers in spite of psychiatry's open opposition and our own often less than stellar strategies and lack of support from our own APA.

Now society wants psychologists to have prescription privileges, so these will be achieved. It is logical that conservatively prescribed medication is often an accompaniment of, not a replacement for, psychotherapy, and the patient need not have to see two doctors to receive both. If psychology integrates pharmacology and retains psychotherapy as preeminent, it will become *the* mental health profession. If it falls prey to the temptation that befell psychiatry, the expedient of the prescription pad over the hard work of psychotherapy, society will look to social work or other mental health professions, rather than to psychology.

REVIEW OF THE PUNDITS

For decades, Budman (Budman & Gurman, 1983) and Cummings (Cummings & Follette, 1968; Follette & Cummings, 1987) have pointed to the growing irrelevance of schools of psychotherapy reporting research indicating that all schools have truth, but no one approach has all the truth. They called for specific treatments designed to ameliorate specific psychological conditions. Cummings was particularly scathing, pointing out that psychotherapy is the only field of health where the patient receives that which the therapist was trained to do, rather than that which one's condition requires (Cummings, 1987). In other words, whether one has a marital problem, a phobia or a job problem, one receives the couch, the painting of pictures, or desensitization, purely on the basis of whether the therapist is a Freudian, Jungian or Behaviorist. Cummings' criticism is admittedly overdrawn, but the point still remains that too often all patients, regardless of presenting complaints, receive essentially the same approach in treatment.

Working independently and on opposite coasts, Budman and Cummings reported research demonstrating that some conditions best respond to dynamic approaches, while others do well with behavioral or systems approaches, but most conditions do best with specific, empirically derived amalgams of all schools of psychotherapy. The admixture varies with the psychological condition. Budman predicted an eventual "blurring" of the boundaries dividing the various approaches, while Cummings foresaw the "melding" of all the schools of psychotherapy into admixtures. Cummings also predicted that instead of keeping a patient in therapy for protracted periods until all problems and potential problems were resolved, the psychotherapist of the future would practice "brief, intermittent psychotherapy throughout the life cycle," not unlike the practice of all the health fields, which treat specific problems as they arise, with continuity for chronic conditions (Cummings, 1990; Cummings, 1992a).

For 30 years, "the mental health complex" (Duhl & Cummings, 1987) has resisted this inevitable trend, each "school" vigorously guarding its own turf and fostering a Babel of idiosyncratic vocabularies that prevented intercommunication and cross-fertilization. Now, in psychology's Centennial year, many of the leaders in psychotherapy who had been showing signs for several years of moving in that direction are flat-out predicting psychotherapy "integration." Diverse clinicians representing a wide range of approaches are predicting not only an (1) integration, but also (2) empirically derived, focused, targeted treatment of specific conditions, (3) emphasis on brief and time-limited interventions, (4) accountability, and even (5) treatment manuals (Austad & Hoyt, 1992; Beck & Haaga, 1992; Coyne & Liddle, 1992; Goldfried & Gastonguay, 1992; Lazarus, Beutler, & Norcross, 1992; Mahrer, 1992). In addition, some of the same authors predict (6) therapies specifically designed to address certain populations. This process will be evolving for years to come, but these predictions are inevitable, because they respond to social and economic forces.

Social and Economic Forces

The exuberance with which the American people espoused psychotherapy immediately after World War II is unparalleled in our history (Cummings, 1975a). It was during that early era that NIMH determined there would never be enough psychiatrists and that it should become involved in sponsoring the training of psychologists. This period also saw the launching of the paraprofessional movement, because it was believed there would never be enough psychiatrists, psychologists or social workers to meet the demand for psychotherapy.

Our own exuberance stemmed from the belief that we were, indeed, following Freud's (1904) exhortation to bring psychotherapy to the people. The fact is, psychotherapy at that time was the penchant of this middle, educated class. There was no third party payment, but out-of-pocket was not a problem with fees of $10 or $15 as standard for a 50-minute hour. As long as middle-class therapists were treating middle-class patients, psychotherapy could remain esoteric, parochial, and splendid.

All of this changed when psychotherapy truly was brought to the people through third-party payment, government inclusion of psychotherapy in its programs (Medicaid, Medicare, CHAMPUS), the community mental health centers movement, and, finally, managed care—which is ultimately catapulting mental health care from a cottage industry into industrialization. The working class and the welfare class do not have the propensity for long-term psychotherapy that characterizes the middle class. And with the shifting of much of the criminal justice system into the mental health system, we are confronted with hundreds of thousands of Axis II patients for whom psychotherapy has been mandated, but who really do not want it at all. Psychotherapy by 1980 could no longer remain splendid.

Yet, historically, psychology has never been hospitable to brief psychotherapy. When Alexander and French (1946) published their *Psychoanalytic Therapy* a half century ago, they unleashed a storm of controversy even though they were conceptualizing "brief" as 150 to 300 sessions. We have become considerably more realistic since then, but the attitude remains ingrained that brief treatment is superficial, longer is better, and the most influential and prestigious practitioners tend to be those who undertake intensive long-term therapy with a very limited number of clients (Bloom, 1991). However, the pressures on the mental health professions by the marketplace for more efficient short-term therapy have become intense. Added to the aforementioned pressures are the economic requirements to tether the runaway inflation rate in mental health and chemical dependency treatment, the so-called cost-containment movement. Planned, short-term therapy is rapidly becoming the treatment modality of the 1990s with outcome research demonstrating a surprising degree of effectiveness (Pallak & Cummings, 1994).

In my own predictions that managed mental health care would sweep the country (Cummings, 1986), I failed to see just how rapid this sweep would be. I had not anticipated the move by employers who, finding they no longer could unilaterally pay the high cost of health care for their employees, shifted much of the burden to the employees themselves. In 1989 and 1990, 78% of labor disputes were related to this move by employers. Once confronted with having to share in the cost of their own health coverage, employees quickly abandoned freedom-of-choice for the value offered by managed care. This one factor accelerated the growth of managed mental health care beyond the rate I had anticipated several years ago.

Psychology and Managed Care

The current heated debate about managed mental health care is not just about money. It is also about "professional prerogatives, about power and about autonomy, things that most mental health professionals value highly but do not often admit" (Feldman, 1992, p. 5). A decade ago, a window of opportunity existed for psychology to initiate and, thereby, own managed mental health care. This was because managed mental health was following the scenario created by medical/surgical managed care. Even eight years later, it still would not have been difficult to accomplish. Rather than seize the moment, psychology and the APA dug in their heels despite warnings and encouragement to do otherwise (Cummings, 1986; Cummings & Fernandez, 1985). A mere handful of psychologists seized the moment and prospered. The majority of the profession went into denial.

As of this writing, the APA has embarked on a stance of what this author has called the ALL-approach: Adversarial, Legislative, and Litigational (Practice Directorate, 1992; Youngstrom, 1992). Undoubtedly, restrictive laws will be passed and disenabling regulations will be written. We are embarking on the path followed by the AMA, when in the 1960s it decided to stop the growth of HMOs by successfully passing a patchwork of inhibiting state laws. But society wanted HMOs, and after millions of dollars spent by the AMA, in the 1970s federal laws were enacted to enable HMO development, thus superseding the inhibiting state laws. There is little question but that the APA will succeed in passing a number of inhibiting laws. These will temporarily slow down the growth of managed mental health care as costs also increase. But society wants managed mental health care and these laws will, after millions in expenditures and much effort, be superseded.

Managed care will evolve in directions no one can adequately predict at this point in time. But whatever the eventual form, health care, once industrialized, will never return to the practitioners' halcyon days as a cottage industry based on fee-for-service. For all time to come, health care delivery will involve those who pay the bills, holding those who deliver the service accountable. If the practitioner can give up the nostalgia about the "good old days" when control was in the hands of the therapist, one might discern that managed care may save psychological practice, because it is an alternative to the current trend just to eliminate the psychotherapy benefit. In addition, it actually increases the amount of money diverted into the private practice of psychotherapy.

Figure 1 demonstrates how, in a population of 100,000 enrollees, with 150 days per 1,000 hospitalization rate and a 4% outpatient penetration, the 95% reduction in the amount of unnecessary hospitalization to 20 days per 1,000 enrollees results in a 50% increase in outpatient psychotherapy. This is because outpatient psychotherapy becomes the appropriate treatment in lieu of inappropriate psychiatric hospitalization. The recipient of this increased volume in outpatient services is most often the psychologist participating in the network and working out of a private office.

THE FUTURE CHALLENGE

Given the realities of the social, economic, and market pressures on psychology, along with the lamentable missed window of opportunity, what can the profession do to meet the challenge of the future? An analysis of where managed mental health care is heading reveals another opportunity which, although not as large as the one that got away, is nonetheless attractive in that it restores some of the autonomy and control that are important to the profession.

The First Generation of managed care, of which almost every reader is now aware, involves telephone utilization review and limited benefits. The Second Generation, which is not as frequent but is growing rapidly, continues telephone utilization review and limited benefits, but adds an unmanaged provider network administered through a negotiated, discounted fee-for-service. The Third Generation of managed care, which is just now beginning, is characterized by expansion of benefits made possible by networks trained in managed care and time-shortened therapy techniques, with clinical case management of outpatient services as well as on-site hospital review, a defined continuum of care, and the inclusion of lifestyle management programs. Within this Third Generation everyone has heard of networks of "preferred providers." There is emerging a new concept that goes beyond "preferred provider" to "prime provider," called "retained provider" in one progressive managed care company. Here is where the opportunity lies.

Retained providers are a group of practitioners who not only are able to deliver the wide range of services required, but have also demonstrated quality, efficiency and effectiveness. These groups of retained providers will contract with the managed care firm to be responsible for all the care to a specified enrolled population, and for a

Figure 1. Diversion of Inpatient Care to Outpatient Care

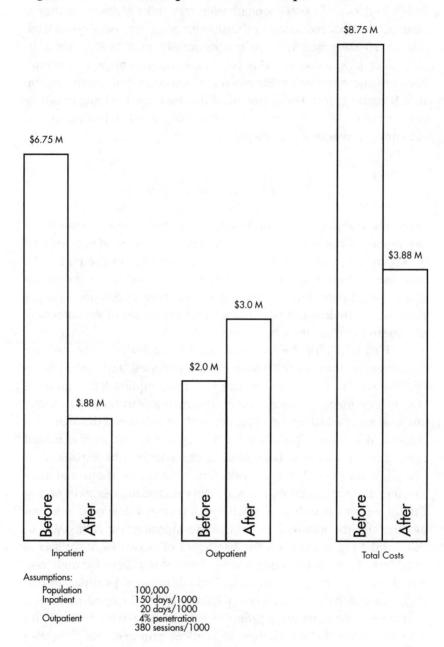

Assumptions:

Population	100,000	
Inpatient	150 days/1000	
	20 days/1000	
Outpatient	4% penetration	
	380 sessions/1000	

prospective reimbursement. Because it has proved its quality, effectiveness, and efficiency, the managed care company no longer case manages the group, and only maintains an arm's-length monitoring to assure that services provided meet the contractual standards. Thus, the managed care company profits by saving the expense of case management, and the practitioners benefit by having their autonomy restored.

The group practices that achieve the status of retained providers will prosper in a climate of relative austerity. These groups will be multifaceted, able to perform the entire range of psychotherapy and lifestyle management services. They will be skilled in focused, targeted interventions and know how to practice brief, intermittent psychotherapy throughout the life cycle (Cummings, 1990). The group practice model, called "the general practice of psychology" and first proposed by Cummings and VandenBos (1979), is still relevant in this new arena, and farsighted psychologists are beginning to move rapidly in that direction on their own initiative. These are the psychologists who will not only survive, but prosper, as they meet the needs of society during an industrial health care revolution.

The Sirens' Song

No look into the future of psychotherapy would be complete without mentioning the fanciful proposal of Kovacs (1991), who suggests that psychologists opt out of the health system, eschew third party reimbursement, and charge the patient out-of-pocket for our services. This proposal has the seductive quality of promising a return to the halcyon days when no one intruded upon the psychotherapist-patient relationship.

One need only look at the data compiled by the government's Health Care Financing Administration (HCFA) in Figure 2 to discern the wish-fulfilling aspects of the Kovacs proposal. In 1960 most of health care was paid out-of-pocket, while the rest was a combination of government and third party payer. By 1990 the situation was reversed, with only about a fourth of health care coming out-of-pocket. When co-payments and other limitations are removed, only 15% of the health care dollar in America is currently a totally noninsured (private or government) phenomenon. When one looks at just psychotherapy, this is reduced to only 7% of the total psychotherapy dollar. In other words, while there are many persons willing to sustain moderate co-

Figure 2. Reimbursement Methods, 1960 vs. 1990

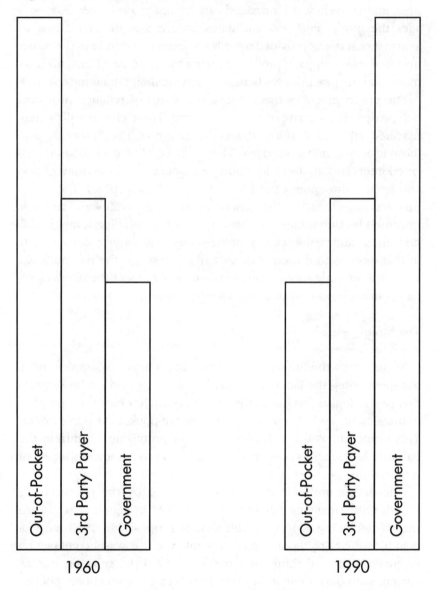

Growth of Medical Coverage (3rd Party Payer and Government) over out-of-pocket reimbursement in the 30 years between 1960 and 1990

Source: HICFA, 1991.

payments, relatively few are willing to pay totally out-of-pocket. This number willing to pay totally out-of-pocket for psychotherapy is less than half that for medicine and surgery.

These data would suggest that the seductiveness of this proposal is like the Sirens' song, from which there is no return. Kovacs is seemingly proposing that we specialize in the diseases of the rich, and even if we were to limit ourselves as he suggests, there is hardly enough revenue to sustain 42,000 professional psychologists and an even larger horde of psychiatrists, social workers, mental health counselors, psychiatric nurse practitioners, and MFCCs.

CONCLUSIONS

In spite of overwhelming opposition from without as well as within, professional psychology prospered because society needed and wanted to make psychotherapy the province of psychology. In those decades from 1945 to 1975, psychology was syntonic with the needs of the society that enabled it, essentially the middle and educated class. With the extension of psychotherapy into the working and welfare classes and to those formerly in the criminal justice system, there are demands on psychotherapy for more efficient, effective treatment. The stressors are also economic now that health care costs, and especially mental health care costs, have gone out of control.

At the present time, professional psychology finds itself dystonic with the needs and demands of society. It missed the window of opportunity to capture managed care, and now it has lost control of its own therapy process, as have all health practitioners. Nonetheless, in spite of its being out of synchrony with social needs, economics, and market forces, professional psychologists are still well positioned to become retained providers and not only prosper, but regain some of their lost autonomy. The pundits seem to have arrived at a consensus that the psychotherapy of the future will be integrated, focused, and targeted to psychological conditions and specific populations, planned short-term accountable and based on empirical research, and that treatment manuals will be standard. The delivery system will favor retained providers who are skilled in the new psychotherapy, and who practice in multifaceted groups whose quality, effectiveness and efficiency relieve them of intrusive scrutiny from the third-party payer.

There will be a shake-down, with many practitioners not surviving because they are unable or unwilling to meet society's challenge. For those that do, the future of psychotherapy is exciting and the future of professional psychology is bullish.

{ 20 }

PSYCHOLOGISTS:
AN ESSENTIAL COMPONENT
TO COST-EFFECTIVE,
INNOVATIVE CARE

ARGUMENTS FOR THE FINANCIAL EFFICACY
OF PSYCHOLOGICAL SERVICES IN HEALTHCARE SETTINGS

THE "HEALTHCARE REVOLUTION" has produced a new array of health and mental health service delivery systems. In light of these changes, a thorough understanding of the evidence for the financial efficacy of psychological services in health settings is critical for the healthcare industry, for service providers, for patients, and for policy-makers.

Psychotherapy Key to Effective Healthcare Planning

Cummings and VandenBos (1981) summarized the twenty-year Kaiser Permanente research experience demonstrating the financial efficacy of psychological services in healthcare settings (see Figure 1). Despite an initial view of mental health services as a less costly "dumping ground for hypochondriacs," twenty-five years of research have led to the conclusion that no comprehensive prepaid system can survive financially without a psychotherapy benefit.

Figure 1. Potential for Reduction in Medical Claims; Decline in Medical Utilization During Year of Intervention.

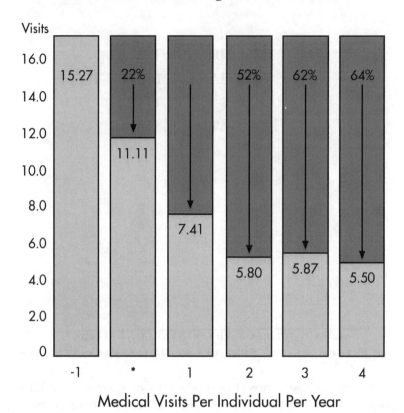

Medical Visits Per Individual Per Year

Kaiser Permanente data
Period 1974-1979
Sample based on 4,166 subscribers
Population sample withdrawn from 187,300

The Somatization Cycle

For example, early investigations confirmed that 60% of all physician visits were for patients without a confirmable physical or biological problem. Add to this figure the visits by patients with stress-related illnesses (e.g., peptic ulcer, ulcerative colitis, hypertension, etc.) and the total approaches 80–90% (cf. Shapiro, 1971). Subsequent research has demonstrated that turning 60–90% of all M.D.'s into psychotherapists (in order to handle the emotionally distressed) was not necessary since a relatively small number of psychotherapists can effectively ameliorate these patients.

Figure 1 (cont.). Potential for Reduction in Medical Claims; Decline in Medical Utilization During Year of Intervention.

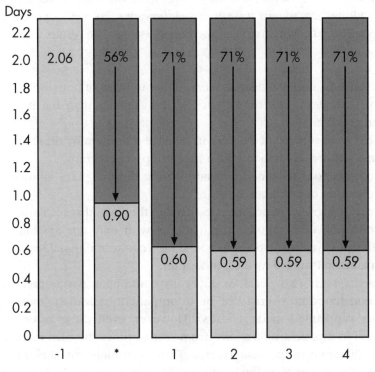

Hospital Days Per Individual Per Year

Once these patients enter the somatization cycle, there is a burgeoning symptomology. This results because the original stress problem still exists despite the physician's best efforts to treat the resulting physical complaint. Patients who enter this cycle move from one physician to another thereby instituting a new round of ineffectual diagnostic tests and medical utilization. In similar fashion, stress may impact an existing physical illness, exacerbating the symptomology and increasing its duration.

The Intertwining of Psychotherapy and Medical Utilization

Follette and Cummings (1967) compared the number and type of medical services used for the year preceding and for five years following psychotherapy for three groups of randomly selected patients: patients who had one interview only, those who were treated by brief therapy (mean of 6.2 interviews), and those who were cared for under a program of long-term therapy (mean of 34 interviews), as well as a control group without therapy based on the initial distress. The results were as follows:

- Persons in emotional distress were higher utilizers of both inpatient (hospitalization) and outpatient medical facilities than the health plan average.
- There were significant declines in medical utilization by those emotionally distressed patients who received psychotherapy.
- These declines remained constant during the five years following termination of psychotherapy.
- The most significant declines occurred in the second year following termination of psychotherapy; patients with only one session or with brief therapy (2–8 sessions) did not require additional sessions to maintain lowered medical utilization.
- Patients seen two years or more in continuous psychotherapy demonstrated no overall decline in outpatient utilization (therapy visits supplanted medical visits). However, even these latter declined in inpatient utilization—from several times the plan average initially down to the plan average. Thus even long-term therapy is cost effective in reducing medical utilization when applied only to those patients that need it and should receive it.
- Cummings and Follette (1968) also concluded that in a prepaid plan that already employs educative techniques to both patients and physicians along with a range of psychological services, the number of subscribers seeking psychotherapy at a given time reaches an optimal level and remains constant thereafter.
- Over a five-year period, 85% of patients were seen for 15 or fewer sessions (mean of 8.6), and achieved a satisfactory state of well-being that continued into the eighth year after termination of therapy.
  The Kaiser Permanente medical cost-offset results have been extensively replicated in a variety of healthcare delivery systems with an overall "best estimate" of between 10% and 30% in cost savings; savings increase as interventions are tailored to the effective treatment of stress.

Psychotherapy and the Physically Ill Patient

In addition to somaticizing patients, there are also patients whose physical illness is either a source of stress, or for whom stress has contributed to or complicates the illness. A third category is the patient who experiences no discomfort, but for whom medical evaluation establishes the existence of illness (e.g., hypertension). Mechanic (1966) estimated that these three categories suggest that 95% of all medical-surgical patients could benefit from psychological interventions resulting in reduced medical costs.

An extensive literature documents the effectiveness of psychological interventions with chronic diseases such as diabetes, ischemic heart disease, airway diseases, and hypertension. These interventions reduce reliance on medications, numbers of hospital days post-surgery, and physician office visits. The potential savings in worker's compensation costs can be even greater as a result of behavioral outpatient pain treatment programs.

In light of the fact that inflation in healthcare is about 9% per year and the fact that inflation in mental healthcare is almost double at 16.5% per year due to increased hospitalization, any health system that does not include comprehensive mental health services will pay for stress-related conditions through over-utilization of its medical services. Psychologists have developed an impressive array of targeted, brief interventions focused on specific psychological conditions that aid in addressing these inflationary trends.

Brief, Targeted Therapy Techniques: Biodyne, a Case Study

Psychologists have developed and innovated brief intermittent therapy throughout the life cycle as a proven outpatient alternative to the over-hospitalization of emotionally disturbed adults, adolescents, and substance abusers. Biodyne, a psychology-driven managed mental health organization, using a wide array of protocols, has achieved what is regarded as the lowest psychiatric and substance abuse hospitalization in the nation while maintaining the highest standards in quality of care. In one market, the 178,000 enrollees averaged 114 hospital days per year per 1000 enrollees. Through application of its managed care techniques and clinical protocols, Biodyne reduced the rate of inpatient days to 4 per 1000 enrollees per year, demonstrating what can be accomplished through the application of state of the art psychological services.

It is important to note that the Biodyne Model of triaging somaticizers out of the medical system was not developed as a cost-containment procedure. Rather it was developed first to bring therapeutic effectiveness and relief from pain, anxiety and depression to the patient in psychological distress. In cases of physical illness, the psychologist accepts the illness as a given and concentrates on the patient's reaction to the condition (depression, rage, despair) and to neurotic conflicts that may be impeding recovery. The Biodyne Model of care was developed as part of an effective comprehensive mental health treatment system, and only then was it discovered that it was also cost-effective in terms of reducing medical costs.

Today, Biodyne provides comprehensive managed mental health-care services as an instrumental part of a comprehensive health plan program to almost two million health plan members throughout the United States.

CONCLUSION

- Persons in emotional distress overutilize medical services
- 60% of all physician visits are by patients with no physical disease
- Psychological intervention can reduce outpatient utilization by 50-65%
- Psychological intervention can reduce medical-surgical hospitalization by 60-75%
- With focused, targeted psychological intervention, 85% of patients can be helped with *brief* therapy

What Went Wrong After I left Biodyne, and the Future of Behavioral Managed Care

When I left Biodyne in 1993, I pleaded with the new owners to keep the clinical focus, and they promised me that they would. After some time, however, all of the clinical work we had done, the protocols we had developed, the methods of training and supervision— all that we had built up over the seven years—began to be dismantled. My daughter, Janet, was there and saw it happening.

J. C.: I stayed for three years after my father left the company. I saw a steady decay over that time until there was nothing left of the original model.

N. C.: If you are not a clinician, it is hard to understand the mission of Biodyne. Businesspeople think very differently. Since they are not tuned into the clinical issues, they go for the short run. When that happens, you do not see the medical cost savings, since the nature of the medical cost offset is that it becomes apparent over time. If you cut corners, you can have a short-term gain. That is what a lot of people do who run managed care companies, and that is why they will eventually fail. We are seeing that today.

L. T.: Once you told me that even when you founded Biodyne, you knew that the carve-out [i.e., the mental health part "carved out" from the rest of healthcare] wouldn't last. In one of your more recent articles, you point out that the usefulness of the carve-out is time-limited (Cummings, 1996).

N. C.: Yes, I predicted that over a decade ago. I said that managed care—or, more precisely, behavioral managed care—was going to have a life span of about ten years, then a three- to five-year period of chaos. Nobody believed me, and when I sold Biodyne, they still did not believe me, even though this prediction is coming true.

J. C.: When you left Biodyne, you were already envisioning that the carve-out would be phased out. Everyone else thought that the *behavioral healthcare model and HMOs were here to stay, and were saying, "Let's get used to it." You were already looking down the road to what the next step in the evolution of healthcare would be.*

N. C.: *The next step will have to be the integration of mental health treatment into medical care. Let's look at the current situation: There are 160 million lives covered under managed behavioral healthcare. Two companies now control 85 million. I find it hard to believe that 60 million lives can be managed properly by anyone. Let's say these companies merge. To manage 160 million lives—I just don't see how it can be done. My prediction is that all of the carve-outs are going to implode. This is going to happen more and more frequently. This kind of debacle will occur because the carve-outs have outlived their usefulness. They saved the mental health benefits from being discarded, they contained costs, and now there is no reason to keep mental health separate from the rest of healthcare. Mental health needs to be brought into all of medical care—which is what we learned at Kaiser over three decades ago.*

I can't predict exactly how these companies will collapse or become dysfunctional; there will be some kind of overall destruction. Managed care, as we know it today, will do itself in. But the overall idea of managed healthcare is never going to go away. The industrialization of healthcare has occurred, and it has to keep evolving. And it will evolve positively. But right now, the carve-out industry is fighting for survival.

L. T.: *What is your reply to all of those people in the American Psychological Association who are saying: "We're winning the battle. Managed care is falling apart. The tide is turning"?*

N. C: *Managed care will fall apart, but only in a sense. The elements that will stay are accountability, a new way of delivering psychological services (some of which are outlined in this book), and keeping a careful eye on the costs of delivering psychological services and overall medical care. Delivering time-effective therapy will remain very important, and long-term psychotherapy will be utilized less and less.*

{ 21 }

THE SOMATIZING PATIENT

THE SETTING

American Biodyne is a mental health maintenance organization (MHMO) that was founded in 1985. It is a privately held Delaware corporation that provides unlimited mental health/chemical dependency outpatient and hospitalization services to enrollees of Blue Cross/Blue Shield, Humana, Lincoln National, and several other health plans in 10 states. It currently serves contracts representing 2.5 million covered lives.

IN THE MID-1950s, the Kaiser Permanente Health Plan, the forerunner of the modern health maintenance organization, was startled to find that 60% of all visits to a physician by its two and a half million enrollees in California were by patients who had no physical illness (Follette & Cummings, 1967). At the time, this surprising figure was thought to reflect a propensity of the HMO: When access to medical services is no longer blocked by limitations, copayments, and deductibles, patients tend to overutilize medical facilities. In those early days, the relationship between stress and physical symptoms that is now known as "the somatization syndrome" was not clearly understood. Yet to label these patients "hypochondriacal," as physicians were likely to do in that era, would have suggested that hypochondria was so widespread as to be nearly universal. The term "No Significant Abnormality" was adopted and was entered as "NSA" in the medical chart by the physician. This term was not satisfactory because of its inaccuracy: These patients did, indeed, have a significant abnormality—the somatization of stress. The term that was adopted years later, and which remains in use, is the "worried well."

The Kaiser Permanente staff believed for many years that the somatization syndrome was peculiar to HMO patients. But in 1976, in his testimony on behalf of the American Medical Association to the U.S. Senate Subcommittee on Health, John Kelly stated that in the United States between 60% and 70% of all patients visiting a physician have no physical disease but are somatizing stress. Why had this figure emerged so early in capitated medicine while it remained obscure and hidden for so many years in fee-for-service medicine?

The answer was obvious. In fee-for-service medicine, the physician must enter an acceptable or suspected diagnosis on the reimbursement form before the third party payer will reimburse for service. The physician who is capitated, as was the case with the Kaiser Permanente HMO, has no need to enter an approximate diagnosis when a definite one does not exist inasmuch as that physician is paid by *prospective* reimbursement to render all subsequent medical care to a group of patient enrollees.

THE HISTORY OF SOMATIZATION

Historically the impact of psychological or emotional problems on physical health was acknowledged intuitively. Not only was the nature of this impact poorly understood, but also it lacked empirical validity. Early experiments in what was termed "psychosomatic medicine" focused on discovering personality types that correlated with certain physical complaints, such as peptic ulcers, migraine headaches, colitis, and so forth (Weiss & English, 1948). These experiments, conducted between 1930 and 1950, failed to find any significant relationship between personality type and physical illness, and interest in psychosomatic medicine waned.

During the same period, other researchers, notably psychologists who were convinced of a relationship between emotional distress and

physical symptoms, continued to research the impact of psychotherapy on people's lives. Identified with this research are such experimenters as Bergin, Luborsky, and Strupp (Bergin & Lambert, 1978).
The major difficulty with this psychotherapy outcome research, as it
came to be called, was the nature of the outcome criteria. A host of
soft outcome variables, such as changes in psychological test scores,
patient reports of "happiness," and measures of being "well adjusted" or
"maladjusted," simply did not discriminate the patient's status before
and after psychotherapy. One of the notable contributions of the
Cummings and Follette studies (1968, 1976) and the Cummings studies (1979, 1983, 1985b, 1985c) was the discovery of a hard measure of
psychotherapy outcome: a reduction in somatization as indicated by a
tabulation of medical utilization before and after psychotherapy
(Budman, Demby, & Feldstein, 1984).

The translation of stress into physical symptoms with consequent
overutilization of medical services was observed in England years before in patients with no physical disease (Balint, 1957). Great Britain,
with its national health care system, began grappling with the problem of the somatizer after the conclusion of World War II. The problem was also discovered in West Germany before it surfaced in the
United States (Jones & Vischi, 1979), and there is some early evidence
that somatization of stress, with consequent overutilization of medical facilities, exists in Japan (M. Sayama, personal communication,
1984).

HOW DOES SOMATIZATION TAKE PLACE?
A CASE ILLUSTRATION

Modern medicine, because of the way it is dispensed, inadvertently
encourages somatization. The physician, trained to find disease, becomes frustrated if he or she cannot find it in the presence of seemingly physical symptoms. Doing the job well requires that the disease
reflected in the symptoms be identified, so evaluations (including laboratory tests, X-rays, and CAT scans) are intensified. Eventually, the
physician gives up, sometimes telling the patient that these symptoms
are imaginary. The patient, convinced that he or she has a physical disease, then seeks out another physician with whom the entire process
is repeated. We have seen patients who serially exhausted over a

dozen physicians in this manner. An example may be helpful in understanding the process:

Bill was in his mid-fifties when the owner of the company where he worked, who was his closest friend, retired. Bill, an accountant, held the title of controller in this firm. The owner's son, fresh from graduate school with his new M.B.A. degree, assumed management of the company. One of his first projects was to computerize the accounting department. Bill, like many people his age, had a fear of computers and was convinced that he could never master them. He worried that he would be on the job market in his mid-fifties, unemployed, and in despair. He began to suffer from a general malaise that included loss of appetite, loss of interest in his surroundings, and inability to sleep. He consulted his physician, who found no physical disease, gave him reassurance, and admonished him that since he was not as young as he used to be, he ought to cut back his work schedule. (Bill was a conscientious man who tended to work long hours.) He was also told to come back in a month if he did not feel better, which Bill did as his malaise steadily increased.

The fact is that Bill was depressed due to his fears of being unemployed and too old to find a new job. He gave his physician a clue when he said at the end of his examination, "You know, Doc, I have this new young boss and he is really on my back." The physician, pressed for time and faced with a waiting room bulging with patients, did not hear this. In a subsequent visit, in which all of the tests again yielded negative results, Bill repeated his remark. "You know, Doc, this young boss is *really* on my back. He's making me nervous." This time Bill said the magic word "nervous" and received a prescription for Valium. Again, he was told to return in a month or two if he did not feel better.

This sequence was repeated a couple more times during which Bill began to complain of low back pain. (Neither he nor the physician recalled at that moment his having said "My boss is on my back.") This time the physician referred Bill to an orthopedist. Over time Bill's backache grew so severe that the specialist signed him out on sick leave. Now Bill did not have to confront the distasteful job situation. By the time the orthopedic surgeon had given up on Bill and referred him to the author for psychotherapy, Bill had an emotional investment in remaining sick and avoiding the job. His was not an easy case, but after six sessions he enrolled in a community college com-

puter class, lost his backache, and returned to work. His medical utilization, which had soared in the past several months, dropped dramatically.

SOMATIZATION AND THE PHYSICIAN

Highly skilled physicians consistently fail to recognize patients with
somatization disorders, in spite of repeated opportunities to diagnose
the behavior. Twenty to 30 physician visits per year might be typical
for a somatizing patient, and over 100 physician visits is not a rare oc-
currence, as reported by a five-year study that tracked a population of
over 100,000 persons (Cummings, Dörken, Pallak, & Henke, 1991,
1993). The medical utilization histories of these patients demonstrate exhaustive physician workups with numerous procedures and
even operations. It is not unusual for such patients to become drug-
dependent since the frustrated physician may rely heavily on overmedication. Iatrogenic exacerbation of their symptoms frequently results from physicians' repeated attempts to find their physical cause.
When an enlightened physician orders yet another laboratory test to
reassure the patient that there is no disease, the net effect is to oper-
antly condition the patient to continue the somatizing behavior and
even escalate the symptoms (Quill, 1985).

Originally, physicians regarded somatization as a form of hysteria.
Later, it was redefined as Briquet's Syndrome, a diagnosis that required the presence of no fewer than 25 of 60 symptoms drawn from
at least 9 of 10 symptom groups lacking in organic explanation.
Further, this multisystemic group of symptoms had to appear before
the patient reached the age of 35 (Quill, 1985). This stringent definition of somatization syndrome seemed to reflect physicians' resistance
to accepting the widespread existence of somatization in the general
population. The third edition of the *Diagnostic and Statistical
Manual of Mental Disorders* (DSM-III) reduced the number of symptoms required to make the diagnosis to 12 for men and 14 for women.
Then, as if to reverse its acceptance of these less stringent criteria,
DSM-III lowered to 30 years the age before which the syndrome of persistent, vague, multisystemic symptoms had to appear (Quill, 1985).
Given such continued resistance to the somatization paradigm, it is no
wonder that skilled physicians continue to underdiagnose the disorder.

A PRAGMATIC DEFINITION OF SOMATIZATION

Somatization is the translation of stress or emotional distress into seemingly physical symptoms where no organic etiology for these symptoms exists. The most frequent symptoms are neurodermatitis, heart palpitations, backaches, chronic headaches, abdominal pains that can change quadrants, chronic malaise, hyperventilation, low blood sugar, unusual allergies, bruxism, hyperemesis, and frequent urination or the inability to urinate freely (Quill, 1985). The somatizer can replicate any symptoms in the medical lexicon, often presenting a baffling array of them. Somatization can occur at any age following a stressful event and at any developmental stage in the life cycle, such as entering school, puberty, adolescence, graduation, adulthood, marriage, parenthood, divorce, bereavement, middle age, old age, and retirement. It can take the form of a single symptom or a group of symptoms that become the focus of the person's life and mask the precipitating stressors. The patient is increasingly convinced, despite all medical findings to the contrary, that the basis for the symptom or symptoms is organic illness and embarks on a never-ending quest for the right physician or the medical procedure that will discover the organic etiology. In the meantime, the psychological stressors go untreated while medical utilization and symptomatology escalate. It is not uncommon for somatizing patients to be hospitalized for an extensive number of medical tests after outpatient procedures have failed to detect organic etiology. If enough of them are administered, one or two inevitably will show marginal findings, as they would with any normal person. This only spurs the frustrated physician to look harder for the elusive, nonexistent organic cause.

Curiously, in spite of the pain and suffering shown by the somatizer, no primary anxiety or depression is present. It is as if the anxiety and depression associated with the stressors have been bound in the somatic symptomatology. Overt anxiety or depression is usually secondary to the somatized condition: "How would you feel if you were sick all the time?"

The author's 30 years of research on somatization have demonstrated that, for most somatizers, the behavior was rewarded in the early days of childhood: "Daddy, I didn't take out the garbage last night because my head was hurting too much from doing my homework." Parents often gave an overabundance of affection and attention when the child was ill, while remaining relatively aloof when the child was physically well. As the offspring of nurses, some somatizers learned in childhood that illness would bring attention from a dedicated caregiver.

THE MEDICAL OFFSET PHENOMENON

The pioneering research at Kaiser Permanente that demonstrated a reduction in medical utilization among somatizers following psychological intervention has been replicated over 30 times with similar results (Jones & Vischi, 1979).

Initially Kaiser Permanente experimented with a number of attempts to provide long-term therapy for all subscribers manifesting emotional distress. These efforts were prompted by the belief that short-term therapy was not as effective as long-term, and by the discovery that providing easily available comprehensive health services as part of a prepaid plan fostered the somatization of emotional problems and the consequent overuse of medical facilities by patients with no physical illness. The result of providing long-term therapy was a long waiting list, a high dropout rate, and only partially successful attempts to reduce the ever-growing waiting list by providing crisis intervention. After several years on such an unsatisfactory course, a series of evaluative studies began that spanned two and a half decades. During this period, an efficient, treatment system emerged that was both therapeutically and financially effective.

In the first of a series of investigations into the relationship between psychological services and medical utilization in a prepaid health care setting, Follette and Cummings (1967) compared the number and type of medical services sought before and after psychotherapeutic intervention in a large group of randomly selected patients. Outpatient and inpatient medical utilization for the year immediately prior to the initial interview in the Department of Psychotherapy, as well as for the five years following it, were studied for three groups of psychotherapy patients. These three groups consisted of patients who had been seen for (a) one therapy session only; (b) brief therapy, with a mean of 6.4 interviews; and (c) long-term therapy with a mean of 33.9 interviews. A "control" group of matched patients demonstrated similar criteria of distress but had not, in the six years under study, been seen in psychotherapy. The findings indicate the following:

1. Persons in emotional distress use both inpatient (hospitalization) and outpatient medical facilities significantly more than average health plan patients.

2. Emotionally distressed individuals who received psychotherapy used medical services significantly less than a "control" group of matched emotionally distressed health plan members who were not accorded psychotherapy.

3. These declines remained constant during the five years following termination of psychotherapy.

4. The most significant declines occurred in the second year after the initial interview; those patients especially who received only one session of brief therapy (two to eight sessions) did not require additional psychotherapy in order to maintain the lower utilization for five years.

5. Patients seen for two years or more in continuous psychotherapy demonstrated no overall decline in total outpatient utilization inasmuch as psychotherapy visits tended to supplant medical visits. However, there was a significant decline in inpatient utilization in this long-term therapy group, from an initial rate several times that of the health plan average to a level comparable to that of the general adult health plan population.

In a subsequent study, Cummings and Follette (1968) found that intensive efforts to increase the number of referrals to psychotherapy by using computerized psychological screening to perform early detection of somatization and alert physicians to its presence did not have that effect. The authors concluded that in a prepaid health plan setting already maximally employing educative techniques to both patients and physicians and already providing a range of prepaid psychological services, the number of subscribers seeking psychotherapy reached an optimal level and remained constant thereafter.

To summarize nearly two decades of prepaid health plan experience, Cummings and Follette (1976) demonstrated that there is no basis for the fear that increased demand for psychotherapy will financially endanger the system. It is not the number of referrals that drives costs upward, but the manner in which psychotherapy services are delivered. The finding that one session only, with no repeat psychological visits, can reduce medical utilization by 60% over the following five years was surprising and totally unexpected. Equally surprising was the 75% reduction in medical utilization over a five-year period by those patients receiving two to eight psychotherapy visits (brief therapy).

In an eighth-year telephone follow-up, Cummings and Follette (1976) sought to answer whether the previously described results could be attributed to therapeutic, deleterious, or extraneous factors. It was hypothesized that if a patient had achieved better understanding of the problem through the psychotherapy sessions, he or she would recall the actual problem rather than the presenting symptom. It was also hypothesized that the presenting symptom would have disappeared and that the patient would be coping more effectively with other problems. The results suggested that the reduction in medical utilization was the consequence of resolving the emotional distress reflected in the symptoms and in the visits to the doctor. The modal patient in the eight-year follow-up can be described as follows: He or she denied ever having consulted a physician about the symptoms for which the referral was originally made. Rather, the underlying problem discussed with the psychotherapist was recalled as the reason for the psychotherapy visit. Although the problem was resolved, this resolution was attributed to the patient's own efforts and no credit was given to the psychotherapist. This affirms the contention that the reduction in medical utilization reflected the diminution in emotional distress that was originally expressed in symptoms presented to the physician.

In their earlier work, Cummings and Follette (1968) addressed the question of cost-effectiveness by demonstrating that savings in medical services offset the cost of providing psychotherapy. However, they insisted that the services provided must also be therapeutic in that they reduce the patient's emotional distress. Therapeutic success was predicted in a model that involved the analysis of transference and resistance, uncovered unconscious conflicts, and had all of the characteristics of long-term therapy except length. In fact, over a five-year period, 84.6% of the psychotherapy patients chose to come for 15 sessions or fewer (with a mean of 8.6). Follow-up showed that, far from being "dropouts," these patients had achieved a satisfactory state of well-being that continued to the eighth year after termination of therapy. Of the remainder, 10.1% were found to be "interminable," in that once they began psychotherapy, they seemingly continued with no indication of termination.

In another study, Cummings (1979) addressed the problem of the interminable patient for whom treatment was neither cost-effective nor therapeutically effective. The concept that some persons may be so emotionally crippled that they may have to be maintained for many years or for life was unacceptable: If 5% of the patients entering psychotherapy were in that category, within a few years a program would be hampered by a monolithic case load. (This has in fact happened in many public clinics where psychotherapy is offered at nominal or no cost.) The hypothesis of the study was that these patients required more intensive intervention, and the frequency of psychotherapy visits was doubled for one experimental group, tripled for another, and held constant for the control group. Surprisingly, the cost-therapeutic effectiveness ratios deteriorated in direct proportion to the increased intensity of treatment: that is, medical utilization increased and the patients manifested greater emotional distress. It was only by reversing the process and seeing these patients at spaced intervals of once every two or three months that the desired cost-therapeutic effect was obtained. These results are surprising in that they seem to disprove traditionally held notions in psychotherapy, but they demonstrate the need for ongoing research, program evaluation, and innovation if psychotherapy is to be made available to everyone.

The Cost-Therapeutic Effectiveness Ratio (Cummings, 1979) and the 38 Criteria of Distress (Follette & Cummings, 1967) have proved to be useful evaluation tools at Kaiser Permanente, American Biodyne, and other large-scale health systems, enabling them to innovate cost-therapeutically effective programs for somatization, alcoholism, drug addiction, the "interminable" patient, chronic psychosis, problems of the elderly, severe character disorders, and other conditions considered by many to be too costly, and, therefore, uninsurable.

METHODS, TOOLS, AND INTERVENTIONS
FOR THE TREATMENT OF SOMATIZERS

"Outreaching" the Somatizer

In testimony before the United States Senate (Cummings, 1985c), it was reported that patients who are experiencing emotional stress generally find "an unsympathetic or uncomprehending ear" when they attempt to discuss their distress with their physician. They quickly begin to translate their problems into the form of X-rays, laboratory tests, prescriptions, and return visits to the primary care specialist. Outreach programs are needed to bring these patients into a psychological service where the causes of their stress can be addressed.

Physician education. The best way to outreach the somatizer is by educating the physician. This task is not as easy as the statement implies. Physicians are trained to find physical disease and are not trained or rewarded for thinking psychologically. Rarely does a physician look for the signs of somatization syndrome. Rather, the typical approach is to eliminate the presence of disease, using exhaustive medical tests. This process only reinforces the patient's belief that he or she has a physical illness while it frustrates the physician, who eventually loses interest in the patient. The patient responds with feelings of hurt and betrayal that are reflected in increased demands on the physician for attention.

Adjusting the system of compensation. The form of compensation often influences practice as it relates to the somatizer. In one large health system where physicians were capitated in the style of the HMO, they identified and referred 83% of their somatizers for psychological intervention, while fee-for-service physicians referred fewer than 6% (Cummings, 1988a; Dörken & Cummings, 1986). In the latter group, there were too many physicians in the community competing for the same patients. Unfortunately, somatizers can represent a substantial portion of a physician's income. This may be true especially of dermatology, where 50% to 60% of patients may suffer from neurodermatitis, a clearly somatized condition. This does not mean that physicians are dishonest or cynical. Rather, it reflects unconscious motivation; the capitated physician has no reward for holding on to the somatizer, while the fee-for-service physician has an unrecognized reward for keeping him or her in the medical system.

Because physicians vary in their ability to identify and refer these patients for psychological intervention, it is often necessary to outreach the patient. Integral to effective treatment is a program that can triage the patient out of the medical system into a psychological system. All patients who have made 20 or more physician visits in one year should be contacted. Of these, somewhat fewer than half generally have a chronic physical illness that requires regular, sustained medical intervention, and more than half will be somatizers. Although some somatizers make fewer than 20 physician visits in one year, this number is the cut-off point at which it is efficient to target outreach. The upper range can exceed 300 such visits in one year, with 32 as the mean and 28 as the mode. Where psychologists have contracted to provide services for an existing health plan, the client organization is usually more than willing to provide a computer print-out of patients who have made more than 50 visits in a 12-month period.

Contact by telephone. Psychiatric nurses are ideal professionals to conduct telephone outreach because they have extensive knowledge of physical illness, are familiar with somatization syndrome, and possess psychotherapeutic skills. Medical social workers have similar knowledge and skills and are an acceptable substitute for psychiatric nurses. Psychologists can also perform telephone outreach if using this level of professional is cost-effective.

The outreach worker is responsible for calling a predetermined number of high medical utilizers. At the time of the phone contact, the patient's belief in the somatic nature of his or her complaints should not be challenged. The patient's interest can usually be aroused by the statement, "Someone who has had as much illness as you certainly must be upset about it." This usually elicits an immediate reaction, ranging from an exposition of symptoms to the complaint that physicians don't seem to understand or to be sympathetic to the patient's plight. After hearing the patient out sufficiently to permit the development of some initial trust, the patient is invited to explore how the counselor (a less threatening term than mental health provider) might be of help. It is suggested that together they can perhaps investigate alternatives to treatments that have not worked, or that the patient can be put in touch with a more sympathetic physician, should the difficulty be better appraised. An initial appointment for psychotherapy is made.

Contact by mail. Periodic mailings is another method used in an attempt to bring somatizing patients into psychotherapy. Brochures or newsletters can remind these high medical utilizers of the services available to them. In addition, the regular newsletter of a health plan can feature articles about a specific somatic complaint in each issue. The condition can be described and discussed, with accompanying recommendations for change, along with the suggestion that an appointment with a counselor may be appropriate.

Community education programs. Outreach personnel are also encouraged to take part in presentations to the community and to local industries in an attempt to further identify high utilizers and encourage their participation in psychotherapy. This allows the prospective patient or potential referer (employer, friend, or coworker) to view the members of the psychological service in vivo and achieve a degree of comfort he or she otherwise might not have.

Triage. Once the patient comes to the office, it is vital that the therapist not challenge the somatization but marshall his or her interviewing skills to detect the underlying problem. Once the problem or set of problems is determined, the therapist treats these without ever directly relating them to the physical symptoms. In fact, most patients conclude therapy with a relief of somatic symptoms and no conscious knowledge of the relationship between psychological factors and previous physical complaints.

It is important to note that our model of triaging somatizers out of the medical system and into a psychological system was not developed as a cost containment measure. Rather, it was developed primarily to bring therapeutic effectiveness and relief of pain, anxiety, and depression to the patient in psychological distress. It became an integral part of a therapeutically effective, comprehensive mental health treatment system, and only then was it discovered to be cost-effective as well.

In cases of any concurrent actual physical illness, the therapist accepts the illness as a given. At that point, the therapist concentrates on the patient's reaction to the condition (depression, rage, despair) and also to any neurotic conflicts that may be impeding recovery. These issues are then addressed in the course of psychotherapy.

Preventive Health Care

Garfield et al. (1976) enunciated a method of triage in which the "worried well" are referred to a health education bypass that is essentially educative, psychological, and behavioral in nature. This relieves the physician of having to identify the somatizer by a process of elimination following weeks, months, and even years of expensive medical diagnosis procedures.

As a result of extensive cumulative research and through the use of the cost–therapeutic effectiveness ratio, a series of focused brief therapy protocols targeted to 68 specific psychological stress conditions have emerged. Along with an outreach system, these protocols enable practitioners to be of real assistance to individuals during stressful points in their lives (Cummings, 1985b). The model that has evolved is called Brief Intermittent Therapy Throughout the Life Cycle. These psychological interventions are not only efficient, in that an average of only 6.4 sessions is required, but also effective, in that problem-solving is highly focused. The interventions are applied only at times of stress, rather than protracted over months and probably years as is done in the traditional model of psychotherapy.

Such stressful periods may coincide not only with developmental milestones, but also with marriage, divorce, births, deaths, bankruptcy, surgery, job changes, geographical relocations, retirement, and so forth. Wide individual variations in handling stressors exist, but the typical maladaptive response in somatization is a dramatic increase in medical utilization. Using a reduction in medical utilization as a measure of resolution of stress, a wide range of preventive health studies have been undertaken. The following examples provide a sample of their findings.

High pediatric utilization. High medical utilization by children often reflects the unhappiness or marital conflict of the parents. An example is the somatization of stress in children whose parents are threatening each other with divorce. The child often learns that his or her "illness" temporarily brings the parents together over concern for the child's health, resulting in an escalation of pediatric utilization as talk of divorce escalates. Psychological intervention with the parents reduced pediatric utilization by 63% the following year. This contrasted with the control group of high pediatric utilizers whose utilization increased slightly but not significantly.

Bereavement. Following the death of a spouse, medical utilization often increases dramatically. In some cases, the symptoms may replicate those of the deceased's terminal illness. Psychologically, this is a way of keeping the deceased "alive" (introjection) or assuaging guilt for negative behavior toward the deceased while still alive. This reaction can represent total somatization, or the promulgation of an actual disease such as cancer, heart disease, or stroke. It has been noted that there is a 20% rise in such actual physical illness following the death of a long-standing spouse. Bereavement counseling reduces medical utilization to expected levels in cases of somatization. An experiment is underway to determine if bereavement counseling can reduce the number of subsequent actual physical illnesses compared with those of a control group.

Surgery. Presurgical counseling by a psychologist can reduce hospitalization by an average of 1.3 days. Similar results have been demonstrated in a number of other studies (Olbrisch, 1977). Typically, this counseling takes place on an outpatient basis before the surgery, but in cases where the need for treatment is sudden, can be conducted in the hospital on the eve of the surgical procedure. Although it is an effective intervention in a number of procedures ranging from appendectomy to henioraphy, it is particularly effective in cases where the procedure has intense psychological meaning to the patient (e.g., hysterectomy) or in cases where the postoperative recovery is long, and accompanying depression is typical (e.g., open heart surgery).

Asthmatic children. Children who have severe asthmatic attacks often are reflecting their parents' marital conflicts. In a typical case, the child might be awakened on a Friday night by the sound of his or her parents quarreling. The parents are tense about having to spend the whole weekend together. Unconsciously, the child has learned that a severe asthmatic attack necessitating an emergency room visit will terminate the quarrel and temporarily bring the parents together. Marital counseling was found to eliminate such emergency room visits, which nonetheless continued for the control group.

Alcoholism. Alcoholics are high utilizers of medical services, but their illness is seldom diagnosed by their primary care physicians, in spite of such severe side effects as cirrhosis, acute pancreatitis, bone fractures, and accidental burns. The medical utilization rates of alcoholics who followed a successful substance abuse program and remained sober during the subsequent year dropped by 77%, and there was a significant reduction in school problems among their children.

Stepparenting. In a search to identify psychosocial stressors, it was noted that a group of high pediatric utilizers had in common the recent acquisition of a stepparent. Group stepparenting counseling with both the natural and stepparents reduced this overutilization by 61% in the year after counseling. The control group maintained its level of pediatric overutilization. The critical factor in the counseling was the subsequent relaxation of the stepparent, who had been trying to achieve the approval and acceptance of the stepchild.

Heart attacks. Parents who suffer myocardial infarction (MI) and who demonstrate signs of depression on a psychological questionnaire return to work weeks later than those patients who do not show those depressive signs (Friedman, Ury, Klatsky, & Siegelaub, 1974). MI patients receiving psychological intervention returned to work significantly sooner than those not receiving such intervention. The sooner the counseling occurred following the MI, the more positive was the outcome.

Retirement. Even though most people look forward to retirement, it is a stressful time of abrupt change. Often the marital equilibrium is upset by a husband who is now constantly at home, yet is reluctant to change his life-style by beginning to perform new behaviors, such as sharing the household chores. Medical utilization, which often shows a sharp increase immediately following retirement, can be maintained at customary levels with preretirement counseling. It is important to prepare not only the retiree but also the spouse for the disequilibrium the new life-style will bring.

Problems and Disadvantages of Outreach Programs

Two caveats are important when using the method of outreaching and triaging the somatizer. The first pertains to resistance that will be engendered on the part of the somatizer if the therapist directly challenges the patient's belief that a physical disease exists. The patient will bolt, only to continue to pursue physical verification through still another physician. Future attempts to reach this patient will be decidedly more difficult. The therapist must win the patient's confidence and address his or her stress without ever challenging the belief that the symptoms represent a physical disease. Most somatizers, once the cause of the stress is ascertained and ameliorated, will abandon the symptomatology and reduce medical utilization. Often, they will leave psychological treatment without ever having made the connection. To insist on linking the symptom with the stress may result in such a loss of self-esteem that gains may be undone.

The second caveat involves the use of overly zealous outreach programs that may result in actual physical disease being overlooked. Cummings (1985a) reports a computerized outreach program that had to be discontinued because it significantly increased the number of medical diagnoses missed by participating physicians. It was almost as if the physicians had so espoused the concept of somatization that they dispensed with the kinds of physical examination and medical tests that would have elicited an existing disease.

CONCLUSION

The most frequent manifestation of stress is somatization. Appropriate medical intervention that treats the stress will result in a dramatic reduction of medical utilization: the so-called medical offset phenomenon. Reduction in medical utilization is a reliable and useful measure of stress resolution. Stress points and stress factors occur throughout the life cycle and are, to some degree, predictable. A com-

bination of triage by the primary care physician and aggressive outreach programs will alleviate the symptoms of stress by directing the
worried-well into problem-solving brief therapy. This results in a preventive health care system that directly promotes the mental health of
individuals and their families.

ADVICE TO HMO PRACTITIONERS

The medical offset literature has demonstrated that somatization can
significantly tax medical resources in any health care system. Through
outreach, HMO psychotherapists are in an excellent position to triage
the somatizer out of the medical system and into a psychological system where the patient will receive relief from suffering and the HMO
will save substantially more than the cost of providing the psychological interventions. Even though the physician compensation structure
in an HMO is conducive to appropriate referral, there is still a need to
educate the physician on how to make the referral without insulting
the patient's belief in the medical nature of the symptom. It is equally
important for the psychotherapist not to challenge the belief system
while still addressing the causes of stress.

An appropriate outreach and treatment program for the somatizing
patient must involve the physician, HMO management, and even the
community. Although the savings in medical costs are an incentive for
the HMO, the therapist's reward is the satisfaction that comes from
the provision of appropriate treatment and the consequent recovery
of a patient whose pain was escalating in response to inappropriate
medical treatment.

{ 22 }

INPATIENT AND OUTPATIENT PSYCHIATRIC TREATMENT: THE EFFECT OF MATCHING PATIENTS TO APPROPRIATE LEVEL OF TREATMENT ON PSYCHIATRIC AND MEDICAL-SURGICAL HOSPITAL DAYS*

ABSTRACT. *The effects of inpatient or outpatient treatment for psychiatric disorder on posttreatment hospital days were examined for 106 Health Maintenance Organization (HMO) patients who initially presented for inpatient treatment. Based on a complete mental status examination and the availability of appropriate treatment alternatives, 15% were admitted to inpatient and 85% were referred for intensive outpatient treatment. In the 12 months following treatment, (a) neither group had further psychiatric hospital days and (b) those treated on an outpatient basis had fewer medical-surgical hospital days. Number of medical-surgical hospital days was lower for patients who completed the full treatment plan. These results complemented experimental research regarding the clinical effectiveness of outpatient treatment alternatives.*

THE RELATIONSHIP BETWEEN inpatient hospitalization and outpatient treatment for psychiatric disorders has become a national policy issue (Grover, 1991; Kiesler & Sibulkin, 1987). Kiesler and Sibulkin

---

* With Michael S. Pallak, Ph.D.

(1987) reviewed literature in which patients were randomly assigned to either inpatient or outpatient treatment. Patients assigned to outpatient mental health treatment did as well or better on most measures of outcome during the following year than did patients assigned to inpatient treatment.

Strumwasser et al. (1991) reviewed 539 psychiatric and substance abuse admissions using a standardized review protocol for appropriateness of admission. Their analysis suggested that about 38% of inpatient days (about 30% for psychiatric and 60% for substance abuse) could have been handled on an outpatient basis. Unnecessary inpatient days were strongly associated with unnecessary inpatient admissions rather than with excessive lengths of stay.

Duhl and Cummings (1987) noted that referral of psychiatric and chemical dependency (CDP) patients to outpatient treatment has gained substantial momentum because of rising costs for inpatient treatment. There was concern, however, that such efforts, if driven only by cost containment motives, may compromise care and treatment. Patients denied appropriate mental health and psychiatric treatment may substitute medical or nonpsychiatric hospitalization when access to appropriate mental health treatment is denied (cf. Cummings & Follette, 1968; Follette & Cummings, 1967; Jones & Vischi, 1979).

Psychiatric patients referred inappropriately from psychiatric hospitalization may seek hospitalization in nonpsychiatric facilities or under nonpsychiatric medical-surgical diagnoses. Patients may deteriorate clinically, medical problems may be exacerbated, and somaticization of the disorder may increase (cf. Cummings & Follette, 1968; Follette & Cummings, 1967). As a result, nonpsychiatric physicians, who may not understand or recognize the emotional and psychiatric components of the patient's condition, may be more likely to admit the patient under medical-surgical diagnoses and into nonpsychiatric units (cf. Kiesler & Sibulkin, 1987).

If so, the potential savings to the healthcare system in reduced psychiatric hospitalization may be attenuated by substituting, and thereby increasing, hospitalization in nonpsychiatric facilities under nonpsychiatric diagnoses. The empirical issue can be assessed by examining patterns of psychiatric and medical-surgical hospitalization following either inpatient psychiatric hospitalization or referral to outpatient treatment.

The present case study included patients who presented for psychiatric hospitalization during a 6-month period that were then tracked in terms of psychiatric and medical hospitalization in the year following the initial treatment episode. Specifically, the study sought to answer the question of whether patients referred to intensive outpatient rather than inpatient treatment were later hospitalized under psychiatric or medical-surgical diagnoses.

A second issue regarding psychiatric inpatient or outpatient treatment is whether or not patients complete the treatment plan (cf. Cummings, 1988a, 1991a, 1991b, 1991c, 1994). Outpatient treatment may be of limited usefulness if patients do not complete the treatment either as the follow-up component to inpatient treatment or as an alternative clinical component of the treatment plan. The rationale for inpatient treatment has often been the potential advantage gained by systematic exposure to treatment and care while in the inpatient facility. Patients who do not complete treatment may be more likely to seek other hospitalization in the same fashion as undertreated patients.

METHOD

The present study examined all patients from a Health Maintenance Organization (HMO) population of 67,000 in a midwestern metropolitan area who presented for inpatient psychiatric hospitalization from July through December 1989. These patients were tracked during the 12 months following the treatment episode in terms of hospital days for psychiatric and medical-surgical diagnoses.

About 20% of the patients studied were evaluated for admission at their request (self-referred) at the HMO Center. The remaining 80% were evaluated in hospital emergency and admitting rooms. In each instance, the mental healthcare provider (a doctoral level psychologist with on-call psychiatric backup as needed) made an immediate, complete mental status examination on site. As part of the evaluation for appropriate level of care, this procedure recognizes that a good predictor of suitability for outpatient therapy is the patient's ability to respond to therapy on site (Cummings, 1990, 1991b, 1991c). Following the on-site evaluation, the mental healthcare provider reported the results and recommendations to the physician who made the formal decision to admit or refer to intensive outpatient treatment.

In all cases of admission, postdischarge outpatient treatment was incorporated in the treatment plan. The treatment approach is fully described elsewhere (Cummings, 1988a, 1991b, 1991c, 1994; Cummings & VandenBos, 1979). The HMO mental health treatment was provided on an exclusive provider organization (EPO) basis, thereby facilitating tracking patients' psychiatric services utilization over time. The intensive outpatient treatment was part of an expanded array of treatment options provided without copayment, without limits on the number of visits, and without deductible requirements (Cummings, 1991a).

RESULTS

A total of 1,259 patients received outpatient or inpatient mental health treatment (MHT) during the 6-month period. These patients represented a 3.76% annual penetration rate for the covered HMO population. Of these treated patients, 106 presented for inpatient psychiatric admission, representing a 0.32% annual rate for all enrollees and a 16.84% annual rate for all patients seeking mental health treatment. Approximately 45% ($n = 48$) were men and 55% ($n = 58$) were women. Mean age for men (33.35% years) did not differ from mean age for women (32.70), and the present analyses are not disaggregated by gender or age.

Inpatient Versus Intensive Outpatient Treatment

Patients who were admitted to inpatient or referred to outpatient treatment are summarized in Table 1 by DSM-III-R diagnosis. Based on the complete mental status examination of 106 patients who presented for admission, 15.09% ($n = 16$) were admitted to inpatient treatment and 84.91% ($n = 90$) were referred to intensive outpatient treatment. Table 1 also summarizes the distribution of diagnoses for patients presenting for admission and the percentage of each diagnosis category admitted or referred to outpatient treatment.

Depression was the diagnosis in 15.09% of those presenting, and 43.75% of these were admitted. Borderline diagnoses represented 11.32% of those presenting, and 33.33% were admitted. Adolescent conduct disorders were diagnosed in 15.09% of those presenting, and 18.75% were admitted. Psychoses were diagnosed in 11.32% of those presenting, and 16.67% were admitted.

Chemical dependency diagnoses and adjustment reactions were seen in 29.24% and 17.92%, respectively, of those presenting, and all

Table 1. *Patients Presenting for Inpatient Psychiatric Admission or Referred to Outpatient Treatment*

			Outcome			
	Presenting		Inpatient		Outpatient	
Diagnosis[a]	n	%[b]	n	%[c]	n	%[c]
ACD	16	15.09	3	18.75	13	81.25
Depression	16	15.09	7	43.75	9	56.00
Borderline	12	11.32	4	33.33	8	66.67
Psychosis	12	11.32	2	16.67	10	83.33
CDP	31	29.24	0		31	100.00
AR	19	17.92	0		19	100.00
Total	106		16		90	

[a]ACD = adolescent conduct disorder; CDP = chemical dependency; AR = adjustment reaction.
[b]Percentage of total patients presenting for treatment.
[c]Percentage of total patients in each diagnosis category.

Table 2. *Distribution of 106 Patients Admitted as Inpatients or Referred to Outpatient Treatment*

	Inpatients (n = 16)		Outpatients (n = 90)	
Diagnosis[a]	n	%[b]	n	%[c]
ACD	3	17.87	13	14.44
Depression	7	43.75	9	10.00
Borderline	4	25.00	8	8.88
Psychosis	2	12.50	10	11.11
CDP	0	0.00	31	34.44
AR	0	0.00	19	21.11

[a]ACD = adolescent conduct disorder; CDP = chemical dependency; AR = adjustment reaction.
[b]Percentage of total inpatient admissions.
[c]Percentage of total outpatient referrals.

of these individuals were referred to outpatient treatment. The results presented in Table 2 summarize by diagnosis the percentages of the total number of patients admitted and the total number of patients referred to outpatient treatment.

Diagnoses of depression were overrepresented among those patients admitted relative to the percentage of those presenting with depression diagnoses (43.75% vs. 15.09%, respectively; $t = 2.41, p < .02$). Borderline diagnoses were overrepresented among those admitted relative to those presenting (25.00% vs. 11.32%, respectively; $t = 1.35$) although the difference was not significant.

Those patients with CDP diagnoses were underrepresented among those admitted relative to the percentage of those presenting (0.00% vs. 29.24%, respectively; $t = 2.94$, $p < .01$). Similarly, adjustment reaction diagnoses were underrepresented among those admitted relative to those presenting (0.00% vs. 17.92%, respectively; $t = 1.94$, $p < .06$).

In short, patients admitted to inpatient treatment were more likely to have depression diagnoses and less likely to have CDP or adjustment reaction diagnoses than the overall distribution of diagnoses among patients presenting for admission. Admissions for patients with the remaining diagnoses (adolescent conduct disorder, borderline personality, or psychoses) were not significantly different in relation to those presenting.

Table 3 summarizes the mean number of inpatient psychiatric treatment days for those admitted, number of outpatient treatment visits for those admitted (follow-up treatment) or referred to outpatient, and the mean number of hospital days under psychiatric and medical-surgical diagnoses in the year following the initial treatment episode. Whether admitted or referred to intensive outpatient treatment, none of the 106 patients presenting for admission had inpa-

Table 3. *Initial Inpatient and Outpatient Psychiatric Treatment and Subsequent Hospitalization During 12-Month Follow-up Period*

Diagnosis[a]	n	Initial Treatment		No. Subsequent Hospital Days	
		No. Inpatient Days	No. Outpatient Visits	Psychiatric	Medical
Inpatients ($N = 16$)					
ACD	3	16.00	0	0	1.00
Depression	7	10.44	11.43	0	0.43
Borderline	4	4.75	0	0	1.25
Psychosis	2	5.00	28.00	0	1.50
CDP	0	—	—	—	—
AR	0	—	—	—	—
Mean		9.00	8.5	0	0.875
Outpatients ($N = 90$)					
ACD	13	0	14.54	0	0.15
Depression	9	0	21.88	0	0.55
Borderline	8	0	26.00	0	0
Psychosis	10	0	19.90	0	0.50
CDP	31	0	19.29	0	0
AR	19	0	3.84	0	0
Mean		0	16.27	0	0.133

Note. Number of days or visits are means for each diagnosis category.
[a]ACD = adolescent conduct disorder; CDP = chemical dependency; AR = adjustment reaction.

tient psychiatric hospital days in the 12 months following the treatment episode. Although the results in Table 3 are presented by diagnosis, the analysis is aggregated over diagnoses because variations among diagnoses were not significant because of relatively small sample sizes.

Patients admitted to inpatient psychiatric treatment (n = 16) had an average of 9.00 inpatient treatment days followed by an average of 8.5 follow-up outpatient treatment visits. Those patients referred to intensive outpatient treatment (n = 90) did not have inpatient treatment days and averaged 16.27 outpatient treatment visits.

In contrast, the 1,153 patients who did not present for hospital admission averaged 4.60 outpatient psychiatric visits over all diagnoses in the same time period. Clearly, those presenting for admission represented a more seriously ill subset of mental health patients in terms of utilization and intensity of treatment needed and received. The absence of further inpatient psychiatric days in the year following the treatment episode suggests that treatment received (inpatient or outpatient) was clinically effective for both subsets of patients.

Patients admitted to inpatient treatment had a total of 14 hospital days under medical-surgical diagnoses (M = 0.875 days per patient) in the year following the treatment episode. In contrast, patients referred to outpatient treatment had a total of 12 days (M = 0.133 days per patient) under medical-surgical diagnoses. The difference in subsequent medical-surgical hospital days between patients initially admitted to inpatient treatment and patients initially referred to outpatient treatment was significant (t = 3.59, p < .01). Thus patients referred to the intensive outpatient treatment alternative had significantly fewer medical-surgical hospital days in the year following treatment than those admitted to inpatient treatment.

Completion of Outpatient Follow-up and Outpatient Treatment

An additional analysis was performed for those patients who, for whatever reason, did not complete the full outpatient treatment plan (either as follow-up to inpatient treatment or as the intensive alternative treatment). Of those admitted to inpatient treatment, 11 of 16 (68.75%) did not complete outpatient follow-up treatment. In contrast, only 8 of 90 (8.89%) of those referred to outpatient treatment did not

complete. This difference in completion rates was highly significant
($t = 4.98, p < .001$).

The mean numbers of medical-surgical hospital days in the year following initial treatment for those patients ($n = 19$) who did not complete outpatient treatment (1.21 days per patient) and for those ($n =
87$) who did complete the outpatient treatment plan (0.03 days per pa-
tient) were significantly different ($t = 6.98, \ p < .001$). An important
issue in further research remains the exploration of variables related to
treatment completion.

DISCUSSION

Patients who presented for inpatient hospitalization ($n = 106$) were
more ill in terms of intensity of treatment needed and received than
were mental health patients in general ($n = 1,153$). Patients who were
admitted after evaluation had an average of 9.00 inpatient days (similar to national averages, Kiesler & Sibulkin, 1987; Pallak, Sibulkin, &
Kiesler, 1987) and 8.5 follow-up outpatient visits. Patients referred to
intensive outpatient used no inpatient days and had 16.27 outpatient
visits. For both subsets of patients, number of outpatient visits was
substantially higher than those for other mental health patients who
did not present for hospitalization.

Neither set of patients had instances of later psychiatric hospitalization in the year following the treatment episode. In studies with randomized assignment to inpatient or to outpatient treatment (Kiesler &
Sibulkin, 1987), patients assigned to outpatient treatment showed
fewer subsequent inpatient psychiatric hospital days than those assigned to inpatient treatment, but the number of days was greater
than zero. A proportion of those randomly assigned to outpatient,
however, may have actually needed inpatient treatment, and outpatient treatment may have been inadequate for the conditions presented, perhaps resulting in subsequent rehospitalization under
psychiatric diagnoses.

The HMO population in the present study may have represented a
less seriously ill group relative to the populations in the randomized
studies. As a result, the inpatient or outpatient treatment would have
been adequate for each patient and would have resulted in the zero rehospitalization under psychiatric diagnoses. Preadmission evaluation

and concurrent review (two factors emphasized by Strumwasser et al., 1991), coupled with the HMO emphasis on initial and intensive treatment, may have enhanced the effectiveness of treatment received by more precisely matching patient to treatment (Cummings, 1991b, 1991c). The exact relationship between these several possible factors is, however, beyond the scope of the present study.

Patients referred to outpatient treatment had fewer subsequent hospital days under medical and surgical diagnoses than did those admitted initially to inpatient treatment. Although this study was conducted under field conditions, our results concerning subsequent rehospitalization are consistent with the implications of randomized experimental studies reviewed by Kiesler and Sibulkin (1987).

The small number of subsequent medical-surgical hospital days in our study does not support the contention that referral to intensive outpatient treatment alternatives may result in either psychiatric rehospitalizations (a "revolving door"; Kiesler & Sibulkin, 1987) or substitution of medical-surgical hospital days because of psychiatric undertreatment. Our results indicate that intensive outpatient treatment was clinically appropriate for those patients that were referred.

Completion of the outpatient treatment plan was significantly related to decreased hospital days under medical-surgical diagnoses whether the patient had been admitted or referred to outpatient treatment. The characteristics of noncompleting patients were not examined, but this issue should be addressed in future studies.

These results are consistent with those of previous research and suggest that comprehensive outpatient treatment may reduce medical-surgical hospitalization among psychiatric patients (cf. Follette & Cummings, 1967). These results are also consistent with the suggestion of Strumwasser et al. (1991) that preadmission evaluation, coupled with concurrent review of inpatient admission, may reduce unnecessary psychiatric admissions by 30% (by 60% for substance abuse patients). All substance abuse (CDP) patients in this study were treated on an outpatient basis, which is consistent with the conclusions reached by Saxe, Dougherty, Esty, and Fine (1983) and Saxe and Goodman (1988). The present results suggest that immediate preadmission evaluation, concurrent review, and referral to clinically appropriate levels of treatment, such as outpatient treatment, may decrease unnecessary inpatient treatment without leading to revolving door hospital readmissions and medical-surgical hospital days. We note, however, that the availability of clinically appropriate treatment alternatives, in addition to the inpatient alternative, is a critical ingredient in matching patient to treatment (Cummings, 1991b, 1991c, 1994, 1996).

Drug-free, Psychoeducational Treatment of Schizophrenics

After I left Kaiser, I became the director of the Mental Research Institute (MRI) in Palo Alto, an office I held from about 1979 to 1981. One project at MRI was a model of helping young schizophrenics, ages 16 to 25, and having them live free of medication in houses in the community. Called the Soteria Communities, they were created by Mark Moser of NIMH and Alma Menn, a social worker at MRI. There were two of these houses. Essentially they were alternatives to hospitalization. Every fourth patient who arrived at the county hospital was sent to Soteria. It was a complete therapeutic community, based on the work of Maxwell Jones in England. He was a psychiatrist in the 1950s who had developed the idea of the therapeutic community.

The Soteria project was in existence for about 10 years. It was floundering financially when I came in, and I was to help turn the project around. We straightened it out and published the reports, some of which was great stuff.

The outcomes were so superior to those of the state hospital system that it was almost unbelievable. But then the budgets were slashed. Unfortunately, the staff at MRI was not interested in continuing this project. They were funded by NIMH, and the project brought in money to MRI. Still, they did not seem to have their hearts in it. To make matters worse, everything was changing to medicalization at NIMH, and the government wanted to support projects that utilized drugs.

L. T.: *The idea of having a community is a wonderful example of dealing with a very difficult disorder that is probably going to be lifelong. To help these people without using drugs is quite an accomplishment.*

N. C.: *It was a good project, and very worthwhile. And it was totally drug-free. No electric shock, no drugs. Then NIMH remedicalized everything. Everything had to be drugs. So we started publishing data like mad, to get the facts into the literature.*

I also realized that it would take me 10 years to turn this project around at MRI. So several of us decided to form an institute, which we called the Institute for Psychosocial Interaction, or IPI. In theory, it was because the Soteria Communities were interactive therapeutic communities. The Hawaii grant was switched to IPI. After some time, I realized that I had the same problems with this new institute—that therapists are not good at the business aspects of our profession—and I eventually formed my own entity, the Biodyne Institute. It was out of this that the Hawaii study operated.

{ 23 }

MEDICAID, MANAGED MENTAL HEALTHCARE, AND MEDICAL COST OFFSET*

Managed mental health treatment (MHT) services were provided in a prospective randomized design to Medicaid recipients and to a comparison population of employed enrollees in a traditional fee-for-service plan. Managed MHT services were an additional benefit to other MHT (OMHT) services available to both populations. Medical costs increased 15% per year (constant dollars) for Medicaid recipients and 22% for the employed comparison population for enrollees who never used mental health treatment (NoMHT). Medicaid recipients who received managed MHT showed a decline in medical costs by 26% to 36% relative to the NoMHT baseline. Managed MHT patients in the employed population showed a decline in costs of 53% to 63% relative to the NoMHT baseline. In contrast, the OMHT patients either did not show a decline (Medicaid group) or

*With Michael S. Pallak, Ph.D.; Herbert Dörken, Ph.D.; and Curtis J. Henke, Ph.D.

Note: This research was supported by Health Care Financing Administration Contract No. 11-C-98344/9 to the State of Hawaii for which the Foundation for Behavioral Health was the subcontractor. While the final report has been accepted by the state and the HCFA, the present conclusions do not necessarily reflect the opinions of either. Preparation of the report was conducted solely by the foundation under the supervision of Michael S. Pallak, Ph.D., Nicholas A. Cummings, Ph.D., and Herbert Dörken, Ph.D., respectively principal and co-principal investigators for the project.

*showed an increase (employed comparison group) in medical costs.
However, OMHT patients without a chronic medical diagnosis of
heart disease, hypertension, airway/respiratory problems or diabetes did show a decline in medical costs. Managed MHT patients
declined in medical costs regardless of medical diagnosis in both
populations. For Medicaid patients, the costs of providing managed
mental health services were recovered in terms of reduced medical
costs within 5 to 21 months, depending on subgroup.*

In an era of mounting attention to healthcare reform, mental health
treatment (MHT) offers a reliable mechanism for restraining medical
costs. Substantial research literature documents reductions in medical
service utilization and cost when patients have access to MHT in
health maintenance organization settings (Follette & Cummings,
1967; Cummings & Follette, 1968; Jones & Vischi, 1979) and in indemnity, fee-for-service settings. (Mumford, Schlesinger, Glass, et al.,
1984; Holder & Blose, 1987). In the present experimental study, we
examined whether managed MHT may result in similar reductions
within a Medicaid population and within an employed comparison
population.

MHT May Reduce Medical Costs for Emotionally Distressed

There are at least two reasons why MHT may reduce medical service
costs—often sufficiently to "offset" the cost of providing MHT. The
first is that patients in emotional distress overutilize medical services
in an attempt to find relief. For example, W. T. Follette and N. A.
Cummings (Follette & Cummings, 1967; Cummings & Follette, 1968)
reported that some 60% of physician office visits did not result in a
confirmed biological or medical diagnosis.

The second reason that MHT may reduce medical service costs is
that patients who somaticize emotional distress continue to evolve
medical symptomatology because the emotional distress remains unrecognized and untreated (Smith, 1991). Appropriate MHT forestalls
evolving symptomatology and increasing medical costs by treating the
underlying emotional distress. MHT reduces medical service utilization to the extent that medical utilization is inappropriate to the emotional condition. As a result, declines in medical costs and utilization

represent a powerful empirical measure of clinical outcome and clinical efficacy for MHT (Pallak & Cummings, 1994).

However, the implications of MHT for medical costs extend beyond issues of referral to appropriate treatment for emotional distress. Emotional distress may exacerbate existing biological and medical conditions (thereby increasing medical utilization), while illness per se may trigger emotional distress that further complicates the medical illness. To the extent that the emotional precursors or sequelae remain untreated, medical utilization and costs continue to increase. MHT directed to these emotional components should forestall or decrease the rise in medical service costs as a result. For example, H. Schlesinger, Mumford, Glass, et al. (1983) found that MHT reliably reduced medical costs (after 3 years) for patients with confirmed chronic medical diagnoses of ischemic heart disease, hypertension, diabetes and/or respiratory problems.

Ironically, the substantial research literature to date regarding the relationship between MHT and medical cost reduction argues for increased access to MHT services rather than restrictions to access. Ideally, in the context of healthcare reform, effective programs could outreach to higher medical utilizing subgroups to encourage MHT utilization.

We note that the policy shift from restricted access to one of increased access holds substantial potential for health policy reform, since almost 40% of the current population may have one of the four chronic medical conditions tracked by Schlesinger et al. These implications extend well beyond the typical 2% to 4% penetration rates for outpatient MHT (Cummings, Pallak, Dörken, & Henke, 1991) or the estimated 5% of medical patients who meet the definition for somatization disorder (Smith, 1991), and they represent much greater potential impact on medical costs as a result.

In light of sharply rising medical and health costs for public programs such as Medicaid, managed care has received increased attention as a strategy for constraining costs while providing clinically effective services through closer coordination of services (Freund & Neuschler, 1986; Hurley & Freund, 1988; Wilensky & Rossiter, 1991). However, at present, the literature concerning MHT and medical costs has been largely derived from employed patient populations. (Holder & Blose, 1987; Mumford, Schlesinger, Glass, et al., 1984). In the present study, the effect of managed mental health services on medical cost was investigated in both a Medicaid and an employed comparison population (federal employees and retirees) in a fee-for-service plan in the State of Hawaii.

METHOD

Managed MHT was provided in a brief therapy model (targeted, focused MHT or TFMHT) described more fully elsewhere (Cummings, Pallak, Dörken, & Henke, 1991; Cummings, 1991a, 1991b, 1991c). As with other managed MHT, TFMHT relies on matching the patient to a level of treatment intensity and duration appropriate to the patient's condition. For example, based on an on-site mental status exam, patients may be admitted to inpatient treatment or referred to intensive outpatient treatment often beginning in the emergency room, if necessary (Pallak & Cummings, 1992). Although services were delivered in a staff model configuration, TFMHT clinical providers were closely case managed as in typical case-managed, preferred provider organization configurations.

Two thirds of enrollees (whether Medicaid or employed) were randomly assigned to eligibility for managed TFMHT services (the experimental group) and one third were not (the control group). Access to TFMHT did not restrict access to other mental health treatment (OMHT) available to either population. The prospective design made possible comparisons between enrollees who used TFMHT services, typical OMHT services or both types of service (BOTH) and enrollees who never used MHT services (NoMHT).

A total of 1,444 Medicaid recipients received mental health services over the 3.5-year project period and about 252 employed patients received services (the latter became available to the project much later in the project time period).

The results summarized here are for enrollees with 30 months of continuous enrollment (Medicaid, N = 711: employed, N = 242). Thus, we compared medical costs for the 12 months preceding and the 12 months following the 6-month period when MHT had been initiated. For NoMHT, the middle 6-month period was designated as the "MHT" period for the purposes of comparing the 12 months pre- and 12 months post-MHT; thereby enabling symmetric distributions over the enrollment period.

CLINICAL DIAGNOSES AND CLINICAL SERVICES UTILIZED

While MHT diagnostic information was not extracted from the claims file for OMHT patients, this information was extracted from the project patient files for TFMHT patients. About 24% of project Medicaid patients had diagnoses of schizophrenia or affective psychoses during the first 6 months of service. This number declined to 4.5% in the last 6 months of the project. The percentage of Medicaid patients diagnosed with depression fluctuated between 16% and 21% and overall represented 19% of all Medicaid patients seen.

In the employed population, schizophrenia and affective psychoses represented only about 2% of all patients, while depression represented 27%. About 16% had diagnoses of adjustment reaction and about 9% had diagnoses of eating disorders.

Only about 44% of all TFMHT procedures involved individual psychotherapy, while group therapy accounted for 20% by the end of the project. About 8% of procedures involved medications primarily for stabilizing psychotic patients. Biofeedback (10%), telephone consultations (9; pc), family therapy (2%) and testing (1%), or combinations thereof, accounted for the rest of services provided.

MEDICAL COST TRENDS IN THE MEDICAID POPULATION

Medical cost trends for Medicaid recipients are summarized in Table 1. We kept the costs of MHT (whether TFMHT or OMHT) disaggregated from medical costs for these analyses and return to them below. Thus results here are for medical costs only, unconfounded by MHT costs (or differences in MHT costs between groups).

- *Pre-MHT Medical Costs*—From Table 1 it can be seen that MHT users (whether OMHT, TFMHT or BOTH) had reliably higher medical cost histories than patients who never used MHT services (NoMHT). OMHT had costs 178% of those for NoMHT ($1,482 v. $848, t = 3.91, p < .001). In turn, due to outreach efforts to high medical utilizers, TFMHT and BOTH project groups had medical cost histories that were 230% of those for NoMHT and 132% of those for OMHT (t = 2.06 to t = 6.84, p < .05 to p < .0001).
- *Change in Medical Costs*—From Table 1 we can also see that medical costs for the NoMHT baseline group reliably increased by

Table 1. *Medicaid Enrollees: Medical Services Costs*

MHT Group	Cost Pre-MHT	Cost Post-MHT	Change in Cost	% Change in Cost
NoMHT (N = 11,236)	$848	$978	+129	+15.21%
OMHT (N = 410)	$1,482	$1,434	−47	−3.17%
TFMHT (N = 369)	$1,958	$1,553	−406	−20.74%
BOTH (N = 342)	$2,774	$2,510	−264	−10.79%

Note: All costs are in 1983 constant dollars and exclude cost of MHT.

15.21% (t = 3.20, p < .01) in constant dollars. While OMHT medical costs declined nominally, the decline was unreliable relative to the NoMHT baseline (−$47 v + $129, t = 1.16).

In contrast, TFMHT and BOTH project group medical costs reliably declined relative to the NoMHT baseline (−$406, −264 v + $129, t = 3.96, p < .007). Despite the relatively small number of people in these groups, these declines were marginally greater than the OMHT (t = 1.55, p < .12). However, the results from the OMHT are discussed later in greater detail.

For the Medicaid population, managed mental health treatment (TFMHT, BOTH, respectively) reduced medical costs by 36% to 26% relative to the NoMHT baseline.

MEDICAL COST TRENDS IN THE EMPLOYED POPULATION

The results from the employed comparison population are summarized in Table 2.

- *Pre-MHT Medical Costs*—For the employed population, OMHT patients had reliably greater medical costs than NoMHT patients ($862 v $464, t = 3.62, p < .01). Similarly, the TFMHT and BOTH groups had reliably greater medical costs than NoMHT ($772 v. $464, t = 2.18, p < .05; $891 v. $464, t = 1.94, p < .06). However, in contrast to the Medicaid results above, there were no differences among the OMHT, TFMHT or BOTH groups in terms of pre-MHT medical costs (t < 1.00).

Table 2. *Employed Comparison Population: Medical Costs in the 30-Month Enrollment Cohort*

MHT Group	12 Months Pre-MHT	12 Months Post-MHT	Change Post-Pre	% Change
NoMHT (N = 26,743)	$464	$568	+$104	+22.39%
OMHT (N = 1,291)	$862	$1,233	+$371	+43.08%
TFMHT (N = 172)	$772	$534	−$238	−30.83%
BOTH (N = 70)	$891	$523	−$368	−41.30%

Note: All cost figures exclude cost of MHT services and are in 1983 constant dollars.

- *Change in Medical Costs*—NoMHT enrollees reliably increased in medical costs in constant dollars by 22% (t = 6.01, p < .001). OMHT patients increased in medical costs by $371, or 43%, reliably greater than in NoMHT (+$371 v. + $104, t = 3.34, p <. 01).

In contrast, TFMHT and BOTH patients declined in medical costs by 31% and 41%, respectively. The declines were reliably different from the increase obtained in NoMHT (−$368, −$238 v. + $104, t = 2.09, p < .05) or in OMHT (−$368, −$238 v. + $371, t = 3.28, p <. 01).

Despite the fact that the employed population had much lower levels of medical cost than the Medicaid population, the patterns of medical cost changes were quite similar. Relative to patients who never used mental health treatment (NoMHT), patients who received managed mental health services (TFMHT, BOTH) declined in medical costs substantially.

In short, the costs to Medicaid of providing managed mental health services were recovered by reduced medical costs in a relatively short period of time.

While OMHT and the TFMHT groups differed initially in level of medical costs prior to MHT (thereby potentially raising issues of regression), in the Medicaid study, there were no differences in pre-MHT medical costs in the employed population. As a result, explanations of these results based on regression seem unlikely for the Medicaid study.

ANALYSES: MANAGED TFMHT AND COST-EFFECTIVENESS

These results demonstrated that provision of managed mental health services produced reliable declines in medical costs. In our analyses we kept the costs of MHT (as in OMHT, TFMHT and BOTH groups) disaggregated from medical costs. This permitted direct comparisons of medical cost trends among the MHT groups and the NoMHT baseline group unconfounded by MHT costs.

We examined the relation between costs of MHT provided and the length of time by which those costs were "offset" by reductions in medical costs. This lets us gauge the length of time in which policy makers might expect to recover costs of managed MHT if these services were included for Medicaid recipients.

During the project, MHT was reimbursed on the average at $48 (constant dollars) per MHT visit. We multiplied the number of MHT visits by $48 as the cost of services in a given unit of time. These costs were divided by the reduction in medical costs for the same unit of time, thereby deriving the number of years or months needed for MHT costs to be recovered or "offset" by medical cost reduction.

The number of MHT visits to either OMHT providers or to TFMHT providers are summarized in Table 3 for the Medicaid study. These data reflect the number of visits in the 6-month period in which MHT was initiated (initiated MHT) and the total MHT visits in the subsequent 12-month period (post-MHT).

TFMHT patients did just visit OMHT providers and OMHT patients did not just visit TFMHT providers. Patients in the BOTH group used services from both providers at some point in the data period.

TFMHT patients averaged a total of 3.75 TFMHT visits in the 18

Table 3. *Medicaid Enrollees: Number of OMHT Visits and TFMHT Visits from the 30-Month Eligibility Cohort*

MHT Group	OMHT Visits			TFMHT Visits		
	Pre-MHT (12 mo) Period	Initiated MHT (6 mo) Period	Post-Pre (12 mo) Period	Pre-MHT (12 mo) Period	Initiated MHT (6 mo) Period	Post-MHT (12 mo) Period
OMHT (N = 410)	0	4.97	7.23	0	0	0
TFMHT (N = 369)	0	0	0	0	2.48	1.27
BOTH	12.77	6.02	11.49	0	4.77	5.02

months (initiated plus post-MHT) data period for a total cost of $180. Medical costs for this group declined by $406 in the post-MHT period (see Table 1). Thus the cost of providing TFMHT services to this group was recovered by medical cost reduction in .44 years ($180/$406 = .44) or about 5.32 months.

The BOTH project group had a total of 12.77 OMHT visits prior to initiation of TFMHT and continued with 6 visits in the 6-month initiation (of TFMHT) period and 11.49 OMHT visits in the post-MHT period. Thus, one additional cost saving to the Medicaid system was the 10% reduction in OMHT visit costs (which we have not factored in here).

The BOTH group had a total of 9.79 TFMHT visits for a cost of $470 (9.79 × $48.00 = $470). These recipients declined in medical costs by $264 (see Table 1) in the post-MHT period. Thus, the costs of TFMHT services were recovered in 1.78 years or 21 months ($470/$264 = 1.78).

In short, the costs to Medicaid of providing managed mental health services were recovered by reduced medical costs in a relatively short period of time. We note also that the lowered medical costs persisted for at least 2 years following the initiation of TFMHT (Cummings, Pallak, Dörken, & Henke, 1991).

OMHT patients used a total of 12.2 OMHT visits for a cost of $586 and declined by $47 in medical costs (see Table 1). Following our logic, 12.45 years would have been needed to recover OMHT costs. However, the results for OMHT are puzzling in light of the research literature and we return to them below.

WHY NO COST OFFSET FOR OMHT?

We were puzzled by the weak results for OMHT. In view of space limitations, we briefly summarize more extensive analyses that were carried out (Cummings, Pallak, Dörken, & Henke, 1991; Pallak, Cummings, Dörken, & Henke, 1993).

We disaggregated by whether patients had one or more of the four chronic medical diagnoses (CMD), i.e., ischemic heart disease, hypertension, diabetes or respiratory problems, as part of the overall project plan. About 27% of the NoMHT Medicaid population had one or more of these diagnoses. The percentage was reliably greater in OMHT (38%) and in the managed TFMHT groups (54%).

For the employed comparison population about 38% of NoMHT and

40% of OMHT fell in the CMD category. About 44% and 50% of the TFMHT and BOTH had a CMD. In short, MHT patients, in general, were more likely to have a CMD than NoMHT in both study populations.

We found several sets of important and corroborating results when we disaggregated the medical cost data by the CMD dimension. The first was that CMD patients had medical costs that were 251% and 223% of the medical costs in the respective Medicaid and employed patient groups.

For Medicaid NoMHT patients, CMD patients showed an increase in medical costs of 27%, while non-CMD patients showed a decline of 3% (recall that the overall average increase in NoMHT was 15%). OMHT patients with a CMD had an increase in medical costs of $300 or 17% (not different from CMD in the NoMHT, t < 1.00). By contrast, TFMHT patients with a CMD showed a decline in medical cost of $528 or 20% (reliably different from the respective NoMHT and OMHT groups).

However, OMHT patients without a CMD (non-CMD) showed a decline of $280 or 24%, about the same as the 27% decline (−$231) shown for non-CMD patients who received TFMHT.

In short, for non-CMD patients, OMHT reduced medical costs about the same as TFMHT although using about three times as many MHT visits. However, the picture was very different for CMD patients in that OMHT-CMD patients continued to increase in medical costs at about the same rate as CMD patients more generally. In contrast, managed TFMHT-CMD patients had absolute declines in medical costs. The same pattern held for the employed comparison population (not presented here).

Traditional mental health services, as in OMHT, resulted in reliable declines in medical costs but only for patients without one of the chronic medical diagnoses. TFMHT services, however, resulted in reliable declines in medical costs for both CMD and non-CMD patients.

DISCUSSION

These results have substantial implications for health and mental health policy reform. Managed mental health services were clinically effective in terms of ameliorating emotional distress as reflected in reduced medical costs. We also examined these results for patients with both shorter and longer periods of eligibility and enrollment. The results were identical in that reductions in medical costs were reliable in the TFMHT group within 6 months after initiation of TFMHT and remained at the lowered level during the 12 (reported here), 18 and 24 months following.

The second implication is that managed MHT, in this case in a brief time-limited format, holds substantial potential for mitigating the effects of the emotional precursors or sequelae of chronic medical conditions. We note that traditionally configured mental health services had no impact on medical costs with this subgroup and that costs continued to increase at the same rate as in the general population. Presumably, if traditional MHT services (as in OMHT) were targeted to this source of emotional distress early in treatment, declines in medical costs would result. We suggest that these results for CMD patients may help to explain instances that failed to find medical cost declines in a Medicaid population (Fiedler & Wright, 1989) in that higher percentages of CMD patients may escalate costs regardless of traditional MHT.

These results argue strongly for the inclusion of managed targeted mental health services within a healthcare system as both clinically effective and cost-effective treatment alternatives. Finally, it seems clear that implementation should include explicit outreach efforts and should encourage early access to services especially for medically high-utilizing subgroups such as the CMD population. Ironically, recent proposals suggest continuing barriers to access to MHT in terms of benefit limits (Frank, Goldman, & McGuire, 1992).

Implementing managed mental health treatment seems an obvious strategy for managing medical costs within Medicaid. However, managed mental health treatment is not a panacea for medical costs and the effect of treatment should be evaluated with some precision.

Patients who present for MHT have histories of substantially higher medical costs. MHT patients, while showing substantial declines, remained at higher levels of medical costs than the overall population, as others have found (Holder & Blose, 1987). A cursory examination of these results in terms of aggregated cost summaries per unit time would only have revealed that MHT patients continued as higher medical utilizing patients. Thus, using the patients as their own control in terms of change in cost relative to initiation of MHT represents a more powerful tool and provides a more accurate picture.

These results argue strongly for the inclusion of managed targeted mental health services within a healthcare system as both clinically effective and cost-effective treatment alternatives.

While higher medical cost patients have medical problems that will continue, it seems clear that emotional components can be cost-effectively addressed with reliable reductions in medical costs as a result. Clearly, managed mental health treatment offers a cost-effective and clinically effective strategy for cost reduction within the context of healthcare reform.

{ 24 }

THE SUCCESSFUL APPLICATION OF MEDICAL OFFSET IN PROGRAM PLANNING AND IN CLINICAL DELIVERY

Medical cost offset was discovered in the health maintenance organization (HMO) setting over 35 years ago and was used not only to justify the earliest instances of the inclusion of mental health treatment as a benefit, but also was used in program design and development. With the new emphasis on outcomes research, medical cost offset remains a viable method of conducting nonintrusive studies of efficacy, efficiency, and quality. Through the use of the research design described, an early HMO delivery system developed 68 focused, target behavioral interventions that years later became the basis for emerging managed mental health care.

SEVERAL DECADES AGO, when I was in psychoanalytic training, I had an encounter with my supervisor, the significance of which was not to impact for a number of years. I was reporting work with a personality disorder patient whose obnoxiousness did not seem to ameliorate with treatment. The training analyst, who was internationally renowned, stated wryly: "If you take a shmuck and analyze him, you end up with a psychoanalyzed shmuck." I was taken aback. The idea that treatment could go on for years with the patient not having a clue as to how to behave as a grown-up (this was long before Woody Allen) was not something I was prepared to accept at that time. Like many analysands I was a convert: psychotherapy was for the inevitable benefit of all.

Eventually I returned to San Francisco and began practicing psychoanalytically oriented psychotherapy, complete with a custom-upholstered couch patterned from a photograph of that which belonged to Freud. It was only a few years before I found myself dissatisfied. Since at that time no health insurance paid for psychotherapy, practitioners were forced to specialize in the diseases of the rich—principally female frigidity and male obsessions. I also realized that I had so honed my craft that by a judiciously placed interpretation I could prevent any patient who was considering termination from doing so. This precipitated a crisis in my life, for I wondered whether I was doing so for the benefit of my patient, or for the benefit of myself. One could always rationalize another six months of therapy on the basis of "self-actualization," a term that to this day has never been adequately defined.

The recollection is still vivid as to how my crisis culminated as I was falling asleep one night. While in the hypnogogic state, I was reviewing the case of an obsessional man who was typical of my caseload. His wife was freezing fresh peaches and ran out of aluminum foil. She sent him to the supermarket for more, where he obsessed for 30 minutes whether he should buy Reynolds Wrap or Kaiser Foil. Not being able to decide, he returned home to ask his wife which he should buy. She exploded into anger, for by this time her peeled, sliced peaches had turned brown. By accepting his obsessional behavior as the problem, the wife could join her husband in denying his intense passive-aggressive expressions of anger toward her. Still half asleep, I wished I could be doing something important, like Doctor Gall who invented the Gall Bladder. The awfulness of this free association jolted me into total wakefulness. I was burned out.

Most psychoanalysts get discouraged with the results of their treatment efforts by midlife, even Freud himself. They deny their burn-out by arranging to do very little actual treatment, while crafting a successful career writing, teaching, training, and consulting. This was of only cold comfort, for I was discouraged at 35! What was I to do?

Fortunately for me, Kaiser Permanente Health Plan was advertising for a chief psychologist who would help create a program to address the 60 percent of physician visits that the nation's prototype of the modern health maintenance organization (HMO) found were primarily responding to somaticized stress rather than physical disease. Sidney Garfield, the physician founder of the Kaiser Permanente Medical Group, conceptualized triaging the somaticizer from the medical system into a psychological system where the cause of the emotional distress would be addressed and ameliorated, thus reducing the overload on the medical system. Research already conducted had demonstrated that repeated visits in which the physician reassured the patient only tended to increase the patient's determination that he or she had a physical disease that in time and with repeated tests would be discovered (Matarazzo, 1984).

In accepting the assignment, I embarked on 25 years of intensive HMO clinical practice and even more intensive outcomes research. Morris Collen, cofounder of the Kaiser Permanente Medical Group and electrical engineer turned physician, made it clear that the effectiveness of any program must be subjected to the most meticulous scientific scrutiny. My predecessor, Timothy Leary, who later became known as the "high priest of LSD," had failed to engage in outcomes research and was discharged. It was made clear that the type of "verification" in vogue among psychotherapists which quoted authorities such as Freud, Jung, and Adler was not acceptable. Unfortunately, the practice of relying on gurus for efficacy has not greatly altered, only the cast of characters quoted has changed. To name only a few among the many gurus, psychotherapists rely upon Haley, Watzlawick, Erickson, Goulding, Kernberg, Sifneos, Masterson, and occasionally (much to my dismay) on Cummings to "prove" the efficacy of their interventions.

The findings indicated that persons in emotional distress were significantly higher users of both inpatient facilities (hospitalization) and outpatient medical facilities than the health plan average.

Since the mission of the newly formed mental health benefit was to triage the somaticizer out of the medical/surgical system, reduction in medical utilization would be a direct measure of success. Thus began a type of outcomes research that subsequently came to be known in the literature as the "medical offset effect." These early studies will be summarized here, for it is the purpose of this article to discuss an application of medical offset in programmatic planning that has never before been reported in the clinical and scientific literature.

THE EFFECT OF PSYCHOTHERAPY ON MEDICAL UTILIZATION

In the first of a series of investigations into the relationship between psychological services and medical utilization in a prepaid health plan setting, Follette and Cummings compared the number and type of medical services sought before and after the intervention of psychotherapy for a large group of randomly selected patients (Follette & Cummings, 1967; Cummings & Follette, 1968). The outpatient and inpatient medical utilization by these patients for the year immediately before their initial interview in the Kaiser Permanente Department of Psychotherapy, as well as for the five years following that intervention, was studied for three groups of psychotherapy patients (one interview only, brief therapy with a mean of 6.2 interviews, and long-term therapy with a mean of 33.9 interviews) and a "control" group of matched patients who demonstrated similar criteria of distress but who were not, in the six years under study, seen in psychotherapy.

The findings indicated that (1) persons in emotional distress were significantly higher users of both inpatient facilities (hospitalization) and outpatient medical facilities than the health plan average; (2) there were significant declines in medical utilization by those emotionally distressed individuals who received psychotherapy, compared to that of the "control" group of matched patients; (3) these declines remained constant during the five years following the termination of psychotherapy; (4) the most significant declines occurred in the second year after the initial interview, and those patients receiving one session only or brief psychotherapy (two to eight sessions) did not require additional psychotherapy to maintain the lower level of medical utilization for five years; and (5) patients seen two years or more in continuous psychotherapy demonstrated no overall decline in total outpatient utilization (inasmuch as psychotherapy visits tended to supplant medical visits). However, even for this group of long-term therapy patients, there was a significant decline in inpatient utilization (hospitalization), from an initial rate several times that of the health plan average to a level comparable to that of the general adult health plan population. Thus, even long-term therapy is cost effective in reducing medical utilization if it is applied only to those patients that need and should receive long-term therapy.

In another study, Cummings and Follette sought to answer, in an eighth-year telephone follow-up, whether the results described previously were a therapeutic effect, were the consequences of extraneous factors, or were a deleterious effect (Cummings & Follette, 1976). It was hypothesized that, if better understanding of the problem had occurred in the psychotherapeutic sessions, the patient would recall the actual problem rather than the presenting symptom and would have lost the presenting symptom and coped more effectively with the real problem. The results suggest that the reduction in medical utilization was the consequence of resolving the emotional distress that was being reflected in the symptoms and in the doctor's visits. The modal patient in this eighth-year follow-up may be described as follows: She or he denied ever having consulted a physician for the symptoms for which the referral was originally made. Rather, the actual problem discussed with the psychotherapist was recalled as the reason for the psychotherapy visit, and although the problem had been resolved, this resolution was attributed to the patient's own efforts, and no credit was given the psychotherapist. These results confirm that the reduction in medical utilization reflected a diminution in the emotional distress that had been expressed in symptoms presented to the physician.

Length of Treatment

Although they demonstrated in this study that savings in medical services do offset the cost of providing psychotherapy, Cummings and Follette insisted that the services provided must also be therapeutic in that they reduce the patient's emotional distress. Both the cost savings and the therapeutic effectiveness demonstrated in the Kaiser Permanente studies were attributed by the authors to the therapists' expectations that emotional distress could be alleviated by brief, active psychotherapy. Such therapy, as Malan pointed out, involves the analysis of transference and resistance and the uncovering of unconscious conflicts and has all the characteristics of long-term therapy, except length (Malen, 1976). Given this orientation, it was found over a five-year period that 84.6 percent of the patients seen in psychotherapy chose to come for 15 sessions or fewer (with a mean of 8.6). Rather than regarding these patients as "dropouts" from treatment, it was found on follow-up that they had achieved a satisfactory state of emotional well-being that had continued into the eighth year after the termination of therapy. Another 10.1 percent of the patients were in moderate-term therapy with a mean of 19.2 sessions, a figure that would probably be regarded as short-term in many traditional clinics. Finally, 5.3 percent of the patients were found to be "interminable," in that, once they had begun psychotherapy, they had continued, seemingly with no indication of termination.

The "Interminable" Patient

In another study, Cummings addressed the problem of the "interminable" patient, for whom treatment is neither cost effective nor therapeutically effective (Cummings, 1977). The concept that some persons are so emotionally crippled that they may have to be maintained for many years or for life was not satisfactory, for if five percent of all patients entering psychotherapy are "interminable," within a few years a program will be hampered by a monolithic caseload, a possibility that has become a fact in many public clinics where psychotherapy is offered at nominal or no cost.

It was originally hypothesized that these "interminable" patients required more intensive intervention, and the frequency of psychotherapy visits was doubled for one experimental group, tripled for another experimental group, and held constant for the control group. Surprisingly, the cost-therapeutic effectiveness ratios deteriorated in direct proportion to the increased intensity; that is, medical utilization increased, and the patients manifested greater emotional distress. It was only by reversing the process and seeing these patients at spaced intervals of once every two or three months that the desired cost-therapeutic effect was obtained. These results are surprising in that they are contrary to traditionally held notions that more therapy is better, but they demonstrate the need for ongoing research, program evaluation, and innovation if psychotherapy is going to be made available to everyone as needed.

Cost Savings

The Kaiser Permanente findings regarding the offsetting of medical-cost savings by providing psychological services have been replicated by others (Goldberg, Krantz, & Locke, 1970; Rosen & Wiens, 1979). In fact, such findings have been replicated in over 20 widely varied health care delivery systems (Jones & Vischi, 1979). Even in the most methodologically rigorous review of the literature on the relationship between the provision of psychotherapy and medical utilization

(Mumford, Schlesinger, & Glass, 1978), the "best estimate" of cost savings is seen to range between 0 percent and 24 percent, with the cost savings increasing as the interventions are tailored to the effective treatment of stress.

In summarizing the 20 years of Kaiser Permanente experience, Cummings and VandenBos concluded that not only is outcomes research useful in programmatic planning, but no comprehensive health plan can afford to be without an effective psychotherapy benefit (Cummings, 1991a). The Kaiser Health Plan went from regarding psychotherapy as an exclusion, to becoming the first large-scale health plan to include psychotherapy as an integral part of its benefit structure. In fact, the absence of a psychotherapy benefit leaves the patient little alternative but to translate stress into physical symptoms that will command the attention of a physician. Even the presence of a copayment for psychotherapy when none exists for medical care will drive the patient toward somaticizing.

DEVELOPING TARGETED, FOCUSED INTERVENTIONS BY USE OF MEDICAL OFFSET RESEARCH

It is not atypical for practitioners to narrowly practice as they were trained, resisting change and evolution. This is more problematic in psychotherapy than in medical practice because psychotherapy has developed few specific treatments for specific conditions. If a practitioner was trained as a Freudian, the couch therapy is applied whether the problem is marital, occupational, or chemical dependency. Should the therapist be a behaviorist, desensitization and behavioral modification become the primary interventions, whatever the condition treated. It is logical to assume that certain conditions will more likely respond to certain types of interventions, while being resistant to others. Discovering these specifics would suggest that psychotherapy could be much more effective and efficient.

Cummings and his colleagues at Kaiser Permanente intuitively observed that certain conditions seemed to respond better to dynamically oriented therapy, others to behavior therapy, and still others to systems approaches. And within the school of therapy, some conditions were more effectively treated in individual therapy, others in group therapy, and still others in psychoeducational programs. They tentatively accepted the premise that all schools and modalities had truth, but none had ultimate truth. The optimal specific could well be an admixture of several approaches, and they set about to test this hypothesis through outcomes research utilizating medical offset as the criterion of efficacy. Since in society persons under stress somaticize their stress, a greater reduction of medical utilization in an aggregate group receiving one type of psychotherapy intervention would be a measure of the effectiveness of the intervention.

The cost-therapeutic effectiveness ratio, also known as the efficiency-effectiveness ratio, was derived by dividing the average (mean) medical utilization for the entire group for the year prior to the intervention by the average (mean) medical utilization plus average (mean) psychotherapy visits for that same group in the year after the intervention:

$$r = \frac{\text{Mean (medical utilization year before)}}{\text{Mean (medical utilization year after)} + \text{Mean (psychotherapy sessions)}}$$

Differentially weighting by cost the various kinds of medical utilization, such as giving an outpatient visit a value of 1 and a day of hospitalization a value of 10, only complicated our computations and neither added precision nor altered outcome. But weighting individual therapy, group therapy, and psychoeducational programs did add precision. The formula adopted was based on psychotherapist time to accomplish a unit. Thus, individual therapy (1 therapist with 1 patient for 45 minutes) received a value of 1, while group therapy (1 therapist with 8 patients for 90 minutes) received a value of .25, and a psychoeducational group (1 therapist with 12 patients for 90 minutes) was given a value of .08. To clarify further, 10 sessions of individual therapy equal 10, the same number of group therapy sessions equals 2.5, and finally 10 sessions of psychoeducational programming yield less than 1. Emergency department visits were weighted 2, which means that 10 emergency department visits had a total value of 20.

To illustrate from actual research, a group of 83 borderline personality disorder patients was placed in individual psychotherapy, with the result that medical utilization declined slightly, but at an enormous expenditure of both individual sessions and emergency room visits:

$$r = \frac{163}{141 + 68} = .8$$

The ratio is low, indicating that interventions were neither thera-peutically efficient (reduction in medical utilization) nor cost efficient (number of mental health units). The staff over time created a focused set of interventions within individual therapy with some improvement in cost efficiency but little impact on therapeutic effectiveness with another group of now 73 borderline personality patients:

$$r = \frac{167}{148 + 51} = .7$$

The overall effectiveness-efficiency ratio actually declined. With an-other population of 76 patients suffering from borderline personality disorder, a great deal of care and effort was expended in designing a 20-session group therapy, augmented with 10 sessions of individual ther-apy, and then with monthly follow-up sessions. Emergency department visits were virtually eliminated, and the ratio rose dramatically:

$$r = \frac{166}{27 + 31} = 2.8$$

Learning a great deal from this group of patients, we sharpened the group therapy to 15 group therapy sessions, followed by 10 psycho-educational sessions, and with subsequent monthly follow-up individ-ual sessions, yielding a ratio and a program that was adopted as both effective and efficient:

$$r = \frac{171}{11 + 12} = 7.8$$

The research team continued to experiment with honing the pro-gram even further, but the work with borderline personality disorder, a category of resistant and highly acting out patients, never achieved the ideal ratio of 9.0 or higher which became the goal or standard. In this way, using medical offset, there were designed 68 focused, tar-geted interventions for 68 psychological/psychiatric conditions that became the methodology in what was termed brief, intermittent psy-chotherapy throughout the life cycle (Cummings & Sayama, 1995), an approach that concentrates on solving the problem in the "here and now" while also giving the patient a greater repertoire of responses to stress. These findings were the backbone of the clinical training and service delivery early at Kaiser Permanente and later at American Biodyne.

FUTURE POSSIBILITIES

Medical offset is being employed in a variety of ways that were never envisaged by the original researchers. In a unique application recently announced by Missouri Blue Cross/Blue Shield, "closer case management will be imposed on the approximately 5% of the members who account for 65% of claims dollars" (*Managed Care Alert*, 1993, p. 8). It is traditional for case managers to handle patients with catastrophic illness or injury, but this plan will go considerably beyond that and impose treatment that is an alternative in a variety of conditions. For example, counseling to improve compliance with medical regimen may be imposed on a diabetic, or an overweight patient complaining of back pain may be required to participate in a weight loss program before surgery is approved. A nurse who suggests counseling alternatives and who also approves all outlays throughout the period of care is expected to reduce unnecessary expenditures and improve effectiveness.

• • •

Medical offset as a type of outcomes research has been employed effectively in both programmatic planning and the development of clinical service models for over 35 years. It has conclusively been demonstrated that no health plan is complete without a comprehensive mental health benefit, the absence of which will result in overutilization of medical/surgical facilities by persons who are somaticizing stress. The Bethesda Consensus Conference on Medical Offset concluded that not only can medical offset be used to improve delivery of services in mental health, but also that improved services subsequently result in greater medical offset (defined as savings in medical/surgical costs over and above the cost of providing the mental health services) (Jones & Vischi, 1980).

There are resistances to the use of medical offset, the principal one being that most health plans do not collect data in such a way that renders medical offset research possible. Another resistance stems from the fact that medical offset research is necessarily tested against contrasting groups (as opposed to control groups) and is retrospective in nature. To do otherwise would require a control group for whom services are denied in the interest of research. This criticism has in large measure been answered by the Hawaii-HCFA-Medicaid research, a seven-year prospective medical offset study.

Much resistance stems from a reluctance to subject one's service delivery system to the intense criteria represented in the medical offset effect. It is easier and safer to do quick patient satisfaction questionnaires whose halo effect will more likely favor the delivery system being studied.

In spite of resistances from many within the health industry and the public policy arena, employers who purchase health insurance know of medical offset and express confidence in the ability of mental health interventions to impact on total health costs. In a unique and courageous published study of consumer attitudes of its own mental health/chemical dependency system, Harvard Community Health Plan reported that "employers believed that expanded mental health coverage would reduce inpatient utilization and decrease overall health care costs" (Pro and con, 1993, p. 11).

{ 25 }

OUTCOMES RESEARCH IN MANAGED BEHAVIORAL HEALTH CARE: ISSUES, STRATEGIES, AND TRENDS*

At least three factors fuel the current wave of enthusiasm for research on clinical outcome and clinical effectiveness in the behavioral health care industry. By far the most important factor is the continuing rise in costs for alcohol, drug abuse, and mental health services—the same cost trends which gave the initial impetus to managed care. A second factor is the perception within the managed care industry that evidence about outcome treatment effectiveness may be useful for marketing purposes in the competition for services contracts. The third factor relates to the increasing availability of useful and practical measurement instruments and strategies which may be adapted to behavioral health services research in managed care settings.

In this chapter, we explore the implications of these factors for clinical outcome research and examine strategies and tools needed to conduct such efforts. Each of the three factors may represent either an impetus or a barrier to empirical evaluation of clinical outcome, depending upon how organizations judge the relative values of the cost of conducting research and the utility of the outcome results for marketing and operating purposes. Each factor may also motivate or en-

*With Michael S. Pallak, Ph.D.

able patients, insurers, and employers to ask more astute questions about whether services provided are in fact clinically effective as well as financially viable. The growing emphasis on outcome and effectiveness data represents a major shift in perspective on the part of buyers of managed behavioral health care services.

INDUSTRY TRENDS: EVOLUTION IN RESPONSE TO COST

Unfortunately, mental health services and related policy have been secondary concerns and poor relations to medical-surgical services and policy for most of this century. The shape of health services delivery and policies affecting their development and implementation has primarily been driven by funding issues related to medical-surgical hospitals rather than by the more comprehensive range of issues which should appropriately affect national health policy and priorities (Klerman, 1985; Stevens, 1989; Kiesler & Sibulkin, 1987). Based on Stevens (1989), Kiesler and Morton (1988) argue that the fact that 70% of each mental health treatment dollar is spent on inpatient services is a result of a long history of policy in which hospitalization is—inappropriately—construed as the primary treatment modality in health as well as mental health.

Cost as a Factor

Costs in both medical and behavioral health care have continued to increase at a rate faster than inflation, population increase, or growth in GNP would predict. In the 1970s and 1980s, cost increases prompted the development by payers of a range of cost containment strategies, most of which were implemented as benefit restrictions and other barriers to care. These strategies failed to control costs of mental health and chemical dependency on a long-term basis (Cummings, 1991a).

The failure of the cost containment strategies led to attempts by payers and service organizations to redefine service delivery models, combining clinical provision of services with a business-oriented management of those services. The business "bottom-line" orientation provided impetus for an outcome perspective in terms of financial profit. The simultaneous desire to "manage" the service delivery led organizations to attempt to address the broader cost-effectiveness question:

Can clinically effective treatment be delivered at lower levels of intensity and, therefore, lower cost?

With this change in perspective came a questioning of the previously unquestioned assumption that usual patterns of treatment were automatically necessary and automatically clinically effective. A more evaluative or outcome-focused orientation came to predominate. The potential for rising costs to erode profitability brought into question, for example, whether the observed clinical outcomes justified the relatively high utilization levels of inpatient treatment.

While the managers were beginning to ask cost-effectiveness questions, researchers were contributing to the shifting perspective by presenting a growing body of empirical research which showed that less costly and less intensive levels of care were generally equally effective in terms of patient outcomes. Kiesler and Sibulkin (1987), for example, reviewed a large number of experimental studies in which mental health patients were randomly assigned either to inpatient treatment or to any one of several outpatient treatment alternatives. Patients assigned to the alternative outpatient treatment did as well as those assigned to the more routinely prescribed inpatient care, almost always at less cost.

In another review, Kiesler and Morton (1988) found that length of stay in an inpatient psychiatric facility was more accurately predicted by variables unrelated (exogenous) to the patient's condition than by endogenous variables such as severity of illness. Kerns and Bradley (1990) provided an extensive and detailed analysis of clinician, patient, and system factors which had been shown to have an impact on the decision to hospitalize. Finally, research on outpatient treatment cast doubt on the cost-effectiveness of anything more than about 24 sessions for the typical psychotherapy or counseling patient (Howard, Kopta, Krause, & Orlinsky, 1986). In short, the growing body of research literature questioned the cost-effectiveness of the more intensive and longer-term services for all but a small percentage of the patients who typically received them.

As sophistication about outcome and efficacy issues increased among payers and service organizations, a primary service objective was reconceptualized as one of matching the patient to the intensity and level of care most appropriate for his or her condition. This was a much more proactive stance than had been typical of these organizations. For example, in one case study, Pallak and Cummings (1992) found that 85% of patients presenting for inpatient admission could be successfully redirected to intensive outpatient treatment.

In this environment, as costs continued to rise and as competition in the marketplace increased, payers and purchasers of health and mental health services became better able and increasingly motivated to routinely ask the outcome questions: *Are the services provided clinically effective?* and *Are there equally effective but less costly alternatives for the patient?* The relatively straightforward goal of reducing or restraining the rate of increase in costs, typically by restricting access to services, gave way to the much more complex task of ensuring that purchased services were cost-effective. Purchasers of mental health services increasingly attempted to base their contracting decisions on consideration of clinical effectiveness as well as cost.

Competition as a Factor

Competition among providers of systems of care is increasingly important as a factor in the managed care industry's move toward providing evidence for the clinical effectiveness of their services. In essence, the question is no longer merely whether a provider organization can mount a program of service delivery for a specific number of covered lives, but also whether the organization will be able to document the clinical effectiveness of those services to the satisfaction of the purchaser. In very simple terms, service organizations must be able to demonstrate in a way that makes sense to the third party payer or (increasingly) the employer that the services make a positive difference in the patient's functional status.

CHALLENGES IN ADDRESSING OUTCOME ISSUES

Managed care companies face three problems when attempting to develop and implement processes to address treatment effectiveness: (1) inertia and orientation of the managed care organization; (2) difficulty in defining outcomes; and (3) difficulty measuring outcome in typical clinical settings in an efficient and easily implemented fashion.

Inertia and Orientation of Managed Care Organization

Certain characteristics shared by most managed care organizations tend to reduce the likelihood that these companies will be either motivated to address outcome issues or capable of doing so.

Inertia Due to Financial Orientation

To the extent that a strict business, accounting, or insurance perspective dominates the managed care organization, an outcome orientation and questions of treatment effectiveness will probably remain relatively distant concerns. The typical industry standard for information in an insurance or other third party program is fairly simple: claims data. Such data are most useful on an actuarial basis for ascertaining how much and what types of treatments were authorized, delivered, and paid for. In this context, the industry simply tracks services which are paid for and leaves judgments about effectiveness and outcome of treatment to the individual provider, the patient, or others. This straightforward approach is primarily geared to financial management to determine, for example, what needs to be charged for the product in the next financial cycle in order to maintain profitability.

A claims data system can, however, be a fundamental element in the process of monitoring and evaluating the service system. Depending on level of detail captured in the data base, claims data can be used to assess factors that shape service utilization and patterns of service delivery. For example, the observed striking variations in patterns of inpatient utilization within the same clinical diagnosis (Kiesler & Morton, 1988) suggest that factors other than the patient's condition drive inpatient service utilization. While even these simple sorts of analyses can be useful in evaluating the services system, they are not likely to be conducted when the information system and staff are oriented solely to claims paid and financial goals.

Inertia Due to a "Simple" QA Orientation

A variety of process-focused review and quality assurance (QA) procedures have evolved within the health services industry. QA procedures and criteria-based review combined with an adequate information system allow tracking of services delivered and assessment of whether "appropriate" (as defined by criteria) care was delivered at appropriate points in time. When combined with information from outcome assessment, such systems provide both a critical monitoring function and a tool by which the process as well as the structure of service provision may be shaped. For example, the review process maintained within an outcome-focused quality assurance program allows the determination of conditions under which morbidity or mortality is more likely to be observed and provides the organization with an empirical basis for making changes in the structure or process of treatment to reduce risk and the probability of adverse consequences.

As typically implemented, however, the QA process represents a partial, but largely inadequate, evaluation of treatment outcome and effectiveness. Under such a process, patterns of treatment are examined, criteria and standards or norms for treatment provision are developed, causes for deviations are analyzed, and changes are implemented to minimize probability of deviations in the future. This "simple" QA system permits aggregation of relevant information across providers, patients, and services settings as a basis for evaluating primarily the *process* of service delivery.

The inherent problem with this type of QA, of course, is that procedural refinements in the process of service delivery do not necessarily translate into better treatment outcomes. This can only happen if appropriate measures of treatment outcome are added to the information routinely collected as part of QA so that the "process-outcome links" can be established. In the most stereotyped example, all the correct steps in the process of treatment provision may have unfolded (according to the criteria), but the average patient may not have improved or been fully restored to functioning. The critical unanswered question is, *What aspects of the process were responsible for the treatment failure?* The situation is particularly problematic in systems where the evidence from the empirical assessment of patient outcome is not routinely available to the QA program, existing, at best, in the unexamined and unquantified case notes contained in the patient's chart and, at worst, only in the mind of the individual service providers.

Inertia Due to a Simple "Selling" Orientation

For service delivery organizations, marketplace issues and the need to be competitive may conflict with the need or desire to evaluate treatment effectiveness. On the one hand, a simple "selling" orientation requires making the best, if not superlative, case for the provider organization and what it offers in terms of services. From this perspective, considerations of treatment effectiveness, which necessarily include analysis of "failures" and variations in outcomes, may not represent the strongest selling position and, as a result, may not be viewed as a priority for allocation of in-house resources.

In contrast, an organization with an outcome orientation focuses on instances of both positive and less than positive outcome as a means to understand the treatment process and the outcome-process relation-ships and to develop more effective clinical procedures. Sophisticated efforts are often necessary to evaluate treatment and clinical outcomes, and organizations which commit to such an approach also must be will-ing to commit sufficient resources to support the activities.

Both selling and outcomes perspectives can be accommodated if the buyer, as well as the managed care company, takes a more analyt-ical approach to the utilization of outcome data. For example, the fact that chemical dependency and substance abuse services are less than 100% effective may lead to a more enlightened discussion about the relative value and necessity of more complex treatment procedures in order to maximize the percentage of patients who remain abstinent at treatment follow-up. Such a discussion could result in more realistic expectations about outcome on the part of the buyer, and to a coop-erative effort between buyer and seller to obtain or develop alterna-tive models of service or support for particular types of patients.

Despite the inertias, the simple computerized data system and QA program maintained by most managed care companies provide a rea-sonable basis from which to develop approaches to the issues of treat-ment outcome and treatment effectiveness in systems of care. At the same time, marketplace trends and competitive pressures in the in-dustry will force increased attention to the more complex issues of pa-tient outcomes. This will be the major focus of development in QA within existing service delivery systems for the next three to five years. The impetus will be the need to answer both the "simple" QA question (*Was the treatment appropriately delivered?*) and the more "complex" questions (*What was the treatment outcome?* and *What aspects of treatment process were related to the outcome?*).

Measuring Treatment Outcome

Given the rather poor record of managed behavioral health care sys-tems in evaluating outcomes, one would be forgiven for believing that the techniques and procedures for doing so have not kept pace with the rapid evolution of the managed systems themselves. In fact, measures and technologies have existed for some time, but only recently have they been adopted or applied, as the importance of quantifying and evaluating treatment outcome has come to be realized within the man-aged care industry (Pallak, 1989). Still, however, the empirical research base for behavioral health services (as for behavioral sciences more generally) has largely remained outside of the business environment, within research and academic settings (Pallak & Kilburg, 1986; Pallak, 1989).

There are a number of factors that have contributed to the absence of research applications to the world of service delivery and policy development in general (Kasschau, Rehm, & Ullman, 1985). In addition, there have been several sources of inertia reinforcing the historical separation between the research "industry" concerned with behavioral health services and the behavioral health service delivery systems themselves.

A major source probably lies with the stereotypes emanating from the psychoanalytic roots of mental health treatment. According to this admittedly simplified view, clinical services of necessity involve intensive treatment (three to five times per week) over several years with the objective of "deep" or "fundamental" personality change, rarely quantifiable (and not easily documented, in any event). In light of these implicit definitions of outcome, any change in personality *function* (that is, changes which could be measured), as opposed to *structure*, in response to treatment was often viewed as evidence of superficial rather than "real change" and not worth measuring in any systematic fashion. For a myriad of reasons, many of these related to the exigencies of health care financing, the psychoanalytic view has lost influence within the mental health community. It has been displaced by new approaches, exemplified by the theories of Aaron Beck (Beck, Hollon, Young, et al., 1985). These new approaches are more structured and directive than psychoanalytic methods, and they are, therefore, much more suited to outcome investigations focused on objective and measurable changes.

Two factors facilitated the movement toward investigations of clinical treatment outcome in applied settings. The first was the growing body of evidence that mental health treatment actually "works." This is best exemplified by the Smith, Glass, and Miller (1980) meta-analytic approach to analyzing therapy outcomes. This research strategy indicated that across a variety of studies, in a variety of settings, using a variety of treatment approaches and measures, patients treated with psychotherapy show improvement relative to controls.

The second factor is the increasing sophistication of psychotherapy research in terms of measures and techniques used to assess outcomes. While some clinical or psychotherapy research studies (Battle et al., 1966) rely on relatively simple measures targeted to the initial problem (indeed, this was the dominant model for many years), more recent studies, typified by the work of Luborsky and his colleagues, involve intensive procedures for data collection and analysis focused on both the process and the outcome of treatment (Luborsky et al., 1988). Combinations of patient questionnaires, provider ratings of clinical progress, ratings by third party clinical judges, and periodic structured interviews have been used to study in depth the process-outcome links. Their results demonstrate that patients improve with treatment, but they also suggest that combinations of patient and provider factors are likely to facilitate or retard clinical improvement. Through efforts of researchers such as Luborsky, the more general debate about whether psychotherapy "works" has been replaced by an evaluative focus on the conditions under which psychotherapy and mental health treatment may be effective (i.e., what combinations of treatment approaches, treatment providers or settings, patients, and problems lead to improvement, and how that improvement can be documented).

The Patient's Perceptions

A patient's perception of his or her progress in coping with problems and restoration of function is a critical measure of clinical effectiveness. For example, Battle et al. (1966) argued that patients seek help with problems and "target" complaints and therefore, just as in medical settings, treatment effectiveness should be judged by whether the patient believes the problem has been alleviated. In their procedure, Battle et al. (1966) asked patients to write in their own words the three problems they most wanted help with and how severe these problems were. At completion of the treatment episode patients were asked again to rate the problems in terms of severity. Change in the patient's rating of the severity was shown to be a useful indicator of patient improvement and clinical effectiveness.

Patients' reactions, judgments, and perceptions of their status and well-being have long been recognized by clinicians themselves as important (perhaps the most important) indicators of clinical effectiveness. For example, in a meeting with some 300 clinical providers of all types during 1991, the clinicians were asked how they knew that their patients improved. The unanimous response was that the patients report improvement directly, in their own words, about developing better coping strategies and about handling problems differently.

A patient's satisfaction with treatment and perception of treatment effectiveness in terms of his or her ability to more effectively deal with problems are critical indicators for a service system. Patients who perceive little progress or report low levels of satisfaction with the services are patients whom we want to know about, since they are the ones most likely to provide the system with information useful in quality improvement efforts.

While there are a variety of general and specific measures of patient outcome, this chapter is not intended as a detailed review or handbook. Rather, the interested reader is referred to resources such as the Health and Psychosocial Instrument (HAPI) data base file (Perloff, 1991), which includes detailed information (reliability, validity, availability, etc.) about a range of specific instruments.

There are a number of short, general measures such as the Client Satisfaction Questionnaire (Nguyen, Attkisson, & Stegner, 1983) which have excellent validity and correlate well with patients' decision to complete treatment. These more general instruments are particularly useful in applied clinical settings, since they may be easily administered in 5–10 minutes (for example, after any treatment session), or can be mailed as follow-up questionnaires after the treatment episode is completed. Periodic administration of brief measures has the advantage of permitting a view of the treatment process over time that may be easily correlated with particular events of clinical interest.

Most questionnaires can be adapted for optically scanned scoring so their results can be directly entered into a data base. This allows the data to be easily summarized and otherwise manipulated as part of, for example, a QA program, and correlated or matched with treatment and other patient information. Organizations such as National Computer Services, Inc. can provide most instruments in optically scannable form along with normative information for the instrument. For any particular patient or subgroup of patients, one can quickly establish clinical functioning in relation to other patient or norm groups, and can track change in functioning either on an "own control" basis (how the patient scores relative to his or her rating at earlier points in time) or relative to other patients with specific characteristics of interest. These scores can be aggregated for the entire service system or for particular components (e.g., for particular provider groups or programs) as one indication of how the service delivery system functions in whole or in part.

Treatment Outcome Measures: New Trends

In recent years there have been two trends of significance in the development of instruments and their application as outcome measures. The first is the use of general "health status" measures to evaluate outcome of behavioral health, as well as other health, treatment. These instruments are exemplified by the Health Status Questionnaire (HSQ) developed initially for the RAND Health Insurance Experiment (Ware, 1991; Brook, Ware, Davies-Avery, et al., 1979). The second trend has been a growing emphasis on evaluating patient functioning and well-being (Ellwood, 1988) by focusing on configurations of problems and patterns of behavior specific to various diagnoses. These two trends have been facilitated by the work of Ellwood's InterStudy group, which has given impetus to a variety of useful measures and strategies in applied health care settings.

The Health Status Questionnaire
The Health Status Questionnaire (Ware & Sherbourne, 1991) consists of 36 items that represent eight dimensions of patient functioning: physical functioning, social functioning, role limitations due to physical problems, role limitations due to emotional problems, general mental health status, vitality, bodily pain, and general perceptions of own health. It is based on the assumption that a person's sense of well-being is impaired by emotional distress and that improvement in well-being is a useful outcome measure in the treatment of mental and emotional problems. The HSQ has excellent validity and involves only a minimum of patient time to complete (about 10–15 minutes). It is sufficiently sensitive to detect changes in patient responses, either in terms of a global factor (well-being) or on more specific dimensions. A score or scores on this measure can be easily added to existing QA data, thereby "closing the loop" in terms of patient outcomes that are easily quantified.

Assessing Patterns of Behavior
Equally exciting are the activities of the InterStudy organization (Ellwood, 1988), which has supported the development of instruments

focused on the assessment of configurations of problems and patterns of behavior more specific to various diagnoses (e.g., alcohol abuse, depression). These TyPE (Technology of Patient Experience) measures have demonstrated substantial potential for measuring outcomes and change due to treatment in most clinical settings. As such, they show promise of becoming a standard industry gauge. InterStudy supports an extensive program of instrument development and refinement and encourages data sharing among organizations using its instruments. The TyPE measures may be used alone or with other measures tailored to particular treatment settings, thereby providing a comprehensive profile of outcomes in terms of national as well as local or specific trends.

Emergence of External Evaluators

Another important development in research in managed care has been the rise of independent groups or firms able to conduct outcome evaluations on a contract basis for organizations which provide services. There are several compelling reasons for the existence of such firms, not the least of which is that managed care companies are often reluctant to devote financial resources to support internal evaluation efforts. Many companies regard research and evaluation activities as inconsistent with their business and marketing-oriented mission. As a result, overhead costs associated with the collection, processing, and interpretation of clinical data are seen as prohibitive to undertaking these activities.

A second reason relates to the lack of rigor with which internal outcome evaluations are often conducted. Much of the outcome data generated internally may be in the form of cases studies, may be descriptive, or may be correlational in nature. If they are not experimental, studies may not be considered rigorous enough to be meaningful. For example, they often would not be acceptable to peer reviewed academic journals. At best, they may require replications which involve additional costs to the managed care company.

Perhaps more important, the data generated internally are considered proprietary and often, of course, reflect at least some outcomes which are less than perfect. Managed care companies (and especially their marketing departments) may well be reluctant to publish data indicating that the services may need improvement.

A final reason for development of external evaluations, and the one which is probably most commonly used publicly as justification for not conducting evaluations internally, is the belief that the objectivity of the results of internal efforts would be questioned—that is, positive results would be seen as self-serving if produced from the managed care company's own internal operations. This is always an issue in the marketplace ruled by fierce competition for service-delivery contracts, and it exemplifies the sharp divergence between the world of business and that of research. In the research world, work is driven by a search for truth. Publication in independently peer-reviewed outlets provides checks and balances on the rigor, quality, and replicability of research studies. In the business world, considerations over and above the search for truth drive decisions about internally supported evaluation—whether to do it, what to do, and whether and where to publish it.

As a consequence of this situation, firms such as Strategic Advantage Inc. (Naditch, 1989) have been organized to provide outcome evaluations on a contract basis. With this type of approach, the client organization need not build the internal capacity to mount its own research or evaluation efforts. While it is argued that these types of externally conducted efforts are more likely to be objective and less likely to be seen as self-serving, there is still some potential for bias if, for example, the outside evaluator wishes to develop a long-term relationship with the client organization.

Considering Medical Offset

Researchers focusing on outcome research in behavioral health services have moved toward a broader definition of outcome. In particular, much attention has been given to investigating the changes in the patient's utilization of medical services which may be related to the need for substance abuse or mental health services (Cummings & Follette, 1968; Jones & Vischi, 1979; Schlesinger, Mumford, Glass, et al., 1983; Pallak, 1989). In general, it has been shown that many patients who seek behavioral health treatment exhibit patterns of increasing medical services utilization leading up to the time of receiving mental health or substance abuse treatment. The use of medical services typically lessens following treatment for the behavioral health problems.

The usual explanation for the "offset" effect is that emotional distress (and, sometimes, associated substance abuse) may exacerbate physical and medical conditions, or may lead to increased somaticization of the distress, thereby leading to increased utilization of medical services. According to this theory, treatment of the distress will result in a decline in medical services utilization and the cost of such services. Therefore, a reduction in medical services utilization following behavioral health treatment may be taken as an indicator of effect of that treatment. This may be particularly true for patients who are high medical utilizers, who have chronic medical conditions, or who have medical conditions exacerbated by high levels of emotional distress. Furthermore, assertively channelling high medical utilizers into behavioral health treatment may represent an area of longer term cost savings particularly for patients with chronic medical diagnoses (Pallak, 1989; Pallak, Cummings, Dörken, & Henke, 1991).

There are some difficulties involved in attempting to use medical services utilization data, such as physician office visits, hospital days, and drug prescriptions, as an index of clinical effectiveness of behavioral health services. A major one is that mental health and substance abuse claim files must be merged with medical services claim files, if, as is often true, they are separate or are managed by different groups under the insurance plan, and utilization must be tracked over time. Second, an effect may not be apparent if data are aggregated into, for example, a single calendar year summary. Rather, medical services utilization needs to be tracked in appropriate units of time before and after the initiation of the behavioral health treatment. The advantage of using medical services utilization data lies in the fact that the data collection process is non-intrusive for the patient, and the data constitute an objective and empirical measure of outcome.

TREATMENT OUTCOMES RESEARCH: SOME OBSERVATIONS

Current measures and technologies make it feasible to assess on a routine basis the outcomes of treatment provided in a wide variety of clinical settings. General measures of the patient's perceptions of treatment outcome as well as measures specific to particular clinical conditions are available, easily implemented, and easily incorporated into computerized data bases and QA systems before, during, and after treatment episodes. Many of these measures are excellent from a psychometric perspective, and they frequently are associated with normative data that can be useful for making judgments about profiles of patients, providers, treatment settings, and other variables of interest. Adding these types of data routinely to QA programs allows the service system to establish a relatively sophisticated picture of the relationship between the clinical process and patient outcomes.

Whether managed care companies exploit the potential of these available tools on a routine basis will be determined by the interaction among several factors. While the development of an outcome approach is feasible given the available technology, system inertias and the resources required to make a commitment to outcomes research act as mitigating factors.

The likely compromise for many managed care companies will be to mount small outcome evaluation efforts conducted by external organizations specializing in applied research and evaluation. Since much of the motivation for conducting outcomes analysis stems from marketplace pressure and business competition, many managed care providers will probably be content with limited short-term projects to demonstrate a commitment to accountability. These studies will be largely conducted for marketing purposes—to enable a provider to claim successful clinical outcomes relative to competitors. Eventually each provider group will probably have a "showcase" study, and potential buyers will be left once again to judge the quality of the results presented and to gauge the implications of the results for their specific beneficiary population or group.

The ultimate gauge of quality of results and, consequently, the value of those results for judging the quality of the services, will be whether or not these studies appear in peer reviewed publication outlets rather than only in marketing presentations. The most likely best outcome for the industry will be represented by managed care companies that invest in a modest but serious routine internal research and evaluation capacity for collection of outcome data, and supplement this with periodic intensive evaluations of those data conducted on a project basis by research and evaluation specialists.

Follow-up on the Early Studies

In the 1967 and 1968 studies Bill Follette and I did at Kaiser, we had good results. But did these results stick? We did a follow-up eight years later, and discovered that the patients had generalized the benefits they had received from therapy. It was also very interesting that they had forgotten what their medical problems were, but remembered the underlying psychological problems. I was surprised that they had generalized the benefits to other parts of their lives. They also did not give credit to the doctors or psychotherapists. They had mobilized their rage in the service of health. Because they thought that the psychotherapists were insulting them, they showed them that they didn't know what they were talking about. So the patients got better.

Budman and Gurman were working on the other side of the country, in the Boston area, and without knowledge of each other's work, we came to the same conclusion—to eliminate the term therapy "dropout." It made no sense to call these people dropouts. Some saw significant improvements in their lives after only one or two sessions. This changed the way in which we looked at the nature of therapy.

{ 26 }

IMPACT OF MANAGED CARE ON EMPLOYMENT AND TRAINING: A PRIMER FOR SURVIVAL

Managed care has become the dominant economic force in health care delivery and has challenged many of professional psychology's training concepts and cherished attitudes. Organized psychology has not kept pace with the rapid industrialization of health care during the past decade and has been overlooked as a participant in health economic decisions. A number of changes need to be made in professional education and training if psychology is to be a major player in the new health systems. Additionally, professional psychologists must reexamine some of their most generally accepted attitudes and beliefs if they are to survive. These are described with a number of recommendations for the survival of an embattled profession.

The illiterate of the future are not those who cannot read or write, but those who cannot learn, unlearn and relearn.
—Alvin Toffler

PSYCHOTHERAPISTS HAVE LONG been conditioned to believe that more is better, "self actualization" is the real goal of psychotherapy, and, consequently, the most prestigious practitioners are those who see a limited number of clients over a long period of time (Bloom, 1991). Managed care, with its emphasis on brief therapy, is changing all of this. A growing body of outcomes research demonstrates that efficient therapy can also be effective therapy (Bennett, 1994). For the past several years, it has been argued that most psychotherapists must receive retraining to become skillful in the efficient–effective therapies (Budman & Gurman, 1983a, 1988). Over the past decade I have retrained literally hundreds of psychiatrists, psychologists, social workers, and counselors in a 130-hour module over a 2-week period and observed that for retraining to be successful, there must be significant changes in the practitioners' attitudes and belief systems. This "enabling attitude" has now only begun to receive the attention of those who are engaged in retraining practitioners (Bennett, 1994; Friedman & Fanger, 1991). Yet this point of view is not new.

Balint (1957), in his monumental work, said.

> A further reason for the failure of traditional courses is that they have not taken into consideration the fact that the acquisition of psychotherapeutic skill does not consist only of learning something new: It inevitably also entails . . . a change in the doctor's personality. (p. 23)

Although Balint was speaking of training the general medical practitioner in psychotherapeutic skills, three and a half decades later Bennett (1994), in addressing the personality changes needed to retrain psychotherapists in efficient–effective interventions, stated that "ironically, much of this involves teaching psychotherapists to become more like general practitioners."

When Cummings and VandenBos (1979) described their "general practice of psychology" and argued that the psychologist should function as a primary care physician not subject to a gatekeeper, they had not anticipated how important these concepts would be in this era of managed care. Their formulations are more appropriate than ever:

> By combining dynamic and behavioral therapies into interventions designed to ameliorate the presenting life problem, using a multimodal group practice, professional psychology can define its own house in which to practice. This general practice of psychology postulates throughout the life span the client has available brief, effective intervention designed to meet specific conditions as these may or may not arise. (p. 438)

And in further describing "brief, intermittent psychotherapy throughout the life cycle," they concluded:

> There is a great need in our society for that now extinct person
> known as the family doctor, a caring human being who heard and
> responded to all of a family's therapeutic needs. Who is better
> equipped to be the family doctor in this age of alienation than the
> psychologist? (p. 439)

THE RESOCIALIZATION OF PSYCHOLOGY

Currently underway is the greatest resocialization of psychologists to
occur since the explosion of clinical psychology in the post–World
War II era. It is being stimulated by the unprecedented growth of managed care, and it is occurring without (until very recently) the help
and guidance of the American Psychological Association (APA). Professional psychology is rapidly changing itself to meet the demands of
survival in spite of the shortsighted assurances of many of professional
psychology's leaders during the past several years that managed care
was paradoxically both a gimmick that would go away and a threat
that would be defeated. This seemingly overnight resocialization of
professional psychology has five aspects.

1. The Stampede Into Group Practices

Recognizing that solo practice is rapidly becoming an endangered
species (Cummings, 1986; Dörken & Cummings, 1986, 1991), psychologists are forming multimodal group practices all over the nation,
and at an astounding rate. In many instances managed care companies
have helped psychologists in their networks to identify exceptionally
skilled colleagues and have encouraged their banding together and facilitated their transition from solo to group practices. The principles of
the general practice of psychology (Cummings & VandenBos, 1979) are
receiving new and intensive interest, and the lines of demarcation
among the various schools of psychology are blurring in favor of psychotherapy integration (Cummings, 1992c). Among those practitioners
so engaged, there is a new vitality, whereas for those who desperately
cling to solo practice or who have waited too long and find the networks closed to new applicants, there is a growing fear and depression.

2. Acquiring the Growing Arsenal of Time-Effective Treatment Techniques and Strategies

Psychology's long-standing resistance to brief psychotherapy is being swept away in the rush to acquire new skills in time-effective interventions. Those who have long been associated with intensive, problem-solving approaches (Bennett, 1994; Budman & Gurman, 1988: Cummings, 1992) are suddenly in demand, and new national companies have been formed in response to the clamor for retraining. One need only peruse the scores of brochures that are coming to practitioners through the mails to see that for every seminar in long-term therapy there are literally dozens of offerings in time-effective or brief therapy. The APA, which would be expected to lead the way in this conceptual revolution, was, under Bryant Welch, curiously aloof. Both the stampede into group practices and the rush to acquire new therapy skills are grass-roots phenomena by psychologists who are in the trenches.

3. A Shift in Values and a Fundamental Redefinition of the Role of a Helper

Practitioners who have long enjoyed a steady, limited stream of fee-for-service clients coming through their comfortable offices will understandably lament the passing of this golden era of psychotherapy. Yet new payment methods such as capitation and prospective reimbursement free the practitioner to perform services needed by the client but previously not covered by fee-for-service insurance. Ultimately, they make possible offices-without-walls, a prospect that is frightening for many and eagerly welcomed by others. Because the shift in attitudes and values is difficult but fundamental to the practitioner who survives, the changes required will be more fully described here later.

4. The Ability to Demonstrate Efficiency and Effectiveness Through Outcomes Research in One's Group Practice

Both practitioner and client are struggling with the new intrusions called *utilization review* and *case management*. Gone are the days when the third-party payor, mystified by what goes on in the inner sanctum of psychotherapy, accepted the word of the practitioner. Gone also are the days when practitioners justified their treatment by quoting gurus, originally those such as Freud, Jung, and Adler, and more recently, to name only a few, Haley, Erickson, Goulding, Masterson, and occasionally (to my dismay) even Cummings. Organized settings make possible sophisticated outcomes research, and soon third-party payors (now the managed care companies) will know more about what goes on in the treatment setting than does the practitioner. Psychotherapists will have to demonstrate their effectiveness as well as their efficiency.

Confidentiality is for the protection of the client and must be zealously guarded. It was never intended to protect the practitioner from inefficiency or ineptitude, but many psychotherapists rationalize confidentiality as a refuge for themselves. As harsh as it may sound, not all practitioners are created equal. Fifty percent are below average by definition! As time-effective techniques continue to reduce the number of psychotherapists needed, managed care companies will want to draw from the upper half of the normal curve of providers. Practitioners will have to justify what they do in outcomes research. This will require a reformulation of confidentiality so that it continues to protect the client yet yields aggregate data that permit research.

Psychologists, with their knowledge and training in research, will have the advantage over other professions that provide psychotherapy and who are not so highly trained. However, psychotherapy outcomes research is a difficult and highly specialized endeavor, and just as retraining in time-effective therapy is needed for most practitioners, the sharpening of research skills will be a must.

5. Regaining Autonomy by Qualifying as Prime (Retrained) Provider

Most psychotherapists who provide treatment services for managed care companies do so in networks of preferred providers. The industry is beginning to identify practitioners whom they call *prime providers* or *retained providers*. These are practitioners who have formed multimodal group practices through which a total array of treatment and diagnostic services can be delivered on a capitated or prospective reimbursement basis. Thus the group named as a prime provider is responsible for a defined population in a geographic area. Prime providers or retained groups have demonstrated exceptional skills in time-effective therapies, and they further demonstrate their continued and growing effectiveness by conducting their own outcomes research. Internally, outcomes research is used to sharpen the focus and effectiveness of their own delivery system.

The innovative vitality of many psychologists has propelled them beyond the prime provider groups to *regional group practices* (RGPs), which are multidisciplinary, involve scores and sometimes even hundreds of practitioners, and serve a wide geographical area and diverse populations. The RGP is undoubtedly the wave of the future and will require purchasing the legal, business, and management skills needed to succeed. Herein lies real autonomy: Contracting with managed care organizations (MCOs), these RGPs possess considerable clout. An MCO can readily replace an individual practitioner and even a small group. A delivery system using a large regional group is not easily replaced, resulting in an increase in bargaining strength for the practitioners.

The advantage of prime provider groups to the managed care companies is in significant savings in utilization review and case management inasmuch as the retained provider group is case managing itself, individually and collectively. The advantage to the practitioner is the regaining of autonomy, for now no one is looking over one's shoulder.

ESSENTIAL PARADIGM SHIFTS

These emerging extended group practices (RGPs) have a special attractiveness to managed care companies other than just the ability to serve large segments of the market—their ability to predict costs—which enables the RGP to enter into capitation agreements and assume risk. It will not be long before group practices that cannot predict costs will be replaced by those that can.

To succeed as a prime provider will require a fundamental and even pervasive shift in values from the traditional approach, which is referred to as the *dyadic model*, to the time-effective approaches, which are referred to here as the *catalyst model*. Drawing on my experiences in retraining literally hundreds of psychotherapists during this past decade. I have chosen to describe this imperative change in values as a series of paradigm shifts. I also acknowledge liberally incorporating the fertile ideas of Bennett (1994) and Budman and Gurman (1988), which in turn are based on their own extensive experiences in retraining.

The need for a fundamental shift in values is no more pronounced than in the expressed attitudes of Cantor (1993), who justified 11 years of semiweekly sessions by the nonsequitur that she had accorded the client a reduced fee, or by Kovacs (in a presentation at the 101st Annual Convention of the APA as cited by Rosofsky, 1993), who acknowledged that he would accept a Woody Allen in 24 years of psychotherapy as the price to be paid for therapist autonomy. Society simply will no longer accept such blatant rationalizations, and because we have lost control over the delivery of our own services, such statements resemble "grandstanding" to our own constituency.

The extreme positions of Cantor and of Kovacs are not reflective of those of most psychologists who nonetheless understandably dislike managed care. Working within it is seen as akin to (borrowing words from the popular motion picture) sleeping with the enemy (Zimet, 1994), not exactly a winning attitude, but one that was nurtured by the unnecessarily strident stance of the APA during the latter part of the 1980s. The APA Practice Directorate has taken a more responsible stance under Russ Newman, developing materials to help psychologists better interact with managed mental health care systems. It has not been easy for psychology, which struggled many years to attain autonomy only to see the rules of the game change just as it became the preeminent psychotherapy profession. All this underscores the importance of the following paradigm shifts.

Paradigm Shift 1

Dyadic model: Few clients are seen, but for lengthy courses of treatment, usually individually.

Catalyst model: Many clients are seen, for brief episodes of treatment, very often in nontraditional modes.

Outcomes research has already begun to demonstrate that many psychological conditions do better in brief episodes of problem-solving therapy (Cummings, 1993). Other examples are group programs designed to teach and facilitate independent living among the chronically mentally ill that maximize effectiveness, whereas continuous individual psychotherapy for these clients is only minimally impactful. Many therapists have found that it is much harder work to see a large volume of patients in brief episodes than to treat a few patients several times a week continuously for several years.

Paradigm Shift 2

Dyadic model: Treatment is continuous, often weekly or even more frequently.

Catalyst model: Treatment is brief and intermittent throughout the life cycle.

Brief, intermittent therapy throughout the life cycle has now been empirically studied for more than 30 years of follow-up (Cummings, 1992c) and has been shown to be more efficient and effective than keeping the patient in treatment beyond the resolution of the life problem presented.

Paradigm Shift 3

Dyadic model: The therapist is the vehicle for change, and emphasis is on treating psychopathology. The aim is a "cure" in some form.

Catalyst model: The therapist is merely a catalyst for the client to change, and the emphasis is on restoring the inevitable drive to growth that has gone awry.

This is decidedly a developmental model that regards growth as the striving of every living organism. The therapist acts as a catalyst so that the client resumes the growth cycle that was temporarily derailed. It broadens the client's repertoire of responses to conflict, stress, or anxiety beyond the typical mode acquired in childhood. The client may, in future years and under exceptional stress, temporarily resort to the old mode, but it is surprising how little intervention is needed to resume growth in these intermittent contacts.

Paradigm Shift 4

Dyadic model: The therapy is the most important event in the client's life, and it is within the treatment span that the client changes.

Catalyst model: The therapy is an artificial situation like an operating room, and significant changes occur and keep occurring long after therapy has been interrupted.

This is especially difficult for therapists who need the narcissistic supplies accorded by grateful clients. It is long-term clients whose dependency has been fostered who are grateful. In the newer model, clients recall the experience as something that was accomplished by themselves.

Paradigm Shift 5

Dyadic model: Therapy continues until healing occurs, and the client is terminated as "cured" to some degree.

Catalyst model: Therapy is yeast for growth outside therapy, and formal treatment is only interrupted. The client has recourse to therapy as needed throughout the life cycle.

The client does not remain in treatment, as many do, for insurance against the fear the problem or symptom will recur. Termination anxiety is diminished or eliminated inasmuch as treatment is only interrupted, and the client is encouraged to return as needed.

Paradigm Shift 6

Dyadic model: Individual and group psychotherapy in the office are the main modalities by which healing takes place.

Catalyst model: Every healing resource in the community is mobilized, often as a better approach than office practice.

Rather than disdaining support groups or self-help programs, the practitioner cooperates with and offers consultation to these resources.

Paradigm Shift 7

Dyadic model: Fee-for-service is the economic base for practice, and the therapist must constantly fight against limitations on benefits.

Catalyst model: Prospective reimbursement or capitation frees the therapist to provide whatever psychological services are needed by the client.

House calls, imperative with house-bound agoraphobics and desirable with the chronic mentally ill, as two examples, become standard. Prevention programs that include such things as stress management, assertiveness groups, healthy lifestyle programs, parenting groups, and vocational and marital counseling, can be provided, whereas they would not be covered in fee-for-service insurance reimbursement.

PSYCHOLOGY AND HEALTH ECONOMICS

Having surmounted the psychological (attitudinal) barriers to a successful future practice, the psychotherapist must now acquire business and management skills. For those psychologists who are like me, this is the most formidable barrier of all. It is as if we gravitated to psychology because we espouse statistics but eschew anything that smacks of business or economics. We no longer have the luxury of our splendid isolation. What follows is our own "reality check."

1. How Did Managed Care Happen?

All goods and services follow the laws of supply and demand: Increased demand over the available supply causes prices to escalate, whereas a glut of supply over demand results in prices falling. The glaring exception has been health care. An overproduction of practitioners should cause fees to drop; instead, the greater the number of health care practitioners, the higher have been the fees. This is because the practitioner controls both the supply and the demand sides. It is the doctor who decides what is to be done, and how and when it will be done, and in the case of psychotherapy, how long it will take. All this is rapidly changing, because those who pay the bills (principally the employers) are taking the economic supply–demand control away from the doctor. As intrusive and arbitrary as managed care can be, when we had the control there was no incentive within our ranks to reduce costs by increasing our efficiency and effectiveness. Health care escalated to 2½ times the inflation rate of the general economy, with mental health and chemical dependency treatment driving the costs disproportionate to their perceived importance by society.

2. The Industrialization of Health Care

After 200 years as a cottage industry, health care is industrializing. The supply–demand control of health care's goods and services has shifted from the practitioner to industrial interests. As in all the industrial revolutions that preceded this one, there are six characteristics that constitute insights as to what lies ahead. (a) Those who make the goods and provide the services (in our case, psychotherapy) lose control of the production of their own goods and services. The control passes to business interests. (b) Because industrialization thrives on cheap labor, the master's-level issue that psychology failed to resolve may well be our demise. In addition, many practitioners have already experienced a reduction in income resulting from the lower fees "negotiated" as part of belonging to an MCO network. (c) Efficiency and effectiveness increase under industrialization, with a consequent reduction in the numbers of practitioners required. For example, 38 HMOs the size and efficiency of Kaiser Permanente can treat 250 million Americans with only 290,000 physicians, half the present number, and with only 5% of the gross national product (GNP) instead of the current 14%. (d) Quality at first suffers, then reaches a new higher level as the industry grows out of its infancy. Practitioners are seeing this wide disparity in quality and will also soon begin to see a stabilization. (e) The increased efficiency of industrialization makes possible distribution to the masses. As an illustration, no one would insist that Levitz furniture is of the quality of Chippendale, but the general population would not have adequate furniture without industrialization. Hence, "managed competition" is the centerpiece of every major health reform proposal under current study. To put it simply, everyone will have shoes, but there will be no more Gucci loafers. (f) Finally, there is a consolidation where the successful companies are buying the unsuccessful ones. This prediction, made years ago (Cummings, 1986), is exceeding all expectations in both intensity and timing. As predicted, the majority of health care in America may be in the hands of 12 to 18 "mega-meds" by the year 2000.

3. The Less Expensive Practitioner

Psychology's failure to find a place for the master's-level practitioner has resulted in the formation of a subdoctoral psychotherapy profession that now has statutory recognition in almost all of the 50 states. The APA has continued to recognize, through the annual publication of a directory (*Graduate Study in Psychology*), over 500 terminal master's programs in psychology, which are producing 6,000 master's-level counselors per year. There are now approximately 130,000 licensed or certified counselors, more than all the licensed or certified counselors, more than the licensed psychologists and psychiatrists combined!

This historical shutting-out of the master's-level counselors while encouraging their training, coupled with our failure to demonstrate that doctoral-level psychotherapists are more effective, are leading the managed care companies to look at the master's-level counselor as a less expensive alternative. The public and the media have already adopted the generic word *therapist*, which cuts across the various professions, whether these be doctoral psychologists, clinical social workers, or master's-level counselors. The generic word is applied even to psychiatrists doing psychotherapy but usually not to those performing medication therapy inasmuch as this is the one activity that excludes nonmedical therapists. Inevitably, most of the psychotherapy of the future will be conducted by master's-level "technicians," and this will further reduce the demand for doctoral-level psychotherapists and redefine the role of the successful doctoral psychologist, as will be described here later.

THE PSYCHOTHERAPY OF THE FUTURE

The most powerful economic arguments for mental health benefits is the evidence that they reduce inappropriate medical care utilization (Cummings, 1991: Goldman & Feldman. 1993). In the 130 million Americans now covered by managed behavioral health care, most of the economic "fat" has been effectively wrung from the mental health system. There remains the far greater economic drain in the medical–surgical sectors resulting from the use of services by the millions of physician visits by somaticizing patients (Cummings, 1993). Thirty years of research have demonstrated the medical-cost offset effect in organized settings: the reduction of inappropriate medical–surgical care by the use of psychological interventions. The current rediscovery of the medical-cost offset phenomenon indicates that the future of the doctoral-level psychologist will be found in health psychology.

The doctorally trained psychologist is in a unique position to plan, research, and implement intervention programs for both the somaticizers and the noncompliant chronically physically ill (Cummings, Dörken, Pallak, & Henke, 1993; Pallak, Cummings, Dörken, & Henke, 1993), as well as behavioral programs for the millions who demonstrate faulty living habits. But in the fact that the interventions of the future will be derived from empirical outcomes research, resulting in treatment protocols, there is an even broader role for the doctoral-level psychologist.

As previously stated, most of the hands-on behavioral treatment will be conducted by master's-level therapists working with empirically derived treatment protocols of targeted, focused interventions. Research, experience, and the nature of human diversity have shown that protocols serve only about 30% to 35% of the persons suffering from each condition being addressed. The master's-level therapists will need the clinical acumen of the doctorally trained therapist for the remaining 65% to 70% of patients.

Outcomes research is beginning to demonstrate that many psychological conditions respond more effectively to group therapy than individual therapy. In addition, there is a growing body of evidence that indicates preventive services in the form of psychoeducational groups reduce the demand for both psychotherapy and inappropriate medical–surgical utilization. These psychoeducational groups range from stress management, parenting programs, and smoking cessation, to programs designed to improve compliance with medical regimens in hypertensives, diabetics, and other chronic diseases where noncompliance is rampant. Outcomes research has identified well over 100 potentially useful psychoeducational approaches.

It is very likely, as a result of empirical findings, that only 25% of the psychotherapy of the future will be individual. It is anticipated that another 25% will be group therapy, whereas half of the psychological interventions will be preventive services in the form of structured psychoeducational programs involving small group participation. The doctoral psychologist will be conducting the empirical research on which the eventual design and implementation of these therapies will rest. It must be reiterated that the 25:25:50 ratio, or something resembling it, will be the result of tested effectiveness and not primarily a drive for further cost-containment.

The most important single characteristic that will define the successful psychologist of the future will be the ability to predict one's costs. This makes the psychologist (i.e., group of psychologists) eligible for capitation and able to assume risk. Without the ability to predict costs, there can be no determination of the capitation rate for which the practitioners will assume the risk to perform all of the services. It also follows that the ability to control (reduce) one's costs makes possible a capitation rate that will be more attractive than that of one's competitors. Only the predictability of costs, therefore, will make the practitioner a participant in the future health care system.

Finally, the successful psychologist will have to market the group's products and services once these have been developed. Unfortunately, space does not permit an extensive discussion of marketing skills. Suffice it to say that most practitioner groups will need to purchase this imperative service.

It would follow from the foregoing that our doctoral programs in professional psychology, including the professional schools, are training excellent practitioners for the 1980s. The skills that future challenges require are not taught in the present curricula. In 1994 the California School of Professional Psychology's Los Angeles campus launched the first managed care track, a historic event that is a harbinger to the doctoral programs that are lagging behind society's demands for the new professional psychologist.

SUMMARY AND CONCLUSION

The prediction that by the year 2000 more than 50% of current psychotherapists will be out of business (Cummings, 1988) is rapidly moving to fulfillment. The losers will be those psychologists who do not or cannot master the foregoing attitudes and skills.

The future professional psychologist will be primarily a health psychologist who will require retraining to acquire an enabling attitude for success and a knowledge of the growing body of efficient–effective therapies. The most likely role will be that of a supervisor to master's-level therapists who are performing from empirically derived protocols of focused, targeted interventions, from which there will be as many as 70% of patients not covered by the intended protocol who will require the benefit of doctoral-level skills.

Furthermore, the future doctoral-level psychologist is in an excellent position to conduct outcomes research and to plan and implement effective and efficient delivery systems in an expanded clinical management role. In summary, the future doctoral practitioner will be an innovative clinician, a creative researcher, an inspired supervisor, a knowledgeable health psychologist, a caring skilled manager, and an astute businessperson.

{ 27 }

Behavioral Health After Managed Care: The Next Golden Opportunity for Professional Psychology

In predicting the rise and consequent course of managed care, and particularly managed behavioral healthcare, it was anticipated it would be only a transition in the new industrialization of healthcare itself (Bevan, 1982; Cummings, 1986, 1988b; Cummings & Fernandez, 1985). As in all of the industrial revolutions preceding it, the industrialization of healthcare would necessarily evolve through a series of steps, albeit in an accelerated manner. Managed care as we know it today is merely the first of these steps.

The American Psychological Association (APA), in its eagerness to deny the important and enduring events which were rapidly unfolding, misinterpreted the nature of these events, and characterized managed care as a "passing fad" (Wright, 1991, 1992). The American Psychiatric Association (ApA), even though it entered the new era in a disadvantageous position to psychology, quickly worked through its own denial and rapidly reached an accommodation with managed care.

By 1994 it was increasingly clear even to the APA that psychology had allowed an unprecedented opportunity to slip through its fingers. As will be indicated below psychology found itself on the inside track when healthcare began to industrialize. Within a short time, however, organized psychiatry overtook and co-opted psychology's advantageous position. Observing this turn of events, and with its denial still strongly in place, the APA leadership implied that psychiatry had been taken over by managed care, a response suggestive of "sour grapes." The fact is no one took over anyone. Sensing the intransigent opposition of psychology's leadership, and welcoming organized psychiatry's eagerness to reach an accommodation, the managed behavioral healthcare industry came to regard organized psychology as irrelevant. Whereas in 1985 professional psychology could have owned managed behavioral healthcare, by 1994 it was all but locked-out. To be certain, many psychologists held important posts in managed care, including senior vice presidencies and C.E.O. positions, but these were more by virtue of their own abilities and entrepreneurship than by any help from the APA.

Rather than lament what might have been, it would be more productive to anticipate the future developments in the industrialization of healthcare, and focus particularly on the next opportunity that will be accorded professional psychology. Our predictions had to await the conclusion of political events on Capitol Hill, where the APA effort was asynchronic and predictably ineffective. The defeat of Clinton-style health reform now makes certain predictions possible, for even though the American people made it clear they did not want a government health bureaucracy, they have also overwhelmingly indicated they do want health reform. Therefore, until there is a single-payor system in the United States, an unlikely event in the foreseeable future, health reform will seek market-oriented solutions. Already events have provided us with a harbinger of what these will be, and although psychology regrettably missed the last opportunity, there will soon be another one if only we will seize it. But in order to comprehend what the next decade will bring and the opportunities that will be accorded psychology, it is important to understand the events of the preceding ten years and the miscalculations that were made. Crying over spilled milk is not the subject of this paper; benefitting from past mistakes is.

A BRIEF HISTORICAL PERSPECTIVE

When literally at the eleventh hour before adjournment several years ago the Congress approved the concept of Diagnosis Related Groups (DRGs) for Medicare and Medicaid, it inadvertently ushered in the era of managed care and the subsequent industrialization of healthcare.

With the limiting of reimbursement by diagnoses, hospitals were hit with adverse financial realities that caused many to become bankrupt. For the first time, armed with support from industry, labor and consumers, the government took a decisive step in slowing down the inflationary spiral in health costs. Accustomed to a "cost-plus" reimbursement, hospitals and particularly charity hospitals could no longer compete and most became proprietary as a way of surviving. Many hospitals experienced 50% empty beds. The new proprietary interests, observing the government's inability to promulgate DRGs in psychiatry, quickly converted the empty beds to psychiatric and chemical dependency treatment. In addition, they launched an unprecedented television campaign to sell these new services, and seemingly overnight many Americans concluded the solution to all emotional and chemical problems was hospitalization at the expense of the insurance carrier. Within a short period, the inflationary cost to the nation for mental hospitalization and chemical dependency rehabilitation soared into the double and triple digits. Adolescent hospitalization, which had been a relatively minor inpatient cost, rapidly became a major cost. Wall Street declared psychiatric and chemical dependency hospitals to be a growth industry, and expanded national chains flourished. Paradoxically, while physicians and surgeons began to feel the loss of income and autonomy, brought on by the early years of managed care, psychologists and psychiatrists were prospering. No wonder denial was rampant when warnings were issued that the same fate that had befallen their medical and surgical colleagues was just around the corner.

The emphasis on economics is purposeful, for it alone explains what next occurred. The acceleration of the inflationary curve would have been slowed dramatically were it not for mental health and chemical dependency costs which were out of control and now driving the inflationary spiral. Having failed to tether psychiatry and chemical dependency costs, the federal government turned private industry loose to do the job by giving emerging managed behavioral healthcare companies encouragement, enabling legislation, and a *de facto* erosion of the laws governing the corporate practice of medicine. Overnight the managed behavioral healthcare industry was launched.

In forming the first psychology driven managed care company, Cummings (Cummings & Fernandez, 1985; Cummings, 1986) offered the blueprint to psychology. He stated that he would cap American Biodyne at one-half million enrollees so as to serve as a demonstration that psychology could have its own delivery system, and he declared that there was room in the United States for fifty such psychology driven systems. He encouraged psychologists to found the other forty-nine, an offer that was accepted by only a handful of psychologists, who subsequently prospered. The majority of psychologists regarded the idea as fanciful, if not grandiose. Organized psychology staunchly opposed and berated the idea. Dispairing, Cummings eventually removed the self-imposed cap on enrollment and American Biodyne (now owned by MedCo, a wholly owned subsidiary of Merck, since Cummings' retirement) soared to fourteen million enrollees in 49 states. This could have been psychology's own house.

THE INDUSTRIALIZATION OF HEALTHCARE

The course of the industrialization of healthcare was not difficult to predict inasmuch as it has followed the same sequence that occurred in every industrialization that preceded it. The only difference is that the steps evolved much more rapidly, not surprising in an age of accelerated technology and communication. These events have been documented elsewhere (Cummings, 1992c) and will only be noted briefly.

1. As in all industrialization, control of the product or services (in our case psychotherapy) passes from those who make the product to business interests.

2. Industrialization thrives on cheap labor, and the incomes of practitioners are depressed. The proliferation of licensed master's-level counselors provides an attractive pool of practitioners who will be doing most of the routine therapy of the future.

3. The product is standardized and delivery is streamlined. In our case we are seeing a rapid integration in psychotherapy (Saunders & Ludwigsen, 1992) with more efficient and effective treatment modalities.

4. With healthcare emerging from a cottage industry to industrialization, the remaining cottage industry can no longer compete. The new industrialization grows at a 20% annual rate for several years, swamping the old system.

5. These resulting economic changes enable the product to be delivered to the masses. Healthcare is gearing for universal delivery.

6. As market opportunities emerge, there is a sudden proliferation of managed mental healthcare companies, not all of which could succeed. There is now the period of consolidation where the successful companies are acquiring smaller and less successful companies, while larger companies are merging so eventually there will be a small number of giants delivering the services.

BEYOND MANAGED CARE

The transition from managed care to the next phase in the industrialization of healthcare has already begun, although it is still in the initial stages. As in all evolutionary development, the transition into the next phase will be uneven and with much overlap. It will be the dominant health economic force by the beginning of the next century. In the meantime, managed behavior healthcare can be expected to continue to grow, but its current rate of 20% will begin to decelerate as the new modes of delivery steadily supplant it. So for those practitioners who will survive the present system, they would do well to heed the survival cogent offered by Shueman, Troy, and Mayhugh (1994), learn to become a prime provider as different from a preferred provider (Cummings, 1995), and make the attitudinal changes necessary to succeed (Friedman & Fanger, 1991). For those who wish to be ahead of the curve, predictions as to the directions healthcare is moving are proferred.

There are a number of reasons why the current era of managed behavioral health is about to be supplanted. Although there is no doubt that managed behavioral healthcare brought mental health and chemical dependency costs under control, most buyers believe that future cost savings will be minimal. Some managed behavioral healthcare companies do not even pass on the savings to their client, believing that having curtailed the inflationary spiral is enough.

Few, if any, behavioral healthcare companies as presently structured will be able to conduct convincing outcomes research that will differentiate their effectiveness from each other in a highly competitive market. Most of the fat has been wrung out of the delivery systems, excepting, of course, the bloat of the behavioral healthcare companies themselves. Demonstrated future health costs savings by behavioral health will be in medicine and surgery through medical cost offset research, showing the impact of psychological intervention on over-utilization of physical health (Cummings, 1994). This will necessitate the integration of current behavioral health carve-outs into the totality of healthcare delivery. Consequently, the managed behavioral healthcare companies as presently structured, as well as their networks, have a limited life expectancy. This leads us to the first of a series of predictions.

Prediction One: Behavioral Health Carve-outs Will Disappear. The primary reason specialized behavioral healthcare companies emerged in the first place is that the health insurers did not know how to control these costs. Now that the technology is available to everyone, carving out behavioral healthcare is unnecessary. The success of managed care has shown that employers/buyers no longer need to be baffled by the practitioner's psycho-babble, or be awed by the so-called sanctity of the client-therapist relationship. The guru has been defrocked, as current buyers know a great deal about our own profession with its frailties, along with its real and potential contributions.

The trend in which large healthcare systems buy the behavioral care carve-outs is well under way. It is also part of the consolidation as a necessary step in industrialization.

Prediction Two: Medical Cost Offset Will Become the Most Regarded Outcomes Research. A recent survey has shown that employers overwhelmingly believe that psychological intervention can significantly impact on medical and surgical costs by addressing effectively the large group of patients who somaticize stress and emotional problems (Oss, 1993). Thirty years of medical cost offset research has demonstrated that the more integrated behavioral care is to the entire health delivery system, the greater the cost offset (Cummings, 1993).

Prediction Three: The Future of Doctoral-Level Psychology Lies in Behavioral Health. With master's-level technicians doing the routine psychotherapy in the future, doctoral-level professional psychologists will become managers, researchers and supervisors of therapy in the integrated behavioral care systems that will dominate our field by the end of the century. Empirically derived treatment protocols will enable master's trained therapists to provide routine care. But as in all protocols, even the best, they are applicable to only about one-third of the patient category they are intended to address. The remaining two-thirds will require the skill and supervision of a doctorally trained psychologist. (See Cummings, 1995, for a more detailed discussion of the future of behavioral health.)

At the present time psychology is the pre-eminent behavioral health profession, but psychiatry is making every attempt to usurp this status. It remains to be seen whether psychology allows yet another opportunity to slip through its fingers. But this need not be mired in another battle over turf. Ideally psychology and psychiatry will work in concert, along with nonpsychiatric physicians, in the behavioral health system of the future.

Prediction Four: Community Consortia Will Emerge and Dictate the Market. These groups will be dominated by the buyers who will insist not only on cost savings, but will monitor the extent and quality of services provided. The consortia will resemble the purchasing alliances proposed in the health reform proposal, but they will not have the force of law along with controversial government sanctions. Rather, they will constitute a market-oriented response with the power of economic force. The negative financial consequences will be severe for those providers who oppose these consortia (Neer, 1994).

Prediction Five: The Delivery Systems of the Future Will Be the Community Accountable Healthcare Networks (CAHNs). The term used is the one proferred by Neer (1994), but it should be expected that other names may emerge as the concept is implemented over the next several years. These networks will be comprehensive and provide *all* health services: outpatient, inpatient and partial care. They will receive prospective reimbursement (capitation) and, as their name implies, they will be accountable to the community consortium which selected them.

Such accountability is not new. When the Kaiser Permanente Health Plan, the precursor to the modern health maintenance organization (HMO), was founded nearly fifty years ago it had strong labor union participation. As the primary buyers, these labor unions met regularly with the health providers and made their expectations known. This phenomenon was often characterized as an unofficial partnership between the doctors and the purchasers of healthcare. A similar participation is anticipated between the community consortium and the accountable network.

The primary examples over the years have been the various regional Permanente Medical Groups (PMGs) which serviced and were accountable to the Kaiser Foundation Health Plan (Cummings & VandenBos, 1981). Many differences exist between the PMGs and what is being envisaged in the future, and a more accurate example may be the Mullikin Group on the West Coast which has been extensively described (DeLafuente, 1993). Of importance is that these CAHNs will restore practitioner autonomy and self-respect, and will eliminate the managed care company as "middleman."

These networks are not easily formed and managed, for a business as well as a caring attitude must prevail. But the astute psychologist will begin talking with like-minded medical and allied health practitioners with the goal of forming such delivery systems so as to be on the ground floor as equal partners with physicians. It is with this goal in mind that the anatomy of the CAHN of the future is described.

THE COMMUNITY ACCOUNTABLE HEALTHCARE NETWORK (CAHN)

The CAHN will be an exclusive provider group, serving a population or a geographical region. This trend is already discernible, as Exclusive Provider Organizations (EPOs) are the newest and fastest growing entities in the current managed care scene. Most follow the network model in delivering services, but there is an increasing interest in the staff-network model, and even the staff model, itself. It is apparent that the network model is not as efficient as the staff model, and as the American people become more accustomed to being managed, there will be a resurgence of the staff model. The group will still bear the name "network" as it will be such in the broadest sense of the term, bringing together not only outpatient clinics, but also hospitals and partial care centers.

Two systems of healthcare will prevail at the turn of the century: the Accountable Healthcare Network (AHN) and the HMO, which is really an extensive group of health providers. The driving force of these systems will be the "physician equity model," a form of participant ownership that should include psychologists in the definition of physician. Forrester (1994) refers to the physician equity model as "the dark horse contender to dominate healthcare delivery in the future." For-profit practitioner groups can "forge an entrepreneurial trail with a zeal and speed" not possible in non-equity systems (Forrester, 1994, p. 1). It is important that psychologists begin now to assure equity in these systems of the future. Those psychologists who succeed will very likely be those who are involved in the initial formations of CAHNs.

The community oversight for these groups has yet to evolve, but current dissatisfactions among employer/buyers will make this inevitable. Distilling out all of the onerous features of the Rodham-Clinton proposed purchasing alliances, advisers to industry are strongly recommending that the buyers take control of the market. With the failure of health reform initiatives in Washington, the way is now open for market-oriented solutions to move rapidly. The next several years will see even greater changes in healthcare than were produced by the last ten years. The CAHNs will have on the boards of oversight committees, community, employers and provider representation.

As of this writing the initiative to form exclusive provider organizations has come essentially from physicians who also possess business foresight and acumen. Psychologists have been important participants, and hopefully in the near future professional psychologists will demonstrate leadership in this regard.

The format for these exclusive provider organizations was enunciated a half century ago by Sidney Garfield, the founder of the Kaiser Permanente health systems and the architect of what was to become the modern HMO: "What makes a cutting-edge health system work is dedicated doctors who believe in the concept and are participant owners" (personal communication, May 1959). At the present time not all of the emerging exclusive provider organizations have participant ownership, but it is very likely that the ones which succeed in the future will manifest this format.

Ownership by the providers does not mean that the CAHN will be a democracy. The landscape was cluttered in the 1980s with the failures of physician-owned managed care. These physicians structured their organizations so that everyone had a voice, overlooking the propensity of providers to obsess any issue to oblivion. Participant ownership requires strong management, with a strict limitation on the providers' ability to meddle in administration.

Prospective reimbursement (caption) will be the only method of payment, and skill in pricing the capitated rate is one of the keys to success. Priced too low, the delivery will fail. On the other hand, pricing it too high makes the delivery system noncompetitive. This will be a new era in pricing, eliminating "low-balling" practices prevalent at the present time. "Low-balling" is merely underpricing one's competitors with the intent of making up the loss by skimping on the delivery of contracted services. The community oversight will closely monitor the extent and quality of what is actually delivered.

Historically the acute care hospitals and their medical staffs have played a pivotal role in the American healthcare delivery system. In the future this will change dramatically with the acute care hospitals becoming equal partners in the accountable healthcare networks. Already we are witnessing the largest proprietary hospital corporation in the country developing all-purpose healthcare networks.

The health systems at the turn of the century must be able to demonstrate efficiency, effectiveness and quality above that offered by their competitors. At the present time there seems to be an inability on the part of managed care companies to do this convincingly.

SUMMARY AND CONCLUSIONS

The industrialization of healthcare, which was initiated in the 1980s with the rapid expansion of managed care, will continue to evolve beyond the types of managed care as it is functioning today. Organized psychology, by seriously misreading the meaning of the events of the past ten years, caused professional psychology to be of minor influence in the developments that occurred. The next series of events between now and the turn of the century present psychology with still one more opportunity to be a major participant.

HMOs, which are essentially exclusive provider networks, and exclusive provider organizations will comprise what has been called the future Community Accountable Healthcare Networks (CAHNs). These will be the predominant managed care companies at the turn of the century (Neer, 1994). The CAHNs will, as a necessity, have a cross section of the community leadership governing the network. The purchasers of healthcare will define the market.

CAHNs will be comprehensive and will offer all healthcare services. Hospitals and other healthcare facilities will be equal partners with the practitioners in these endeavors. It is predicted that the most effective and successful of the CAHNs will have participating-ownership, termed "physician equity," so it is imperative that professional psychologists become active with entrepreneurial physicians and allied health professionals in forming such exclusive provider organizations.

The future of doctoral-level professional psychology lies in behavioral health, conceptualizing and implementing programs in behavioral medicine. They will serve as supervisors of the master's-level therapists who will be performing the routine psychotherapy, and they will be the leadership in the new wave of outcomes research. Many will be managers, and some will even be senior managers. There will be a serious impact on the oversupply of psychologists, and many will not survive the transition. It is anticipated that this time, for the sake of an already embattled profession, the leadership of organized psychology will read the signs correctly and promote professional psychology's participation.

EPILOGUE

Predictably, only about 15 to 20% of practicing psychologists will have the foresight, energy and adaptability to become equity participants in the HMOs and CAHNs which will dominate the healthcare landscape in the next century. The fate of the majority of psychologists will depend on whether psychology succeeds in becoming a primary care profession as Cummings and VandenBos advocated a decade and a half ago (see "The General Practice of Psychology," *Professional Psychology*, 1979, 430–440). Two forces are important in this struggle: *prescription privileges* and the *leadership of the National Register*.

If psychology obtains the ability to prescribe psychotropic drugs, status in primary care will be enhanced. Furthermore, the prediction that the profession is destined to lose 50% of its doctoral-level practitioners will be cut to 25%. The other 25% attrition will be made up by losses in psychiatry, for with psychologists able to prescribe, the demand for more costly psychiatrists will diminish.

With the APA essentially regarded as irrelevant by the industry, the role of the National Register becomes very significant. Unfortunately, after years of shortsighted and needless polemics, the APA has locked itself out of the decision making process in the market oriented healthcare arena. Having bet on the losing horses in the national healthcare debate, it is now turning its resources toward promulgating restrictive, regulatory legislation in the states. This will only hasten the industry's contracting with the accountable healthcare networks as a way around such restrictions. The National Register has risen to the need and assumed the leadership in educating its registrants in a balanced approach to the realities, advantages and disadvantages of the new healthcare climate. As the oldest meaningful credentialing organization in psychology, the National Register is poised to help managed care companies in their search for qualified, competent practitioners. It is respected by the industry, as well as its members because it has taken the high ground. Failing in its attempts to open a dialogue with the APA, the industry will welcome the National Register which it regards not only as a sane voice, but also as a strong advocate in promoting professional psychology.

{ 28 }

PRACTITIONER-DRIVEN MANAGED CARE: THE QUALITY SOLUTION

This telephone has too many shortcomings to be seriously considered as a means of communication.
President, Western Union Internal Memo, 1876

IN 1876, THE telegraph was state-of-the-art communication, and Western Union Telegraph Company was at the very top of the game. Smug in its success, Western Union rebuffed Alexander Graham Bell who was desperately attempting to sell his invention. Today, as Western Union struggles, after several restructurings, to survive as a small business that instantaneously wires money, this telephone industry, despite the government's breakup of the Bell System, which created an array of competing companies, remains one of the nation's largest businesses. Interestingly, Western Union could have incorporated the telephone easily, by using existing cross-country poles and by slightly modifying input into thousands of miles of already strung wire. But that day in 1876, it elected to commit slow suicide.

More than a century later when Cummings (1986) offered psychology an entire new industry soon to be known as managed behavioral care, the American Psychological Association (APA) was also at the top of its game. After 30 years of struggle as the underdog, psychology had emerged as the nation's preeminent mental health profession. Psychiatry had remedicalized and accorded psychotherapy to psychology. This war between psychology and psychiatry would have ended had psychology not decided to expand into its natural frontiers: hospitalization privileges and prescription privileges. Now the APA is a fractionated, economically irrelevant association whose members are embittered and struggling to survive in outmoded solo practices. In contrast, managed care now comprises 75% of the insured population and continues to grow at 20% per year (Oliver, 1996).

A recent survey (Saeman, 1996) reveals that psychologists over age 50 are contemplating early retirement, young psychologists are looking for salaried jobs, and those in between are working longer and longer hours to maintain a semblance of their previous incomes. Most state their practices are declining, while 25% report things are better. Although this is a decided minority, the figure is probably twice as high as it was two years ago, indicating more and more psychologists are adapting to healthcare industrialization and prospering. This essentially has been accomplished by self-determination and without the help of their professional societies, which are finally showing signs of emerging from a decade of denial.

PSYCHOLOGY AND HEALTH ECONOMICS

How did psychology permit this opportunity to slip through its fingers when, as the preeminent psychotherapy profession, it could have easily incorporated the growing arsenal of efficient and effective psychotherapies and managed behavior healthcare much better than the present companies are doing? First, most practitioners are not versed in economics and failed to see that after 200 years as a cottage industry, healthcare in the United States was industrializing (Cummings, 1988b). The question is not why healthcare industrialized, but why it took so long. Manufacturing was well on its way at the turn of the 20th century, and retail goods and services had achieved the status of full industrialization by the 1930s, trailing such pioneering giants as Sears, Roebuck and Montgomery Ward. And while psychologists are reeling under the impact of the belated industrialization of healthcare, the remainder of our society is in the beginning stages of the Information Age, which will eclipse the Industrial Age.

Although Western Union failed to see industrialization as a constantly evolving process in which the telegraph would be replaced by the telephone, the telephone industry is not making that mistake. It has seen to it that it owns cellular phones, space satellite transmissions, fiber-optics, the fax, computer modems, and every communications discovery that might come along. In contrast, practitioners are like Western Union, seeing managed care as a "thing" to be opposed or discarded.

The APA is typical of practitioner responses. Its governing system was sensitive to a powerful constituency of established solo practitioners who supported a Practice Directorate that told them what they wanted to hear. Managed care was characterized as "a passing fad," a system "so antithetical to practice that it will be defeated" (Wright, 1991, 1992). Managed care itself was made politically incorrect, and all who aspired to political office within our professional societies had to declare themselves a St. George who would slay the dragon. At the present time, the APA is divided between the old guard that continues its grip on governence and would rather bring down the entire system than change, and those who support the new practice directorate, which is aggressively and realistically addressing the issues. This later effort is difficult inasmuch as the Kevorkianization of psychology was all but completed.

Just as the telegraph was an early stage in the industrialization of communication, current managed care is only an evolutionary step in the industrialization of healthcare. Once industrialization begins, however, it cannot be reversed. It proceeds unrelentingly, and Henry Ford's first assembly line has little resemblance to space technology other than as a historical precedent. Similarly, industrialized healthcare 20 years from now will little resemble what exists today. This chapter is intended not for those 50% of practitioners who will disappear with the cottage industry (Cummings, 1995), but for those who will accommodate to industrialization as it will steadily evolve, and not only will survive, but also will prosper. To help them, the remainder of this chapter is devoted to a series of predictions as to what will occur in the next decade (Cummings, 1996). Practitioners who heed the trends can become a part of the continued healthcare evolution.

THE RENAISSANCE OF THE PRACTITIONER

In addressing the question of whether practitioners can manage healthcare, the first answer is a resounding, "They could not do worse than the present managed care organizations (MCOs) are doing."

As Pigott (1996) has aptly pointed out, today's "managed healthcare" is a misnomer. The MCO's fundamental role is that of an arbitrageur, or broker, between buyers and sellers of healthcare services. Given healthcare's trillion-dollar-per-year cottage industry, which had virtually no internal oversight mechanisms, it was easy for the arbitrageurs to save money. Despite complaints from providers, services were not adversely affected, and in some few cases they actually improved. There was such an excess of capacity that prices plunged once controls were in place and practitioners no longer determined either supply or demand. The buyers were happy, the MCOs made money, and the providers went into decline, economically and emotionally.

In all of this, however, the MCOs lost their clinical focus. With the founding of American Biodyne, a clinically driven MCO, Cummings demonstrated that if providers learned to predict and control costs, abandoned outmoded attitudes by making appropriate paradigm shifts (Cummings, 1995), and learned business principles, they could curtail the inflationary spiral and deliver superior services. American Biodyne flourished for seven years, and a number of merging MCOs that adopted the Biodyne model also did well. Eventually, Cummings, then well past retirement age, grew weary of the shortsightedness of the professional societies and their constant onslaught. He sold the company to business interests that understood finances, but knew nothing of practice. Clinical dominance was lost, arbitrageurs took over, and managed care became business driven.

There are a number of reasons the current era of managed behavioral health is about to be supplanted. Although managed behavioral healthcare undoubtedly brought mental health and chemical dependency costs under control, most buyers believe that future cost savings will be minimal. Some managed behavioral healthcare companies do not even pass on the savings to their client, believing that having curtailed the inflationary spiral is enough.

Few, if any, behavioral healthcare companies as presently structured will be able to conduct convincing outcomes research that will differentiate their effectiveness from each other in a highly competitive market. Most of the fat has been wrung out of the delivery systems, excepting the bloat of the behavioral healthcare companies themselves. Perhaps inevitably, cost containment has befallen the cost cutters. Demonstrated future health costs carvings by behavioral health will be in medicine and surgery through medical cost offset research, showing the impact of psychological intervention on overutilization of physical health (Cummings, 1994). This will necessitate the integration of current behavioral health carve-outs into total healthcare delivery. Consequently, the managed behavioral healthcare companies as presently structured, as well as their networks, have a limited life expectancy.

THE PRACTITIONER ADVANTAGE

The American people like their doctors. Collectively, the professions must learn to take advantage of the high degree of professionalism in the United States that has won patients' respect and loyalty. But there is a difference between utilizing this loyalty versus relying on it. Those practitioners who believe that patient loyalty does not also depend on other, mostly economic, factors are scheduled for loss of practice. Over and over again, doctors have been shocked to hear from a departing longtime patient, "Doctor, I love you. But if I come to you there is a large co-payment. If I go to the managed care plan my company has contracted with, it is free" (Cummings, 1996, p. 9).

Surveys repeatedly demonstrate overwhelming patient satisfaction with practitioners. In fact, most patient satisfaction surveys conducted by health plans actually reflect attitudes toward the caretaker, not the insurer. When practitioner and health plan are separated, surprisingly, the patients rate the doctor high even when they rate the health plan low. An excellent example is the survey conducted by the Pacific Business Group, one of the largest and most active purchasing alliances in the nation (Hall, 1995). This survey found that even when patients rate the health plan as unsatisfactory or marginally satisfactory, they rate the doctors very highly.

Now that purchasing alliances have made possible contracting directly with practitioner owned/managed groups, thus bypassing the managed care companies, the practitioners have the advantage of wide public acceptance along with the ability to better contain costs by eliminating the "middleman," the managed care organizations (MCOs). The latter is the key; despite having obvious advantages, the practitioner groups must learn to predict and control costs. Without this ability, one is not a player in the health system today.

The MCOs are well aware of this edge held by practitioners, and they are now relying on practitioner inertia and their unwillingness to change to win the race that is evolving. Knowing that practitioners can now compete directly, the MCOs are frantically buying up group practices so they can proffer their own captives in the struggle for contracts. Many successful group practices are selling to the MCOs, unable to resist "cashing in" and erroneously believing they can continue their autonomous environment under the masters (Cummings, 1996).

The next two or three years will determine who will win this race. Practitioners who want to create a congenial career environment where they can practice with self-respect must act now to form practitioner-equity group practices. This leads us to the first of a series of predictions to help providers form these practitioner-equity group practices. These predictions, which were recently published, have been modified to accommodate evolved changes since that time (Cummings, 1995, 1996).

Prediction 1. Behavioral Health Carve-outs Will Disappear.

The primary reason specialized behavioral healthcare companies emerged in the first place is that the health insurers did not know how to control these costs. Now that the technology is available to everyone, carving out behavioral healthcare is unnecessary. The success of managed care has shown that employers/buyers no longer need to be baffled by the practitioner's psycho-babble, or be awed by the so-called sanctity of the client-therapist relationship. The guru has been defrocked, as current buyers know a great deal about our own profession with its frailties along with its real and potential contributions.

The trend in which large healthcare systems buy the behavioral care carve-outs is well under way. It is also part of the consolidation as a necessary step in industrialization.

Prediction 2. Medical Cost Offset Will Become the Most Regarded Outcomes Research.

A recent survey has shown that employers overwhelmingly believe that psychological intervention can significantly impact on medical and surgical costs by addressing effectively the large group of patients who somaticize stress and emotional problems (Oss, 1993). Thirty years of medical cost offset research have demonstrated that the more integrated behavioral care is to the entire health delivery system, the greater the cost offset (Cummings, 1993).

Prediction 3. The Future of Doctoral-Level Psychology Lies in Behavioral Health.

With master's-level technicians doing the routine psychotherapy in the future, doctoral-level professional psychologists will become managers, researchers and supervisors of therapy in the integrated behavioral care systems that will dominate our field by the end of the century. Empirically derived treatment protocols will enable master's-trained therapists to provide routine care. But as in all protocols, even the best, they are applicable to only about one-third of the patient category they are intended to address. The remaining two-thirds will require the skill and supervision of a doctorally trained psychologist. (See Cummings, 1995, for a more detailed discussion of the future of behavioral health.)

At the present time psychology is the pre-eminent behavioral health profession, but psychiatry is making every attempt to usurp this status. It remains to be seen whether psychology allows yet another opportunity to slip through its fingers. But this need not be mired in another battle over turf. Ideally psychology and psychiatry will work in concert, along with non-psychiatric physicians, in the behavioral health system of the future.

Prediction 4. Community Consortia Will Emerge and Dictate the Market.

These groups will be dominated by the buyers, who not only will insist on cost savings, but will monitor the extent and quality of services provided. The consortia will resemble the purchasing alliances proposed in the health reform proposal, but they will not have the force of law along with controversial government sanctions. Rather, they will constitute a market-oriented response with the power of economic force. The negative financial consequences will be severe for those providers who oppose these consortia (Neer, 1994).

Prediction 5. The Delivery Systems of the Future Will Be the Community Accountable Healthcare Networks (CAHNs).

The term used is the one proffered by Neer (1994), but other names are likely to emerge as the concept is implemented over the next several years. These networks will be comprehensive and provide *all* health services: outpatients, inpatient, and partial care. They will receive prospective reimbursement (capitation) and as their name implies, they will be accountable to the community consortium that selected them.

Such accountability is not new. When the Kaiser Permanente Health Plan, the precursor to the modern health maintenance organization (HMO), was founded nearly 50 years ago, it had strong labor union participation. As the primary buyers, these labor unions met regularly with the health providers and made their expectations known. This phenomenon was often characterized as an unofficial partnership between the doctors and the purchasers of healthcare, and a similar participation is anticipated between the community consortium and the accountable network.

The primary examples over the years have been the various regional Permanente Medical Groups (PMGs) that serviced and were accountable to the Kaiser Foundation Health Plan (Cummings & VandenBos, 1981). Many differences exist between the PMGs and what is being envisaged in the future, and a more accurate example may be the Mullikin Group on the West Coast, which has been extensively described (DeLafuente, 1993). Of importance is that these CAHNs will restore practitioner autonomy and self-respect, and will eliminate the managed care company as middleman.

These networks are not easily formed and managed, for a business as well as a caring attitude must prevail. But the astute psychologist will begin talking with like-minded medical and allied health practitioners with the goal of forming such delivery systems so as to be on the ground floor as equal partners with physicians. The providers today have the advantage over their predecessors in that there now exist physician management companies that help practitioners form such groups, and to manage their costs thereafter. This has prevented a repetition of the casualty rate of the 1980s when physicians formed equity groups without any ability to predict and control costs. Less than 5% of such groups survived the decade, with most being acquired by managed care organizations at a bargain price.

Prediction 6. The Eventual Return of the Staff Model.

The CAHN will be an exclusive provider group, serving a population or a geographic region. This trend is already discernible, as exclusive provider organization (EPOs) are the newest and fastest growing entities in the current managed care scene. Most follow the network model in delivering services, but there is an increasing interest in the staff-network model, and even the staff model itself. It is apparent that as the American people become more accustomed to being managed, there will be a resurgence of the staff model. The group will still bear the name "network" as it will be such in the broadest sense of the term, bringing together not only outpatient clinics, but also hospitals and partial care centers.

Prediction 7. The Hospital Will No Longer Be Pivotal.

Historically, the acute care hospitals and their medical staffs have played a pivotal role in the American healthcare delivery system. In the future, this will change dramatically with the acute care hospitals becoming equal partners in the accountable healthcare networks. Already we are witnessing the largest proprietary hospital corporation in the country developing all-purpose healthcare networks.

To stop the steady decline of the hospital, while recognizing that ambulatory care will increasingly be the treatment of choice, the physicians formed alliances with many hospitals throughout the nation. These "provider hospital organizations" (PHOs) seldom fared well inasmuch as hospital management has difficulty changing from its "bricks and mortar" mentality. The hospital's objective remains that of filling empty beds, the very antithesis of the national trend of shifting costs from inpatient to ambulatory care.

Other physicians formed their own delivery systems apart from the hospital, preferring to independently contract with the latter only for needed inpatient services, and thus avoiding the enormous overhead and other liabilities that plague hospital administration. The objective was to move the industry toward physician-owned managed care. These physicians structured their organizations so that everyone had a voice, overlooking the propensity of providers to obsess any issue to oblivion. Participant ownership requires strong management, with a strict limitation on the providers' ability to meddle in administration.

Prediction 8. Behavioral Care Will Integrate with Primary Care.

The concept of the carve-out was initially necessary to save the mental health benefit as insurers were deleting it from health coverage because of skyrocketing costs. In his initial prediction, Cummings (1986) stated that the life span of the "carve-out" should not exceed 10 to 12 years. All of the financial "fat" has essentially been wrung out of the mental health system and the future cost savings will come out of the enormous expenditures that patients with psychological distress require of the medical-surgical system.

The carve-outs have grown to encompass 75% of the insured population, and do not want to change. But as long as medicine and behavioral care remain separate delivery systems, medical cost offset research is hampered or rendered impossible. It is through savings in primary care through psychological interventions that behavioral health will be accorded its rightfully important role in the U.S. health system.

Prediction 9. Prospective Reimbursement Will Predominate.

Prospective reimbursement (capitation) will be the only method of payment, and skill in pricing the capitate rate is one of the keys to success. Priced too low, the delivery will fail. On the other hand, pricing it too high makes the delivery system noncompetitive. This will be a new era in pricing that eliminates the low-balling practices prevalent at the present time. Low-balling is merely underpricing one's competitors with the intent of making up the loss by skimping on the delivery of contracted services. The community oversight will closely monitor the extent and quality of what is actually delivered.

For the interim that MCOs continue, steadily decreasing case rates will prevail over capitation. The reason is that most groups are not yet sophisticated enough to undertake capitation, but those that can prepare themselves early will get the contracts. Those groups remaining on case rates will feel the pinch as MCOs have no alternative in today's market but to squeeze the providers.

Fee-for-service, already regarded as an endangered species, should disappear by the end of the century.

Prediction 10. The Standardization of Psychotherapy.

Practioners' long-standing resistance to brief psychotherapy is being swept away in the rush to acquire new skills in time-effective interventions. Those who have long been associated with intensive, problem-solving approaches (Bennett, 1994; Budman & Gurman, 1988; Cummings, 1992) are suddenly in demand and new national companies have been formed in response to the clamor for retraining. One need only peruse the scores of brochures coming to practitioners through the mails to see that for every seminar in long-term therapy there are literally dozens of offerings in time-effective or brief therapy.

Organized healthcare makes possible the intensity of outcomes research that was not contemplated until recently. Computers and millions of patients as potential subjects are coming together in a way that will facilitate standardization—one of the prime characteristics of industrialization. Effective, efficient protocols will be rapidly developed and will be extensively available by the turn of the century (Edley, 1996; Morrison, 1996). In addition, a national newsletter is being planned that will publish protocols and encourage providers to test their effectiveness and provide feedback (Thomas, 1996). Finally, even the APA has a new task force on standardization, a surprising move for a professional society that has demonstrated so much resistance to change in the recent past.

Seven years of experience and research at American Biodyne (Cummings, 1994, 1995, 1996) indicate that so many psychological conditions respond better to group psychotherapy that only 25% of the psychotherapy of the future will be individual. Another 25% will be group psychotherapy, while at least 50% will be psychoeducational programs based on behavioral health models. These latter groups not only have been demonstrated as impacting effectively on stress and unhealthy lifestyles, perhaps the leading escalators of health costs, but also they appropriately reduce the demand for individual psychotherapy.

SUMMARY AND CONCLUSIONS

Lacking understanding of economic principles, providers angrily reacted to managed care as a static "thing." Rather, it is only the first phase of healthcare's industrialization, an evolving process that will render healthcare delivery in 20 years to bear as little resemblance to the MCOs of today as Henry Ford's Model T has to space technology.

In this evolutionary process, the MCOs seem to have outlived their usefulness as arbitrageur, or broker between the buyers and sellers of healthcare, and an era of opportunity is opening that could well herald the renaissance of practice. This would resupport the clinically driven managed care system as conceived and implemented by Cummings (1986), replacing the outmoded MCOs that have succeeded in removing all the fat from behavioral health except for their own bloated bureaucracies.

Scrambling to differentiate themselves from their competitors in a time characterized by downward pressure on prices, the MCOs are looking for quality. It is doubtful if any can produce convincing outcomes research that will differentiate one from another, and they haven't a clue as to how to regain their clinical focus. In counterproductive desperation, they are squeezing the providers with even smaller case and capitation rates, a sure way to achieve even poorer quality.

On the other hand, the providers who can now market directly to the purchasing alliances, bypassing the MCOs, are in a position to replace the managed care companies if they respond rapidly and aggressively to 10 already discernible trends. These predictions could well define the course of behavioral healthcare in the first decade of the next century:

1. Behavioral health will become an integral part of the healthcare system as carve-outs disappear. Carve-outs are out; carve-ins are in.

2. Medical cost offset research will position behavioral healthcare to impact on medical/surgical costs, establishing its rightful place in primary care.

3. The future of doctoral-level mental health practitioners lies in behavioral health, as master's-level personnel will provide most of the psychotherapy.

4. Community consortia, or purchasing alliances, will enable the consumer to make intelligent buying decisions.

5. Practitioner-driven networks will emerge that will be accountable to the consumer.

6. As the American people become more accustomed to being managed, there will be a resurgence of the more efficient staff model.

7. The hospital will no longer be pivotal to the health system, and will be just another segment of the network.

8. There will be a preeminence of the physician-equity model, and since healthcare will be in the hands of all-service health groups, it is imperative that behavioral health providers become owners in these emerging groups.

9. Prospective reimbursement will predominate, and case rates will in time give way to capitation.

10. Psychotherapy will be standardized.

The MCOs recognize the practitioner advantage and are in a race to buy up group practices so that they can own the next generation of managed care. They are relying on practitioner inertia. The next two or three years will determine whether behavioral care providers seize the moment and own their own destinies, or whether they will remand themselves to work for the "company store."

The Importance of the Psychodynamic Formulation

Although some people call me a "strategic therapist," in my book Focused Psychotherapy, *I stress that psychodynamics are the road map of the treatment plan. That is the way I formulate the case.*

L. T.: *Could you drop the psychodynamics and still get the same results?*

N. C.: *I don't think so. I admit that the psychoanalytic approach we were using during the early Kaiser years was different from that of anyone else. This was the mobilization of rage in the service of health. And that's what seemed to be the factor that made our one-session people have such good results.*

L. T.: *In one of the studies, a remarkable result was that a single session actually seemed to decrease medical use over time. It seems the person keeps resolving his or her psychological issues—without therapy! Do you think the psychodynamic formulation, regardless of whether it is obvious or not, contributed that part?*

N. C.: *I think that is right.*

L. T.: *Were there therapists at Biodyne who never believed in the psychodynamics but whom you hired anyway? And how did they do compared with those who did the psychodynamics?*

J. C.: *They never did as well.*

N. C.: *This is why I have said repeatedly: the best therapists are those who have had tremendous training in psychodynamics and are able to divorce it from the "psycho-religion" of psychanalysis. The therapists who did not do the psychodynamic formulation did not do as well. This is why I invented the garlic and onion chart and started teaching those who didn't understand psychodynamics.*

J. C.: The people at Biodyne who had no background whatsoever in psychodynamics were the ones who kept attempting to remediate, and they either weeded themselves out or eventually a clinical manager would ask them to leave because they just weren't getting it.

N. C.: And Janet was in the middle of it. She was a staff psychologist and was working the trenches. This wasn't something I perceived from the top.

J. C.: I saw several people leave on their own or be asked to go and work somewhere else for the simple reason that they were never able to grasp the psychodynamics, or, in Biodyne terms, the onion and garlic. They were never able to grasp the operational diagnosis, the implicit contract—the things that were central to the Biodyne model. And those who were trained strictly as behavioral psychologists, or cognitive behavioral, with no background in psychodynamics, got weeded out along the line. A few of them managed to learn about this level of analysis, but most of them didn't learn and didn't stay.

{ 29 }

THE BEHAVIORAL HEALTH PRACTITIONER OF THE FUTURE: THE EFFICACY OF PSYCHOEDUCATIONAL PROGRAMS IN INTEGRATED PRIMARY CARE*

IN THE PAST 20 years, and especially during the last decade, there has been a surprisingly rapid emergence of psychoeducational programs that combine treatment, information dissemination, and behavioral techniques directed at inducing life-style changes, all within a time-limited group model. Early research, to be discussed below, strongly suggests that these programs are effective with a number of psychological and medical conditions and may replace much of the work that is currently conducted in one-on-one psychotherapy. Not only does the research indicate that many of these targeted group models are more effective with a surprisingly wide range of emotional reactions and physical diseases, they also cost significantly less than does individual psychotherapy, and even brief individual psychotherapy, for the same conditions.

In this era of cost containment, when psychotherapists' practices are experiencing serious economic downturns, any efforts to render psychotherapy more efficient are viewed with suspicion and even alarm by practitioners. Yet several psychotherapist researchers who predate the current cost-conscious climate have held that the respon-

*With Janet L. Cummings, Psy.D.

sibility of the practitioner is to render our interventions more effective and efficient for the sake of the patient, and that effective therapy results in cost containment without making economics the primary focus (Balint, 1957; Budman & Gurman, 1988; Cummings, 1977; Cummings & Follette, 1968; Cummings & VandenBos, 1979; Davanloo, 1978; Erickson, 1980; Follette & Cummings, 1967; Hoyt, 1995; Malan, 1976; Sifneos, 1987). Effective–efficient practitioner driven psychotherapy systems are seen as the quality solution against which business driven systems cannot successfully compete (Cummings, 1996c, 1966d). Cummings and Sayama (1995) make explicit that the therapist's obligation is to bring relief from pain, anxiety, and depression to the patient in the shortest time possible. This requires honing one's skills and striving to make this outcome a reality with every patient that is treated.

Several movements converged to produce the current enthusiasm for psychoeducational programs: brief psychotherapy, time-limited group therapy, and skills training. It is worthwhile to trace the historical precursors to the present movement, and to examine a few examples of research through which psychoeducational programs are being developed. This discussion will review the necessary characteristics and ingredients of successful psychoeducational programs and present several diverse, but effective models.

HISTORICAL PERSPECTIVE

Time-Sensitive Psychotherapy

Early efforts to render therapy more efficient and effective were largely directed toward individual therapy and have not abated. Alexander and French (1946) were considered outlandish when they suggested that in many instances psychoanalysis could be concluded within 150 sessions. They angered the psychotherapeutic community with their contention that Freud discovered brief psychotherapy when he eliminated Bruno Walter's psychic pain in his conducting arm in just 6 sessions and "cured" Gustav Mahler's sex problem during a 3-hour walk.

Bloom (1991) traced the history of short-term therapy and concluded that the field has never been hospitable to the notion of time-sensitive approaches. Most psychotherapists not only prefer long-term therapy, but they continue to see patients as long as they are willing to come in, and as long as insurance will pay for it, ignoring what might be identified as therapeutic drift. Bloom indicates that recently many psychotherapists have escalated their hostility to short-term therapy as these techniques have impacted negatively on their previously flourishing practices.

Origins and Development of Group Therapy

Balint (1957) unleashed a storm of controversy when he envisaged group psychotherapy as filling the gap created by the shortage of psychotherapists. Since that time, critics of group therapy have continued to see this method as an expedient, while advocates take strong issue with that attribution. Actually, long before Balint, Freud (1921/1955) outlined a group therapy model that is still quite meaningful. He stated that, in a way, all psychology is essentially group psychology, and group psychology is the original and oldest psychology. He spoke of a group of two, and thus was able to link individual and group psychotherapy together. Freud emphasized that a collection of people is not a group, but it can develop as such with the introduction of leadership. Traditional group therapy has consisted of "open groups" in which patients who are generally comparable in goals and problems enter a group, participate for a few months to a few years, and then move on. The group and the group leader have a perpetuity of their own. Most often group members are recruited from the psychotherapist's individual therapy practice, but a smaller number of prestigious group therapists who exclusively conduct groups receive referrals from a broad array of colleagues.

Historically, group psychotherapy received its greatest impetus in the United Kingdom after World War II. Following a lukewarm reception throughout most of the world's psychotherapeutic community, the nationalization of health care in Great Britain created a demand for group therapy because the need for treatment exceeded the number of practitioners who could provide one-on-one therapy. Within a relatively short time clinical research demonstrated that group therapy was not only expedient, it was also effective (Balint, 1957).

More recently, the perpetual nature of traditional group psychotherapy has been challenged. Two highly respected long-term group psychotherapists discovered that 40% of their patients left before the end of the first year, 75% left before the end of 2 years, and 90% left before the end of 4 years (Rutan & Stone, 1984; Stone & Rutan, 1984). Only 10% of the group therapy patients fulfilled the traditional notions of perpetuity. Similarly, Klein and Carroll (1986) found that in a community mental health center 52% of patients entering group therapy left by the twelfth session, and the mean number of sessions for all patients was 18.8, while the mode was a single visit. Following a number of similar researches, Budman and Gurman (1988) developed their generic model of short-term experiential group psychotherapy. Its demonstrated effectiveness, along with its markedly increased efficiency, has made it an attractive alternative to more traditional models.

Much earlier clinical research revealed that certain conditions are more responsive to group therapy than to individual therapy. For example, early work at Kaiser Permanente indicated that group psychotherapy was highly effective with addictions, while individual psychotherapy was relatively ineffective (Cummings, 1979). Addicts require the group culture of enforced abstinence as a potent force, a feature absent in one-on-one therapy where they seem to settle for becoming a "comfortable loser" (Peele, 1978). For different reasons, agoraphobics were found to recover much more rapidly in specially designed groups, benefiting from the reinforced desensitization as well as the realization that others share their fears and that they are not "insane" or about to have a fatal heart attack (Hardy, 1970). Since these early reports, there has been a proliferation of groups designed to address specific conditions. A number of trends are rapidly converging to forge the new group psychotherapies.

From Skills Training to Psychoeducation

Paralleling the development of short-term group therapy, and actually preceding it, is the large body of research in skills training. This has been reviewed extensively by O'Donohue and Krasner (1995), beginning with Jacobsen's relaxation training at the beginning of the century, through the social skills training of both children and adults, assertiveness training, parenting skills training, marital skills training, and even such issues as self-appraisal skills training and employment skills training. Throughout these groups, skills were emphasized. However, they never really became part of the health system (until at least very recently), and the term *psychoeducational* only rarely appeared and was overlooked in favor of skills training.

Third-party payors took the experimenters and clinicians who were involved in skills training at their own word, concluding they were not treatment per se, and excluded such approaches from insurance reimbursement. With a few notable exceptions, it remained for the emergence of organized health settings, and particularly capitated ones, before there was a widespread use of these kinds of groups which, once in an organized behavioral health care setting, began very quickly to be known as psychoeducational programs.

The Influence of Organized Settings

It is not surprising that, given the rapid development of protocols for individual psychotherapy, there is a decided movement toward the rapid development of group protocols. There is a new definition of group cohesion, for now groups are being formed in direct response to patients suffering from a specific psychological or medical condition, including severe mental illness and chronic physical disease. Programs addressing chronic populations have been especially useful and popular in the emerging integration of behavioral health and primary care.

Currently there are available over 200 psychoeducational programs targeting specific populations. Examples range from survivors of incest to bipolar disorder, and from hypertension to rheumatoid arthritis. Unfortunately, only a few are the results of either empirical research or clinical demonstrations. Many seem to resemble pop psychology, while others have been subjected to rigorous study. In the future, only the latter will be part of the repertoire of our mental and behavioral care delivery systems. Managed care companies and HMOs have no incentive to finance ineffective therapies in which reliving childhood trauma is supposed to undo adult personality problems (Seligman, 1994), or to subject themselves to malpractice suits resulting from unsound treatment techniques. They do have a need for effective and efficient group therapy protocols, empirically derived.

If some clinically driven organized settings are harbingers, there are drastic changes about to take place in the delivery of behavioral health services. In its seventh year of operation nationally, American Biodyne's mental health and chemical dependency services were only 25% individual psychotherapy; another 25% was time-limited group therapy, while fully 50% were psychoeducational programs emanating from empirically derived protocols. The behavioral care system at the Santa Teresa Kaiser Permanente Medical Center is rapidly approaching a similar experience.

Research is beginning to demonstrate the optimal number of group sessions for each condition (Budman & Gurman, 1988). The group protocols are as few as 5 sessions and as many as 60, again depending on the specific psychological or medical condition being addressed.

Most experienced HMO therapists find a length of 60 sessions excessive, and prefer allowing the one or two patients from each group who could benefit from additional treatment to repeat the series rather than prolong the original series. In addition to parsimony, this also has the advantage of having one or two group members in the new group who are "seasoned" by a previous group experience.

It is difficult, if not impossible, for solo practitioners to attain the critical mass necessary to form a number of specific groups. On the other hand, organized delivery systems such as HMOs and managed care networks can offer a wide array of specific, time-limited groups. There are solo practitioners who specialize in a circumscribed population, such as patients suffering from repressed memories of child abuse or multiple personality disorder, to name only two of the most common. The danger here is the tendency of some such practitioners to overly diagnose the condition that absorbs their interest, and represents the majority of their practice and livelihood. Organized settings, having the capacity to address the universe of psychological conditions, have no incentive to overly diagnose certain conditions. One delivery setting has available over 70 specific group protocols (Cummings, 1985b) as covered benefits, making it unnecessary to funnel patients into a small repertoire of special groups.

PSYCHOEDUCATIONAL PROGRAMS

The senior author and his colleagues first began experimenting with psychoeducational programs in the late 1960s and early 1970s at the Kaiser Permanente Health Plan in the San Francisco Bay Area (Cummings & VandenBos, 1981). Those early years required seeking out or developing sophisticated programs, because there was a paucity of information and data. Four highly developed group protocols were available: (1) the agoraphobia desensitization program having wide dissemination throughout the Terrap National Network (Hardy, 1970) and adapted by the authors for their use; (2) a highly successful internally generated program to teach abstinence life-styles to addicts (Cummings, 1979); (3) a relaxation program which was the precursor to a more sophisticated stress management protocol that came later; (4) a smoking cessation program that attracted many referrals, as the Surgeon General had just issued his first warning on smoking.

During the ensuing years, more programs were empirically developed as a result of highly encouraging early determinations of effectiveness. By the early 1980s, there were 68 psychoeducational programs in various stages of development ready to be field tested in the Hawaii Medicaid Project (Cummings et al., 1993; Pallak et al., 1994). The research methodology employed to construct these protocols was the medical cost offset outcome methodology previously and extensively reported (Cummings, 1994). Although the efficiency and effectiveness of these programs were demonstrated in Hawaii, these findings were part of an overall evaluation revealing the superiority of a prospectively reimbursed, organized, and focused psychotherapy system over the traditional, disjointed fee-for-service system of local solo practitioners. An additional study was needed which would render a direct comparison between individual therapy effectively delivered as the control group, and a comparable population diverted from individual psychotherapy to specific psychoeducational programs as the experimental group.

Methodology

Two new Biodyne Centers established in the same city in the late 1980s were designated for the study. Center A (experimental) implemented several psychoeducational programs and every patient who presented during two successive periods of 6 months, and who fell into any of five categories, was assigned to the corresponding psychoeducational program. These programs with designated patients were as follows: (1) adult children of alcoholics; (2) agoraphobia and multiple phobias; (3) borderline personality; (4) independent living for chronic schizophrenia; (5) perfectionistic personality life-style.

In center B (control), every patient falling into any of the above five categories was routinely assigned to individual psychotherapy for two successive periods of 6 months each. All of the study patients in both centers were followed for a period of 2 years after their 6 months in treatment. Although there was not a randomized assignment of patients to the control and experimental conditions because this would be tantamount to denying available services in center A, the two groups from the two centers were comparable in all demographic characteristics (age, gender, socioeconomic level, education, ethnicity). Further, this arrangement permitted direct comparison between individual psychotherapy and psychoeducational programs which was not possible within the randomized assignment of patients in the Hawaii Medicaid Project.

As noted, there were two different periods of patient selection of 6 months' duration each in both centers. All patients had a 2-year follow-up after the initial 6 months. The total time of experiment was 3 years, but only 2½ years for each particular group. Because center A was larger, there were 151 patients in the experimental group, while smaller center B yielded 84 patients for the control group.

Results

The results are shown in Table 1, which reveals that for these five categories, the average number of psychoeducational sessions (experimental group) was only two more than the average number of individual sessions in the control group. Not even taking into account the cost differential (individual ratio 1:1 between patients and therapists, psychoeducational 1:8 to 15), this resulted in a 90% reduction in demand for individual therapy, a 95% reduction in hospital days, a 97% reduction in emergency services (including emergency room visits and drop-in sessions), a 70% reduction in prescriptions for medication, and an 85% reduction in return visits.

Table 1. *A Comparison in the Use of Various Behavioral Health Services Between an Experimental Group Assigned to a Psychoeducational Model and the Control Group Assigned to the Traditional Model*

	N		Group Sessions		Individual Sessions		Hospital Days		Emergency		Perscript		Return Visits	
	Ex	Co	Ex	Co	Ex	Co	Ex	Co	Ex	Co	Ex	Co	Ex	Co
ACOA	38	12	570	46	76	132	1	11	6	8	16	24	53	38
Agoraphobia	23	8	460	0	46	122	14	21	9	37	26	28	38	63
Borderline	42	29	840	109	5	609	3	145	0	289	38	87	22	493
Indep. Living	22	18	422	315	21	72	26	183	4	51	41	68	251	488
Perfectionism	26	17	390	0	24	401	0	19	0	23	14	39	13	208
TOTALS	151	84	2682	480	172	1336	44	379	19	398	135	246	377	1290
MEANS			17.8	5.7	1.2	15.9	0.2	4.5	0.1	4.7	0.9	2.9	2.5	15.4

Legend:
ACOA: Adult Children of Alcoholics 15-session program
Agoraphobia and Multiple Phobias 20-Session program
Borderline Personality Disorder 20-Session program
Independent Living for Chronic Schizophrenics 25-Session program
Perfectionism Leading to Disabling Episodes 15-Session program
Note: Group therapy sessions for the control group were in traditional (i.e., nonpsycho educational) groups, while group sessions for the experimental group were all in psychoeducational programs.

For illustrative purposes, these findings can be translated into economic terms. Assuming an hour of individual psychotherapy costs $100, the cost of 1½ hours of a psychoeducational program per patient would be $150 divided by the average patient group of 10, which equals $15 per patient. What is startling, this $15 per patient unit investment then goes on to save between 70 and 97% in hospitalization, individual therapy, emergency room visits, medication prescriptions, and return visits.

Discussion

These results do not indicate that all patients would do better in psychoeducational programs rather than individual therapy. Quite the contrary, what these results reveal is that for certain psychological conditions, a well-designed, empirically derived psychoeducational program may well be the treatment of choice. It must be emphasized that a good psychoeducational protocol is not the product of armchair speculation, but the outcome of fastidious empirical research (see again the description of the research methodology in Cummings [1994]).

Case Illustration

Loni was a 38-year-old married mother of three children. Her husband was a highly paid vice-president for a large corporation, while she ran a successful financial planning business out of her home. She delighted in her three beautiful children who were excelling in school, her attentive executive husband, and a business that allowed her to set her own hours. Her large home in exurbia reflected a high degree of success and her excellent taste. She could not understand why every 1½ to 2 years she would be unable to cope and would need psychotherapy.

The first breakdown came in college when Loni was unable to turn in her term papers and other homework assignments because she saw her work as inadequate. She became suicidal and was successfully treated in the university counseling center. Since that time, she experienced 11 more episodes, approximately 1½ to 2 years apart, necessitating treatment which was always effective within 2 to 4 months. These episodes were typically bouts of severe depression, or disabling obsessive-compulsive symptoms. Twice she became agoraphobic, and struggled to leave the house.

Loni was a perfectionist, the perfect daughter of a perfectionistic father. When she became dysfunctional again at age 38, instead of treating her depression, she was referred to the Perfectionistic Lifestyle Group. Highly resistant at first, she quickly took hold and by the 15th and last session, she had drastically altered her life-style. She no longer subjected herself to unattainable standards, and her husband's perfectionistic demands, which sometimes seemed to replicate those of her deceased father, no longer bothered her. She became more relaxed with her three children, and especially toward the daughter she heretofore was certain "would turn out neurotic like me." As of this writing, it is over 5 years since her last recurring episode.

CHARACTERISTICS AND UTILITY OF PSYCHOEDUCATIONAL MODELS

Psychoeducational programs serve three functions with varying degrees among the various programs as to which is the primary function in a specific model: treatment, prevention, and management.

Treatment

The surprising feature of psychoeducation is that it can be therapeutic, and for some conditions, more effective than traditional modes. Our preliminary results indicate that the greatest therapeutic effect is most likely to be with life-styles which reflect the patient's overscrupulousness: perfectionists, agoraphobics, adult children of alcoholics, and other conditions in which the patient suffers from overbearing neurotic guilt. These patients keep their appointments, engage themselves attentively, respect the authority of the professional, and always do their homework.

A lesser therapeutic effect is seen in personality disorders, such as borderline personalities, addicts, and other patients who are rebellious, challenge authority, are likely to thwart appointments, and avoid homework assignments. These are the patients who do not suffer from direct feelings of guilt, and their main distress is the result of their own chaotic life-styles. It is important that personality disorders not be placed in groups where the patients are neurotically guilt-ridden, as they will literally wreck the group and drive the other program participants to despair. This often happens because personality disorders can become depressed, phobic, or anxious, while borderline patients can mimic just about any psychological condition. The primary diagnosis of personality disorder must prevail over the dual diagnosis reflecting the secondary condition.

In chronic physical conditions such as asthma, emphysema, diabetes, rheumatoid arthritis, essential hypertension, and other diseases, the goal is not to cure that which cannot be cured. This does not mean that reductions in pain and morbidity are not in themselves therapeutic; the emphasis, however, is in disease management.

Management

It is precisely with these kinds of intractable conditions, both medical and psychological, that management is important. In the psychological conditions (e.g., borderline personalities, addicts, chronic schizophrenics, impulse disorders, and most "Axis II" patients), every practitioner is painfully aware of the constant, clawing demands and acting out that are so characteristic. Yet these patients, including the borderline personality, become manageable and less vulnerable to the consequences of their own emotional lability, constant rage, and impulsiveness. (For a full description of the borderline protocol, see Cummings & Sayama [1995, pp. 241-248]).

The independent living programs are conducted in various critical places in the environment, and teach chronic schizophrenics how to accomplish such frightening tasks as purchasing underwear, ordering a meal, or buying a bus ticket without being overcome with psychotic anxiety. Although the psychotic thought disorder is incurable, the patient suffers fewer and fewer "crises" which provoke acute exacerbations of the kinds of ideation and behavior which result in restraint and hospitalization.

With chronic medical diseases, psychoeducational programs can increase coping, especially regarding the management of pain and physical limitations, as well as enhance compliance with the medical regimen.

Prevention

The remarkable finding is that for appropriate patients assigned to appropriate psychoeducational programs, the demand for more intrusive services is significantly, if not dramatically, diminished. This is true prevention: services are no longer needed (i.e., the "demand" side in health economics), as contrasted with reducing services as found in most cost-containment (i.e., the "supply" side in health economics). Those patients who are prone to abuse hospitalization or emergency rooms by threatening suicide, such as borderline personalities, learn to manage their lives without such drastic recourse. Chronic schizophrenics who require frequent and sometimes protracted hospitalizations learn to avoid the exacerbations which trigger this need for hospitalization or restraint by medication.

Reducing costs by reducing demand is certainly more desirable than rationing care, and is the very essence of both prevention and cost-containment. In fact, the impetus for developing the independent living programs was a direct result of the discovery that the first capitated behavioral health Medicare contract of 140,000 covered lives, along with the elderly, had 8,000 persons in their thirties who were on Social Security by virtue of disabling mental illness. Their average hospitalization rate of nearly 50 days a year could have bankrupted the coverage for the entire cohort of which the vast majority were elderly Social Security recipients. A series of independent living programs rescued the entire contracted system by drastically reducing the need for hospitalization (Cummings, 1997).

Hospital days utilized can also be reduced in populations suffering from chronic medical conditions, along with significant reduction in emergency room visits and invasive procedures (Mumford, Schlesinger, & Glass, 1982; Schlesinger et al., 1983).

ELEMENTS OF PSYCHOEDUCATIONAL PROTOCOLS

There are a number of elements that psychoeducational programs have in common, although not every protocol will contain each and every one of the following:

An *Educational Component* from which the patient learns a great deal about the medical or psychological condition, as well as the interplay between one's body and emotions.

Pain Management for those populations suffering from chronic pain. This includes help in reducing undue reliance on pain medication and addressing any problems of iatrogenic addiction.

Relaxation Techniques, which include meditation and guided imagery.

Stress Management, adjusted to meet the needs of specific conditions and populations.

A *Support System* which includes not only the group milieu, but also the presence of "veterans" who have been through the program. A useful modification of this element is the pairing of patients into a "buddy system" that allows them to call each other, meet for desensitization or other homework, and generally be there for each other in time of need.

A *Self-Evaluation* component which not only enables the patient to assess how well he or she is doing psychologically, but also teaches the patient to monitor such critical features as blood pressure, diet, insulin, and other signs important in chronic illness.

Homework is assigned after every session. The homework is carefully designed to move the patient to the next step of self-mastery, and may include desensitization, behavioral exercises, planned encounters with one's relationships or environment, readings, and other assignments which are critical to the well-being of the patient. The homework is never perfunctory. It is always relevant to the condition being treated and well timed to enhance development.

Timing, Length, and Number of Sessions vary from protocol to protocol, reflecting the needs of each population or condition, and in accordance with research and experience.

Treatment of Depression for those patients whose severely altered mood is interfering with their ability to participate in the program.

Self-Efficacy (after Bandura, 1977a, 1977b) refers to the belief that one can perform a specific action or complete a task. Although this involves self-confidence in general, it is the confidence to perform a specific task. Positive changes can be traced to an increase in self-efficacy brought about by a carefully designed protocol that will advance the sense of self-efficacy.

Learned Helplessness (after Seligman, 1975) is a concept that holds helplessness is learned and can be unlearned. Some patients with chronic illnesses fall into a state of feeling helpless in the face of their disease. A well-designed protocol will enable a patient to confront and unlearn helplessness.

A *Sense of Coherence* (after Antonovsky, 1987) is required for a person to make sense out of adversity. Patients with chronic physical or mental illnesses feel not only that their circumstances do not make sense, but neither does their life. The ability to cope often depends on the presence or absence of this sense of coherence, and the protocol should be designed to enhance it.

Exercise is an essential component of every protocol, and is the feature that is most often neglected by patients. Exercise helps ameliorate depression, raises the sense of self-efficacy, and promotes coping behavior. The patient should be encouraged to plan and implement his or her own exercise regimen, and then to stick to it.

Modular Formatting enables a protocol to serve different but similar populations and conditions by inserting or substituting condition-specific modules. An example of this is the chronic illness self-help program discussed below.

PSYCHOEDUCATIONAL PROTOCOLS

As of this writing the senior author has identified approximately 200 psychoeducational–psychotherapeutic protocols, many of which have an impressive empirical base (Beck, Steer, & Garbin, 1988), while others reflect extensive clinical experience and judgment (Beckfield, 1994). Some are proprietary and for sale, while still others are in the public domain even though they may be in use within specific settings (Cummings & Sayama, 1995).

Two examples will be discussed. The first illustrates the modular format whereby mixing and matching one basic protocol serves a number of chronic diseases. It is based on the Arthritis Self-Help Course first developed by Lorig in 1978, and subjected to considerable later research and experience (Lorig & Fries, 1990). It was extensively utilized in the 7-year Hawaii Medicaid Project (Cummings et al., 1993) and subsequently within the American Biodyne behavioral care system nationwide.

The second example is illustrative of a single-purpose, but highly effective, bereavement program for widowed older adults that was developed and subjected to research verification in a cohort of 140,000 managed Medicare recipients in Florida (Cummings, 1997).

The Chronic Disease Self-Help Program

Target Population: Adults suffering from asthma, emphysema, diabetes, ischemic heart disease, hypertension, rheumatoid arthritis.

Sessions:	Eight 2-hour sessions spaced as follows: six weekly sessions followed by two monthly sessions.
Group Members:	Eight to 10 adults in each group, with each group limited to one medical condition.
Specific Education:	There is one educational module for each of the six conditions, and the appropriate module is inserted for each group. Each patient learns a great deal about his or her medical condition. Although comprehensive, it is presented simply and with clarity.
General Education:	This educational component imparts knowledge as to how emotions and stress affect the body, and what kinds of psychological factors exacerbate a physical condition or act as triggers for relapse.
Self-Evaluation:	Patients are taught and encouraged to monitor their own important signs and their own medication. Each monitors his or her pertinent signs (e.g., blood pressure, blood sugar, etc.).
Exercise:	Exercise is mandatory and tailored to the patient's condition. Each patient is encouraged to design and implement his or her own exercise program and to stick to it.
Pain Management:	Extensive use is made of the best of pain management techniques, along with
Relaxation:	Relaxation techniques, guided imagery, meditation, and stress management.
Readings:	Self-help books on both the medical condition and psychological factors are assigned throughout the program. Patients are encouraged to discuss how what they read applies to themselves.
Support System:	The group is structured to be highly supportive. In addition, the patients are paired into a "buddy system" and encouraged to meet during the week, do their homework together, and practice their exercises together.
Homework:	Homework is given at the end of each session. There are two types: general homework which addresses common problems, and special home-

work designed to help the patient with difficult problems.

Self-Efficacy:
: Much of the content and homework of the program is designed to restore confidence in performing specific tasks originally restricted by the patient's physical limitations, increasing coping behavior by reducing the sense of helplessness, and restoring the sense of meaning to life in spite of one's circumstances.

Depression:
: Patients who are suffering from clinical depression of the magnitude that prevents full participation in the program are referred for treatment of that severe mood disorder. After the depression has improved sufficiently, the patient may undertake the program. Since some degree of depression may accompany many patients with chronic medical conditions, it has been found that the milder depressions are best treated within the program.

The Bereavement Program for Widowed Older Adults

Target Population:
: Widowed older adults (over 62) who have recently lost a spouse, usually after many years of marriage.

Outreach:
: An aggressive outreach program within the health plan identifies the patient shortly after the death of a spouse. Empathic telephone contact invites the individual to the first session only.

Sessions:
: Total of 14 sessions of 2 hours each, and spaced as follows: four semiweekly sessions, followed by six weekly sessions, and concluding with four monthly sessions.

Group Members:
: At least five and not more than eight patients are assigned to each group. An even number is desirable as the patients are paired in a "buddy" support system.

Screening:
: In addition to the usual bonding, the first session is used to screen out patients who reveal

severe depression rather than uncomplicated mourning. Reactive depression reflecting internalized rage for years of marital unhappiness interferes with the healing process of mourning and is treated separately.

Medication: Patients are helped to use antidepressants sparingly or not at all. These medications retard the process of healing and prolong and even postpone bereavement.

Education: The patient learns a great deal about the process of mourning and its painful, but healing sequence. The grieving person is encouraged to cry, is given permission to spend a lot of time alone in spite of well-meaning friends, and rewarded for reflecting on a lifetime with the deceased, recalling all the good and bad moments. It is normal to miss the deceased very much!

Self-Efficacy: The patient learns to cope with being alone, and if the widowed patient was unduly dependent on the deceased in certain matters (finances, initiative, etc.), he or she is taught to unlearn the helplessness.

Support System: The pairing into a buddy system is particularly important for these patients who at times would rather be with someone who is also mourning than to be with well-meaning friends who often do not know what to say. The patient is also taught how to make friends more comfortable by releasing them from their self-imposed duty to make the mourner feel better. This results in making it possible for patient and friends to comfortably spend more time with each other.

The Veteran: One or two patients who complete each group need additional support and wish to go on to a second group. They are encouraged to do so. Additionally, the presence of one or two "veterans" in each group is additional help and sup-

Homework:

port to the newer patients. Their ability to say, "I remember when I felt exactly as you do, and this is what I did," is of inestimable value.

Since these patients spend a lot of time alone, appropriate reading assignments are welcomed. Not as welcomed is the homework to exercise, and they often must be cajoled into getting out and doing brisk walking. Once they try it, however, they feel so much better that they become fairly consistent in exercising. Mall walking early in the morning is a common older adult activity, so these patients do not feel out of place engaging in that form of exercise.

At the appropriate time homework involving a *moderate* amount of social activity is assigned. This must be carefully tailored to the needs and abilities of each individual.

SUMMARY AND CONCLUSIONS

Several historical movements have converged to make the current interest in psychoeducational programs possible. The development of brief psychotherapy, the emergence of time-limited group psychotherapy, and decades of research in skills training all joined with the rapid emergence of organized settings where the critical mass existed, and the need in primary care was apparent.

Over 25 years of research in three disparate prepaid, organized health settings have demonstrated that selected psychological conditions respond well to empirically derived psychoeducation programs, and for these patients such programs are the treatment of choice over individual psychotherapy or more traditional group psychotherapy. The programs are directed toward faulty life-styles and do not replace the need for either individual or group psychotherapy. These psychoeducational programs are utilitarian in that they accomplish treatment, patient management, and prevention of future need, with varying degrees among the various programs. Finally, psychoeducational programs yield true cost containment by reducing the need for more costly and intrusive services, such as individual therapy, hospitalization, emergency services, medication, and return visits. Rationing of care is thus avoided.

Although psychoeducation will never fully replace individual psychotherapy, years of experience with health delivery would predict the following proportions of psychotherapeutic services in the not too distant future: 25% individual psychotherapy, 25% time-limited group psychotherapy, and as much as 50% psychoeducational programs (Cummings, 1996c). Several health care settings are already reflecting this configuration.

A Secret of Behavioral Health Integration: The Handoff

We learned by experience at Kaiser that a good model is to have health professionals organize themselves into disease-based groups, such as a Low Back Pain Clinic or a Diabetes Clinic. In this way, the behavioral health-care specialists, or psychologists, would be integrated with the other health care practitioners. The psychologist would learn the particular disorder very well, and address the behavioral issues peculiar to that disorder. We also noticed that the doctors would have 15-minute interviews. In the integrated system, the physician would see that a certain patient had a psychological issue, and might profit by seeing the psychologist. So the physician would say, "Let's go see Dr. Cummings," and there would be a handoff to the psychologist. Now this is the subtlety we discovered, and one that can make all the difference in the world as to whether the patient will continue in treatment with the psychologist. The primary care physician stays in the room while the psychotherapist starts the informal session with the patient.

L. T.: So this technique is something like "log rolling." That is, you have one foot on the log you are leaving and the other foot on the log you are going toward. You have a foot on each log at the same time. So you also have two doctors in a room at once, holding the patient's hand, so to speak, until it comes time to leave the patient with the behavioral health-care professional.

N. C.: Yes, that's how it was done. And that difference helped the patient continue with the behavioral treatment. Without this seemingly simple touch, patient compliance was not very good, but with this idea of the handoff, compliance jumped to 90 percent. And the saving in medical costs was tremendous. This became part of the fabric of the health system at Kaiser.

In other medical care systems, the doctors do not want to bother with the psychological problems of their patient. Most often they *don't know what to do even if they do see the problem. In an en-lightened place, perhaps 40 percent of the patients needing a psy-chologist are recognized and referred, and of these, only 10 percent get into therapy. Contrast this with an integrated system in which 90 percent of those who need psychological help would be referred or handed off, and 80 percent would continue in treatment. Thus, in the integrated system, there would be a lot more efficiency in having the patient get the correct treatment.*

In contrast, the carve-out has heightened the problem, since the patient is going not only to a different building, but to a different company. This makes patients reconsider whether or not they want to see a "shrink." Most choose to avoid seeing the psychotherapist. Also, having the patient accept psychological help is only half the battle. The other half is making sure that the psychotherapist can deal with these patients in a flexible way.

I learned a very important lesson during this developmental time at Kaiser: You need to hire the right people up front. Many psychol-ogists did not want to work in such an integrated setting because they felt that they were losing their identity. It was difficult to train them into this more integrated and flexible model, to have them ad-just their point of view toward doing psychological work in ways they had not previously learned.

References

Alexander, F. & French, T. M. (1946). *Psychoanalytic therapy: Principles and applications.* New York: Ronald Press.

Albee, G. W. (1977). Does including psychotherapy in health insurance represent a subsidy to the rich from the poor? *American Psychologist, 32,* 719–721.

Albee, G. W. (1992). The future of psychotherapy. *Psychotherapy, 29,* 139–140.

American Psychiatric Association. (1980). *Diagnostic and statistical manual of mental disorders* (3rd ed.). Washington, DC: Author.

American Psychiatric Association. (1994). *Diagnostic and statistical manual of mental disorders* (4th ed.). Washington, DC: American Psychiatric Press.

Annis, H. (1987, October). Effective treatment for drug and alcohol problems: Do we know? Paper presented at the Annual Meeting of the Institute of Medicine, National Academy of Sciences, Washington, D.C.

Antonovsky, A. (1987). *Unraveling the mystery of health: How people manage stress and stay well.* San Francisco: Jossey-Bass.

Austad, C. S. & Hoyt, M. F. (1992). The managed care movement and the future of psychotherapy. *Psychotherapy, 29,* 109–118.

Avnet, H. H. (1962). *Psychiatric insurance: Financing short term ambulatory treatment.* New York: Group Health Insurance, Inc.

Balint, M. (1957). *The doctor, his patient and the illness.* New York: International Universities Press.

Balint, M. & Balint, E. (1961). *Psychotherapeutic techniques in medicine.* London: Tavistock Publications.

Bandura, A. (1977a). Self-efficacy: Toward a unifying theory of behavioral change. *Psychological Review, 84,* 191–215.

Bandura, A. (1977b). *Social learning theory.* Englewood Cliffs, NJ: Prentice-Hall.

Bandura, A. (1991). Self-efficacy mechanism in physiological activation and health-promoting behavior. In J. Madden (Ed.), *Neurobiology of learning, emotion and affect.* New York: Raven Press.

Battle, C., Imber, S. D., Hoehn-Saric, L. A., Stone, A. R., Nash, E. H., & Frank, J. D. (1966). Target complaints as criteria of improvement. *American Journal of Psychotherapy, 20,* 184–192.

Bean, E. (1985, March 15). Doctors find a dose of marketing can cure pain of sluggish practice. *Wall Street Journal,* 27.

Beck, A. T. & Haaga, D. A. F. (1992). The future of cognitive therapy. *Psychotherapy, 29*(1), 34–38.

Beck, A. T., Hollon, S. D., Young, J. E., et al. (1985). Treatment of depression with cognitive therapy and amitriptyline. *Archives of General Psychiatry, 42,* 142–148.

Beck, A. T., Steer, R. A., & Garbin, M. G. (1988). Psychometric properties of the Beck Depression Inventory: Twenty-five years of evaluation. *Clinical Psychology Review, 8,* 77–100.

Beckfield, D. F. (1994). *Master your panic and take back your life! Twelve treatment sessions to overcome high anxiety.* San Luis Obispo, CA: Impact.

Bennett, M. J. (1994). Can competing psychotherapists be managed? *Managed Care Quarterly, 2,* 29–35.

Bergin, A. E. & Lambert, M. J. (1978). The evaluation of therapeutic outcome. In S. Garfield & A. E. Bergin. (Eds.), *Handbook of psychotherapy and behavior change* (pp. 330–343). New York: Wiley.

Bevan, W. (1982). Human welfare and national policy: A conversation with Stuart Eizenstat. *American Psychologist, 37,* 1128–1135.

Bloom, B. S. (1991). *Planned, short-term psychotherapy: A clinical handbook.* Needham Heights, MA: Allyn & Bacon.

Blum, R. H., et al. (1972). *Horatio Alger's children.* San Francisco: Jossey-Bass.

Bradley, D. D., Wingerd, J., Petitti, D. B., Krauss, R. M., & Ramcharan, S. (1978). Serum high-density lipoprotein cholesterol in women using oral contraceptives, estrogens and progestins. *New England Journal of Medicine, 299.*

Breslow, L. (1973). An historical review of multiphasic screening. *Preventive Medicine, 2.*

Brook, R. H., Ware, J. E., Davies-Avery, A., et al. (1979). Overview of adult health status measures fielded in RAND's health insurance study. *Medical Care, 19,* 787.

Buck, K. & Miller, W. R. (1986). Minimal intervention in the treatment of problem drinkers: A controlled study. Unpublished manuscript as quoted in Miller, W. R. & Hester, R. K., Inpatient alcoholism treatment. *American Psychologist, 41,* 794–805.

Budman, S., Demby, A., & Feldstein, M. L. (1994). Insight into reduced use of medical services after psychotherapy. *Professional Psychology: Research and Practice, 15*, 353-361.

Budman, S. & Gurman, A. (1983a). The practice of brief therapy. *Professional Psychology, 14*, 277-292.

Budman, S. H. & Gurman, A. S. (1983b). *The practice of brief therapy.* New York: Guilford Press.

Budman, S. H. & Gurman, A. S. (1988). *Theory and practice of brief therapy.* New York: Guilford Press.

Budman, S. H., Hoyt, M. F., & Friedman, S. (Eds.). (1992). *The first session of brief therapy.* New York: Guilford Press.

Canelo, C. K., Bissell, D. M., Abrams, H., & Breslow, L. A. (1949). A multiphasic screening survey in San Jose. *California Medicine, 71.*

Cantor, D. (1993, August). Will the solo independent practitioner be extinct by the year 2000? Presented at the APA Practice Directorate Miniconvention of the 101st Annual Convention of the American Psychological Association, Toronto, Ont., Canada.

Casey, T. & Siegel, H. (1982, June). Compensation and benefits: Health care cost containment. *Personnel Journal*, 410-411.

Chapman, P. & Huygens, I. (1988). An evaluation of three treatment programs for alcoholism: An experimental study with 6 and 18 month follow-ups. *British Journal of Addiction, 83*, 67-81.

Chein, I., Gerard, D., Lee, R., & Rosenfeld, E. (1964). *The road to H.* New York: Basic Books.

Collen, M. F. (1966). Periodic health examinations using an automated multitest laboratory. *Journal of the American Medical Association, 195.*

Collen, M. F. (1973). Introduction to health testing forum. *Preventive Medicine, 2.*

Collen, M. F., Feldman, R., Soghikian, K., & Garfield, S. R. (1973). The educational adjunct to multiphasic testing. *Preventive Medicine, 2.*

Collen, M. F. & Linden, C. (1955). Screening in a group practice prepaid medical care plan. *Journal of Chronic Disability, 2.*

Collen, M. F., Rubin, L., Neyman, J., Dantzig, G. B., Baer, R. M., & Siegelaub, A. B. (1964). Automated multiphasic screening and diagnosis. *American Journal of Public Health, 54*, 741.

Collen, M. F. & Soghikian, K. (1974). Health exhibits accentuate the positive. *Hospitals, 48.*

Coyne, J. C. & Liddle, H. A. (1992). The future of systems therapy: Shedding myths and facing opportunities. *Psychotherapy, 29*, 44-50.

Cummings, N. A. (1969, September 4). Exclusion therapy: An alternative to going after the drug cult adolescent. Paper presented at the meeting of the American Psychological Association, Washington, D.C.

Cummings, N. A. (1970, September 7). Exclusion therapy II. Paper presented at the meeting of the American Psychological Association, Miami.

Cummings, N. A. (1975a). The health model as entrée to the human services model in psychotherapy. *Clinical Psychologist, 29*(1), 19–21.

Cummings, N. A. (1975b). Survey of addictive characteristics of a random sampling of patients presenting themselves for psychotherapy. (In-house paper.) San Francisco: Kaiser Permanente.

Cummings, N. A. (1977). Prolonged (ideal) versus short-term (realistic) psychotherapy. *Professional Psychology, 8,* 491–501.

Cummings, N. A. (1979). Turning bread into stones: Our modern antimiracle. *American Psychologist, 34*(12), 1119–1129.

Cummings, N. A. (1983). *Biodyne training manual of brief, intermittent psychotherapy throughout the life cycle.* San Francisco: Biodyne Institute.

Cummings, N. A. (1984). The new mental health care delivery system and psychology's new role. Invited Awards Address to the American Psychological Association Annual Meeting, Los Angeles.

Cummings, N. A. (1985a). Assessing the computer's impact: Professional concerns. *Computers in Human Behavior, 1,* 293–300.

Cummings, N. A. (1985b). *Biodyne training manual* (2nd ed.). San Francisco: Foundation for Behavioral Health.

Cummings, N. A. (1985c). Testimony to U.S. Senate. *Congressional Record—Senate,* June 24, 1985, S 8656-S 8659.

Cummings, N. A. (1986). The dismantling of our health system: Strategies for the survival of psychological practice. *American Psychologist, 41,* 426–431.

Cummings, N. A. (1987). The future of psychotherapy: One psychologist's perspective. *American Journal of Psychotherapy, 61,* 349–360.

Cummings, N. A. (1988a). Brief, intermittent psychotherapy throughout the life cycle. *News from EFPPA* (European Federation of Professional Psychologists Association), *2*(3), 4–11.

Cummings, N. A. (1988b). Emergence of the mental health complex: Adaptive and maladaptive responses. *Psychology: Research and Practice, 19*(3), 308–315.

Cummings, N. A. (1990). Brief, intermittent psychotherapy throughout the life cycle. In J. K. Zeig & S. G. Gilligan (Eds.), *Brief therapy: Myths, methods, and metaphors* (pp. 169-184). New York: Brunner/Mazel.

Cummings, N. A. (1991a). Arguments for the financial efficacy of psychological services in health care settings. In J. J. Sweet, R. G. Rozensky, & S. M. Tovian (Eds.), *Handbook of clinical psychology in medical settings* (pp. 113-126). New York: Plenum.

Cummings, N. A. (1991b). Brief, intermittent therapy throughout the life cycle. In C. Austad & W. H. Berman (Eds.), *Psychotherapy in HMOs: The practice of mental health in managed care*. Washington, DC: American Psychological Association.

Cummings, N. A. (1991c). Brief, intermittent psychotherapy throughout the life cycle. In J. K. Zeig & S. G. Gilligan (Eds.), *Brief therapy: Myths, methods and metaphors*. New York: Brunner/Mazel.

Cummings, N. A. (1991d). Ten ways to spot mismanaged mental health care. *Psychotherapy in Private Practice, 9,* 31-33.

Cummings, N. A. (1992a). Brief intermittent therapy throughout the life cycle. In C. S. Austad & W. H. Berman (Eds.), *Psychotherapy in managed care* (pp. 232-244). Washington, DC: American Psychological Association.

Cummings, N. A. (1992b). Professional psychology's fifty year centennial. *American Psychologist, 47*(7), 845-846.

Cummings, N. A. (1992c). The future of psychotherapy: Society's charge to professional psychology. *Independent Practitioner, 21*(3), 126-130.

Cummings, N. A. (1993). Somatization: When physical symptoms have no medical cause. In D. Goleman & J. Gurin (Eds.), *Mind-body medicine* (pp. 221-232). Yonkers, NY: Consumer Reports.

Cummings, N. A. (1994). The successful application of medical offset in program planning and in clinical delivery. *Managed Care Quarterly, 2*(2), 1-6.

Cummings, N. A. (1995). Impact of managed care on employment and training: A primer for survival. *Professional Psychology: Research and Practice, 26* (1), 10-15.

Cummings, N. A. (1996a). Does managed mental health care offset costs related to medical treatment? In A. Lazarus (Ed.), *Controversies in managed mental health care* (pp. 213-227). Washington, DC: American Psychiatric Press.

Cummings, N. A. (1996b). The impact of managed care on employment and professional training: A primer for survival. In N. A. Cummings, M. S. Pallak, & J. L. Cummings (Eds.), *Surviving the demise of solo practice: Mental health practitioners prospering in the era of managed care* (pp. 11-26). Madison, CT: Psychosocial Press.

Cummings, N. A. (1996c). The new structure of health care and a role for psychology. In R. A. Resnick & R. H. Rozensky (Eds.), *Health psychology through the life span* (pp. 27-37). Washington, DC: American Psychological Association.

Cummings, N. A. (1996d). The resocialization of behavioral care practice. In N. A. Cummings, M. S. Pallak, & J. L. Cummings (Eds.), *Surviving the demise of solo practice: Mental health practitioners prospering in the era of managed care* (pp. 3-10). Madison, CT: Psychosocial Press.

Cummings, N. A. (1997). Approaches in prevention in the behavioral health of older adults. In P. Hartman-Stein (Ed.), *Innovative behavioral healthcare for older adults: A guide-book for changing times* (pp. 1-23). San Francisco: Jossey-Bass.

Cummings, N. A. & Bragman, J. I. (1988). Taking the "somaticizer" out of the medical system into a psychological system. In E. M. Steven & V. E. Steven (Eds.), *The psychotherapy patient* (pp. 109-112). Binghamton, NY: Syracuse University Press.

Cummings, N. A. & Dörken, H. (1986). Corporations, networks, and service plans: Economically sound models of practice. In H. Dörken & Associates (Eds.), *Professional psychology in transition* (pp. 165-174). San Francisco: Jossey-Bass.

Cummings, N. A., Dörken, H., Pallak, M. S., & Henke, C. J. (1991). The impact of psychological intervention on health care costs and utilization. The Hawaii Medicaid Project. *HCFA Contract Report no. 11-C-983344/9.*

Cummings, N. A., Dörken, H., Pallak, M. S., & Henke, C. J. (1993). The impact of psychological intervention on health care costs and utilization: The Hawaii Medicaid Project. In N. A. Cummings & M. S. Pallak (Eds.), *Medicaid, managed behavioral health and implications for public policy, Vol. 2: Healthcare and utilization cost series.* New York: Springer.

Cummings, N. A. & Duhl, L. J. (1987). The new delivery system. In L. J. Duhl & N. A. Cummings (Eds.), *The future of mental health services: Coping with crisis* (pp. 85-88). New York: Springer.

Cummings, N. A. & Fernandez, L. E. (1985, March). Exciting future possibilities for psychologists in the marketplace. *Independent Practitioner*, 38-42.

Cummings, N. A. & Follette, W. T. (1968). Psychiatric services and medical utilization in a prepaid health plan setting: Part II. *Medical Care, 6,* 31–41.

Cummings, N. A. & Follette, W. T. (1976). Brief psychotherapy and medical utilization: An eight-year follow-up. In H. Dörken & Associates (Eds.), *The professional psychologist today: New developments in law, health insurance, and health practice.* San Francisco: Jossey-Bass.

Cummings, N. A., Kahn, B. I., & Sparkman, B. (1962). *Psychotherapy and medical utilization: A pilot study.* Oakland, CA: Annual Reports of Kaiser Permanente Research Projects.

Cummings, N. A., Kahn, B. I., & Sparkman, B. (1964). Psychotherapy and medical utilization. As cited in M. Greenfield, *Providing for mental illness.* Berkeley, CA: Berkeley Institute of Governmental Studies, University of California, Berkeley.

Cummings, N. A., Pallak, M. S., Dörken, H., & Henke, C. J. (1991). *The impact of psychological services on medical utilization HCFA contract no. 11-C-98344 report.* Baltimore, MD: HCFA.

Cummings, N. & Sayama, M. (1995). *Focused psychotherapy: A casebook of brief intermittent psychotherapy throughout the life cycle.* New York: Brunner/Mazel.

Cummings, N. A., Siegelaub, A., Follette, W., & Collen, M. F. (1963). *An automated psychological screening test as part of an automated multiphasic screening.* Oakland, CA: Annual Reports of Kaiser Permanente Research Projects.

Cummings, N. A. & VandenBos G. R. (1978). The general practice of psychology. *Professional Psychology, 10,* 30–40.

Cummings, N. A. & VandenBos, G. R. (1981). The twenty years Kaiser Permanente experience with psychotherapy and medical utilization: Implications for national health policy and national health insurance. *Health Policy Quarterly, 1*(2), 159–175.

Cummings, N. A. & Wright, R. H. (1991, Spring). Managed mental health care: Two perspectives. *AAP Advance Plan, 1,* 14–16.

Cutler, J. L. (1973). Multiphasic checkup evaluation study. *Preventive Medicine, 2.*

Dales, L. G. (1973). Multiphasic checkup evaluation study: Outpatient clinic utilization. *Preventive Medicine, 2.*

Dales, L. G., Friedman, G. D., Ury, H. K., Grossman, S., & Williams, S. (1978). A case-control study of relationships of diet and other traits to colorectal cancer in American blacks. *American Journal of Epidemiology, 109.*

Davanloo, H. (1978). *Basic principles and techniques in short-term dynamic psychotherapy.* New York: Spectrum.

DeLafuente, D. (1993, June). California groups join for survival: Mullikin Healthcare Partners exemplify trend. *Modern Healthcare, 21,* 24–26.

DeLeon, P. H., VandenBos, G. R., & Cummings, N. A. (1983). Psychotherapy: Is it safe, effective, and appropriate? The beginning of an evolutionary dialogue. *American Psychologist, 38,* 907–911.

Ditman, K. S., Crawford, G. G., Forgy, E. W., Moskowitz, H., & MacAndrew, C. (1967). A controlled experiment on the use of court probation for drunk arrests. *American Journal of Psychiatry, 124,* 160.

Dörken, H. (1960). Minnesota's progressive community mental health services. *Mental Hygiene, 44,* 442–444.

Dörken, H. (1962a). Behind the scenes in community mental health. *American Journal of Psychiatry, 119,* 328–335.

Dörken, H. (1962b). Problems in administration and the establishment of community mental health services. *Mental Hygiene, 46,* 498–509.

Dörken, H. (1971). A dimensional strategy for community focused mental health services. In G. Rosenblum (Ed.), *Issues in community psychology and preventive mental health.* New York: Behavioral Publications.

Dörken, H. (1977). CHAMPUS ten-state claim experience for mental disorder: Fiscal year 1975. *American Psychologist, 32,* 697–710.

Dörken, H. (1983). Advocacy and the legislative process: Representation in a changing world. *American Psychologist, 38,* 1210–1215.

Dörken, H. & Cummings, N. A. (1986). The impact of medical referral on outpatient psychological services. *Professional Psychology: Research and Practice, 17*(5), 431–436,

Dörken, H. & Cummings, N. A. (1991). The potential effect on private practice training in targeted focused mental health treatment for a specific population: A brief report. *Psychotherapy in Private Practice, 9,* 45–51.

Dörken, H., VandenBos, G. R., Henke, C., Cummings, N. A., & Pallak, M. S. (1993). Impact of law and regulation on professional practice. *Professional Psychology: Research and Practice, 24*(3), 256–265.

Duhl, L. & Cummings, N. A. (1985, Fall). Mental health: A whole new ballgame. *Annals of Psychiatry,* Special Issues I & II.

Duhl, L. J. & Cummings, N. A. (1987a). The emergence of the mental health complex. In L. J. Duhl & N. A. Cummings (Eds.), *The future of mental health services: Coping with crisis.* New York: Springer.

Duhl, L. J. & Cummings, N. A. (Eds.). (1987b). *The future of mental health services: Coping with crisis.* New York: Springer.

Edley, R. S. (1996). The practitioner as owner. In N. A. Cummings, M. S. Pallak, & J. L. Cummings (Eds.), *Surviving the demise of solo practice: Mental health practitioners prospering in the era of managed care.* Madison, CT: Psychosocial Press.

Edwards, G., Orford, J., Egert, S., Guthrie, S., Hawker, A., Hensman, C., Mitcheson, M., Oppenheimer, E., & Taylor, C. (1977). Alcoholism: A controlled trial of "treatment" and "advice." *Journal of Studies on Alcohol, 38,* 1004–1031.

Ellwood, P. M. (1988). Outcomes management: A technology of patient experience. *New England Journal of Medicine, 318,* 1549.

Elpers, J. R. (1977). Unpublished report of the Program Chief, Orange County Department of Mental Health, Santa Ana, Calif.

Erickson, M. H. (1980). In E. Rossi (Ed.), *Collected papers (Vols. 1–4).* New York: Irvington.

Eysenck, H. J. (1966). *The effects of psychotherapy.* New York: International Universities Press.

Fahrion, S. (1990). Cost effectiveness in biobehavioral treatment of hypertension. *Biofeedback and Self-Regulation, 14,* 131–152.

Fahrion, S., Norris, P., Green, E., & Schnar, R. (1987). Behavioral treatment of hypertension: A group outcome study. *Biofeedback and Self-Regulation, 11,* 257–278.

Feldman, D. J., Pattison, E. M., Sobell, L. C., Graham, T., & Sobell, M. B. (1975). Outpatient alcohol detoxification: Initial findings on 564 patients. *American Journal of Psychiatry, 132,* 407–412.

Feldman, R., Taller, S. L., Garfield, S. R., Collen, M. F., Richart, R. H., Cella, R., & Sender, A. J. (1977). Nurse practitioner multiphasic health checkups. *Preventive Medicine, 6.*

Feldman, S. (1992). Managed mental health services: Ideas and issues. In S. Feldman (Ed.), *Managed mental health services.* Springfield, IL: Charles C Thomas.

Fiedler, J. L. & Wright, R. B. (1989). *The medical offset effect and public health policy.* New York: Praeger.

Flor, H., Haag, G., Turk, D., & Koehler, H. (1983). Efficacy of biofeedback, pseudotherapy, and conventional medical treatment for chronic rheumatic back pain. *Pain, 17,* 21–31.

Follette, W. T. & Cummings, N. A. (1962). Psychiatry and medical utilization. An unpublished pilot project.

Follette, W. T. & Cummings, N. A. (1967). Psychiatric services and medical utilization in a prepaid health plan setting. *Medical Care, 5,* 25-35.

Forrester, D. (1994, March). The "physician equity model." *Integrated Healthcare Report,* 1-4.

Forsham, P. H. (1959). Lecture before the Permanente Medical Group, San Francisco.

Fox, R. E. (1992, Spring). Health care planning poses major threats to mental health and psychology: A call to battle. *AAP Advance Plan, 1,* 15.

Frank, R. G., Goldman, H. H., & McGuire, T. G. (1992, Fall). A model mental health benefit in private health insurance. *Health Affairs,* 98-117.

Freud, S. (1904/1950). On psychotherapy. Reprinted in E. Jones (Ed.), *Collected papers of Sigmund Freud, Vol. I* (pp. 249-263). London: Hogarth Press.

Freud S. (1921/1955). Group psychology and the analysis of the ego. Reprinted in J. Strachey (Ed.), *The standard edition of the complete psychological works of Sigmund Freud, Vol. 18* (pp. 63-143). London: Hogarth Press.

Freund, D. A. & Neuschler, E. (1986). Overview of Medicaid capitation and case-management initiatives. *Health Care Financing Review Annual Supplement,* 21-30.

Friedman, G. D., Dales, L. G., & Ury, H. K. (1979). Mortality in middle-aged smokers and nonsmokers. *New England Journal of Medicine, 300.*

Friedman, G. D., Ury, H. K., Klatsky, A. L., & Siegelaub, A. B. (1974). A psychological questionnaire predictive of myocardial infarction: Results from the Kaiser Permanente epidemiologic study of myocardial infarction. *Psychosomatic Medicine, 36.*

Friedman, S. & Fanger, M. T. (1991). *Expanding therapeutic possibilities: Getting results in brief psychotherapy.* Lexington, MA: Lexington Books.

Gallant, D. M., Bishop, M. P., Mouledoux, A., Faulkner, M. A., Brisolara, A., & Swanson, W. A. (1973). The revolving-door alcoholic: An impasse in the treatment of the chronic alcoholic. *Archives of General Psychiatry, 28,* 633-635.

Gamblin, J. (1975). Claims are up, but payments are down for insurer's health maintenance plans. *Business Insurance*, 55-56.

Garfield, S. R. (1976). Evolving new model for health-care delivery. *Orthopaedic Review, 5*, 21-24.

Garfield, S. R., Collen, M. F., Feldman, R., Soghikian, K., Richardt, R. H., & Duncan, J. H. (1976). Evaluation of an ambulatory medical-care delivery system. *New England Journal of Medicine*, 294-302.

Goldberg, I. D., Krantz, G., & Locke, B. Z. (1970). Effect of a short-term outpatient psychiatric therapy benefit on the utilization of medical services in a prepaid group practice medical program. *Medical Care, 8*, 419-428.

Goldfried, M. R. & Gastonquay, L. G. (1992). The future of psychotherapy integration. *Psychotherapy, 29*, 4-10.

Goldman, W. & Feldman, S. (Eds.). (1993). Managed mental health care. *New Directions for Mental Health Services, 59*, 1-112.

Gonick, U., Farrow, I., Meier, M., Ostmand, G., & Frolick, L. (1981). Cost effectiveness of behavioral medicine procedures in the treatment of stress-related disorders. *American Journal of Clinical Biofeedback, 4*, 16-24.

Griffith, W. K. & Madero, B. (1973). Primary hypertension patients' learning needs. *Journal of Nursing, 73*.

Grover, P. L. (1991). Is appropriate hospital care an inevitable component of the health care system? *Medical Care, 29* (Aug. suppl.), AS1-AS4.

Haley, J. (1976). *Problem solving therapy*. San Francisco: Jossey-Bass.

Hall, C. T. (1995, October 25). Customers rate health plans. *San Francisco Chronicle*, B1, B8.

Hardy, A. (1970). *The Terrap manual for the treatment of agoraphobia*. Menlo Park, CA: Terrap.

Harrington, R. (1977). Unpublished report to the Executive Committee of the Permanente Medical Group. San Jose, CA: Kaiser Permanente Medical Center.

Hayashida, M., Alterman, A. I., McClellan, A. T., O'Brien, C. P., Purtill, J. J., Volpicelli, J. R., Raphaelson, A. H., & Hall, C. P. (1989, February 9). Comparative effectiveness and costs of inpatient detoxification of patients with mild-to-moderate alcohol withdrawal syndrome. *New England Journal of Medicine*, 358-365.

Hodges, A. & Dörken, H. (1961). Location and out-patient psychiatric care. *Public Health Reports, 76*, 239-241.

Holder, H. D. & Blose, J. O. (1985). Mental health treatment and the reduction of healthcare costs: A four-year study of U.S. federal employees enrollment with the Aetna Life Insurance Company. In S. Sharfstein & A. Beigel (Eds.), *The new economics and psychiatric care* (pp. 102–116). Washington, DC: American Psychiatric Press.

Holder, H. D. & Blose, J. O. (1987). Medical health treatment and the reduction of healthcare costs: A four-year study of U.S. federal employees enrollment with the Aetna Life Insurance Company. In R. M. Schleffler & L. F. Rossiter (Eds.), *Advances in health economics and health services research, Vol. 8.* Greenwich, CT: JAI Press.

Hollingshead, A. B. & Redlich, F. C. (1958). *Social class and mental illness.* New York: Wiley.

Holser, M. A. (1979). A socialization program for chronic alcoholics. *International Journal of the Addictions, 14,* 657–674.

Howard, K., Kopta, S., Krause, M., & Orlinsky, D. (1986). The dose-effect relationship in psychotherapy. *American Psychologist, 41,* 159–164.

Hoyt, M. F. (1995). *Brief psychotherapy and managed care.* San Francisco: Jossey-Bass.

Humphreys, L. (1973, September/October). Should psychotherapy be included in National Health Insurance? No! *APA Monitor,* 8.

Hurley, R. E. & Freund, D. A. (1988). A typology of Medicaid managed care. *Medical Care, 26,* 764–774.

Jacobs, D. (1988). Cost-effectiveness of specialized psychological programs for reducing hospital stays and outpatient visits. *Journal of Clinical Psychology, 21,* 23–49.

Jameson, J., Shuman, L., & Young, L. (1976, December). The effects of outpatient psychiatric utilization on the costs of providing third-party coverage. (Research Service Report 118.) Blue Cross of Western Pennsylvania.

Jones, K. & Vischi, T. (1978). Impact of alcohol, drug, and mental health treatment on medical care expenditures. ADAMHA/NIMH.

Jones, K. R. & Vischi, T. R. (1979). The impact of alcohol, drug abuse, and mental health treatment on medical care utilization: A review of the research literature. *Medical Care, 17*(12, suppl.), 43–131.

Jones, K. R. & Vischi, T. R. (1980). The Bethesda Consensus Conference on Medical Offset. Alcohol, drug abuse, and mental health administration report. Rockville, MD.: Alcohol, Drug Abuse, and Mental Health Administration.

Julien, R. M. (1978). *A primer of drug action* (2nd ed.). San Francisco: Freeman.

Kandel, E. R. (1976). *Cellular basis of behavior*. San Francisco: Freeman.

Karon, B. P. & VandenBos, G. R. (1972). The consequences of psychotherapy for schizophrenic patients. *Psychotherapy: Theory, Research and Practice, 9,* 111–119.

Karon, B. P. & VandenBos, G. R. (1975). Treatment costs of psychotherapy as compared to medication for schizophrenia. *Professional Psychology, 6,* 293–298.

Karon, B. P. & VandenBos, G. R. (1976). Cost/benefit analysis: Psychologist versus psychiatrist for schizophrenics. *Professional Psychology, 7,* 107–111.

Karon, B. P. & VandenBos, G. R. (1977). Psychotherapeutic technique and the economically poor patient. *Psychotherapy: Theory, Research and Practice, 14,* 169–180.

Kasschau, R. A., Rehm, L. P., & Ullman, L. P. (1985). *Psychology research, public policy and practice*. New York: Praeger.

Kaufman, M. (1989, April 24). Cancer: Facts vs feelings. *Newsweek,* 10.

Kerns, L. L. & Bradley, W. J. (1990, September/October). Factors influencing psychiatric hospitalization. *EAP Digest,* 28–65.

Kiesler, C. A. (1982a). Mental hospitals and alternative care: Noninstitutionalization as potential public policy for mental patients. *American Psychologist, 37,* 349–360.

Kiesler, C. A. (1982b). Public and professional myths about mental hospitalization: An empirical reassessment of policy related beliefs. *American Psychologist, 37,* 1323–1339.

Kiesler, C. A., Cummings, N. A., & VandenBos, G. R. (Eds.). (1979). *Psychology and National Health Insurance*. Washington, DC: American Psychological Association.

Kiesler, C. A. & Morton, T. L. (1988). Psychology and public policy in the "health care revolution." *American Psychology, 43*(12), 993–1003.

Kiesler, C. A. & Sibulkin, A. (1987). *Mental hospitalization: Myths and facts about a national crisis*. Newbury Park, CA: Sage.

Kissin, B., Platz, A., & Su, W. H. (1970). Social and psychological factors in the treatment of chronic alcoholism. *Journal of Psychiatric Research, 8,* 13–27.

Klatsky, A. L., Friedman, G. D., & Siegelaub, A. B. (1981). Alcohol and mortality: A ten-year Kaiser Permanente experience. *Annals of Internal Medicine, 95.*

Klein, R. H. & Carroll, R. (1986). Patient characteristics and attendance patterns in outpatient group psychotherapy. *International Journal of Group Psychotherapy, 36,* 115–132.

Klerman, G. L. (1985). The role of the federal government in mental health services. In R. A. Kasschau, L. P. Rehm, & L. P. Ullman (Eds.), *Psychology research, public policy and practice.* New York: Praeger.

Kovacs, A. L. (1991). Escaping managed care—the use of brief therapeutic strategies to build fee-for-service practices. Presented at the meeting of the American Psychological Association Continuing Education Workshop no. 108, San Francisco.

Kramon, G. (1989, January 8,). Taking a scalpel to health costs. *New York Times,* 1, 9–10.

Kulka, R. A., Veroff, J., & Douvan, E. (1957/1979). Social class and the use of professional help for personal problems (Reprint). *Journal of Health and Social Behavior, 20,* 2–17.

Lazarus, A. A., Beutler, L. E., & Norcross, J. C. (1992). The future of technical eclecticism. *Psychotherapy, 29,* 11–20.

Lech, S. V., Friedman, G. D., & Ury, H. K. (1975). Characteristics of heavy users of outpatient prescription drugs. *Clinical Toxicology, 8.*

Levenson, A. (1983). Issues surrounding the ownership of private psychiatric hospitals by investor-owned hospital chains. *Hospital and Community Psychiatry, 34,* 1127–1131.

Lichtenstein, H. (1961). Identity and sexuality. *Journal of the American Psychological Association, 9,* 1979.

Lorig, K. & Fries, J. (1990). *Arthritis helpbook* (3rd ed.). Reading, MA: Addison-Wesley.

Luborsky, L., Crits-Christoph, P., Mintz, J., & Auerbach, A. (1988). *Who will benefit from psychotherapy? Predicting therapeutic outcomes.* New York: Basic Books.

Magaro, P. (1985). Fourth revolution in the treatment of mental disorders: Rehabilitative entrepreneurship. *Professional Psychology, 16,* 540–552.

Mahrer, A. R. (1992). Shaping the future of psychotherapy by making changes in the present. *Psychotherapy, 29,* 104–108.

Managed Core Alert (1993).

Malan, D. H. (1963). *A study of brief psychotherapy.* New York: Plenum.

Malan, D. H. (1976). *The frontier of brief psychotherapy.* New York: Plenum.

Mann, J. (1973). *Time-limited psychotherapy*. Cambridge, MA: Harvard University Press.

Matarazzo, J. D., et al. (Eds.). (1984). *Behavioral health: A handbook of health enhancement and disease prevention*. New York: Wiley.

McClellan, A. T., Luborsky, L., Woody, G. E., O'Brien, C. P., & Druley, K. A. (1983). Predicting response to alcohol and drug abuse treatments: Role of psychiatric severity. *Archives of General Psychiatry, 40,* 620-625.

McCrady, B., Longabaugh, R., Fink, E., Stout, R., Beattie, M., & Ruggieri-Authelet, A. (1986). Cost effectiveness of alcoholism treatment in partial hospital versus inpatient settings after brief inpatient treatment: 12 month outcomes. *Journal of Counseling and Clinical Psychology, 54,* 708-713.

McCrady, B., Noel, N., Abrams, D., Stout, R., Nelson, H., & Hay, W. (1986). Comparative effectiveness of three types of spouse involvement in outpatient behavioral alcoholism treatment. *Journal of Studies on Alcohol, 47,* 459-467.

McLachlan, J. F. C. & Stein, R. L. (1982). Evaluation of a day clinic for alcoholics. *Journal of Studies on Alcohol, 43,* 261-272.

Mechanic, D. (1966). Response factors in illness: The study of illness behavior. *Social Psychiatry, 1,* 52-73.

Mercer, W. (1980). Mental health and medical cost containment. *Mercer Bulletin, 6*(5), unnumbered pages.

Miller, W. R. (1985). Motivation for treatment: A review with special emphasis on alcoholism. *Psychological Bulletin, 98,* 84-107.

Miller, W. R. & Baca, L. M. (1983). Two-year follow-up of bibliotherapy and therapist-directed controlled drinking training for problem drinkers. *Behavior Therapy, 14,* 441-448.

Miller, W. R., Gribskov, C. J., & Mortell, R. L. (1981). Effectiveness of a self-control manual for problem drinkers with and without therapist contact. *International Journal of the Addictions, 16,* 827-837.

Miller, W. R. & Hester, R. K. (1986). Inpatient alcoholism treatment. *American Psychologist, 41,* 794-805.

Miller, W. R. & Hester, R. K. (1987a). Matching problem drinkers with optimal treatments. In W. R. Miller & N. Heather (Eds.), *Treating addictive behaviors: Processes of change*. New York: Plenum Press.

Miller, W. R. & Hester, R. K. (1987b). The effectiveness of alcoholism treatment methods: What research reveals. In W. R. Miller & N.

Heather (Eds.), *Treating addictive behaviors: Processes of change*. New York: Plenum Press.

Morrison, D. P. (1906). The practitioner as informatics expert. In N. A. Cummings, M. S. Pallak, & J. L. Cummings (Eds.), *Surviving the demise of solo practice: Mental health practitioners prospering in the era of managed care*. Madison, CT: Psychosocial Press.

Mosher, V., Davis, J., Mulligan, D., & Iber, F. L. (1975). Comparison of outcome in a 9-day and 30-day alcoholism treatment program. *Journal of Studies on Alcohol, 36*, 1277–1281.

Mullen, P. (1988, December 27). Big increases in health premiums. *Healthweek, 2*(25), 1, 26.

Mullen, P. (1989, November). Increases in health premiums continue. *Healthweek, 3* (22).

Mumford, E., Schlesinger, H. J., & Glass, G. V. (1978). A critical review and indexed bibliography of the literature up to 1978 on the effects of psychotherapy on medical utilization. Report to NIMH under Contract no. 278-77-0049-M.H.

Mumford, E., Schlesinger, H. J., & Glass, G. V. (1982). The effects of psychological intervention on recovery from surgery and heart attacks: An analysis of the literature. *American Journal of Public Health, 72*, 141–151.

Mumford, E., Schlesinger, H. J., Glass, G. V., Patrick, C., & Cuerdon, T. (1984). A new look at evidence about reduced cost of medical utilization following mental health treatment. *American Journal of Psychiatry, 141*, 1145–1158.

Naditch, M. P. (1989, September). Measuring up: The dawning era of outcome management. *American Journal of Preventive Psychiatry and Neurology, 2*(1), 154–162.

National Institute of Alcoholism and Alcohol Abuse. (1978). *1975 statistical report*. Washington, DC: Alcohol, Drug Abuse, and Mental Health Administration Clearinghouse.

National Institute of Drug Abuse. (1978). *1975 statistical report*. Washington, DC: Alcohol, Drug Abuse, and Mental Health Administration Clearinghouse.

National Institute of Mental Health. (1976). Federal employees health benefits (FEHB). In draft report: The financing, utilization, and quality of mental health care in the United States. Rockville, MD: NIMH.

Neer, H. M. (1994, July). The future of occupational medicine. Address to the National Workers' Compensation and Occupational Medicine Seminar, Hyannis, Mass.

Nguyen, T. D., Attkinsson, C. C., & Stegner, B. L. (1983). Assessment of patient satisfaction: Development and refinement of a service evaluation questionnaire. *Evaluation and Program Planning, 6,* 299-314.

O'Briant, R., Petersen, N. W., & Heacock, D. (1977). How safe is social setting detoxification? *Alcohol Health and Research World, 1*(2), 22-27.

O'Donohue, W. & Krasner, L. (1995). *Handbook of psychological skills training.* Needham Heights, MA: Allyn & Bacon.

Olbrisch, M. (1981). Evaluation of a stress management program. *Medical Care, 19,* 153-159.

Olbrisch, M. E. (1977). Psychotherapeutic interventions in physical health: Effectiveness and economic efficiency. *American Psychologist, 32,* 761-777.

Oliver, S. (1996, January 22). Doctor downsizing. *Forbes,* 104-106.

Orford, J., Oppenheimer, E., & Edwards, G. (1976). Abstinence or control: The outcome for excessive drinkers two years after consultation. *Behavior Research and Therapy, 14,* 409-418.

Oss, M. (1993, June). Pro and con: A look at Harvard's new mental health and chemical dependency benefit plan. *Open Minds, 7,* 3-4.

Page, R. D. & Schaub, L. H. (1979). Efficacy of three- versus five-week alcohol treatment program. *International Journal of the Addictions, 14,* 697-714.

Pallak, M. S. (1989). Defining and delivering effective and cost-effective mental health services. Invited address, Behavioral Healthcare Tomorrow Conference, Washington, D.C.

Pallak, M. S. & Cummings, N. A. (1992). Inpatient and outpatient psychiatric treatment: The effect of matching patients to appropriate level of treatment on psychiatric and medical-surgical hospital days. *Applied and Preventive Psychology: Current Scientific Perspectives, 1,* 83-87.

Pallak, M. S. & Cummings, N. A. (1994). Outcomes research in managed mental health care: Issues, strategies and trends. In S. A. Shueman, S. L. Mayhugh, & B. S. Gould (Eds.), *Managed behavioral health care: A search for precision* (pp. 205-221). Springfield, IL: Charles C Thomas.

Pallak, M. S., & N. A., Dörken, H. D., & Henke, C. J. (1991). The impact of psychological intervention on health care costs and utilization: The Hawaii Medicaid Project. Contract Report no. 11-C-98344/9, HCFA.

Pallak, M. S., Cummings, N. A., Dörken, H., & Henke, C. J. (1993, Fall).

Managed mental health, Medicaid, and medical cost offset. *New Directions for Mental Health Services, 59,* 27–40.

Pallak, M. S., Cummings, N. A., Dörken, H., & Henke, C. J. (1994). Medical costs, Medicaid, and managed mental health treatment: The Hawaii study. *Managed Care Quarterly, 2,* 64–70.

Pallak, M. S., & Kilburg, R. K. (1986). Psychology, public affairs and public policy: A strategy and review. *American Psychologist, 41,* 933–940.

Pallak, M. S., Sibulkin, A. E., & Kiesler, C. A. (1987). Hospitalization for mental disorder in general hospitals. *American Behavioral Scientist, 30,* 231–245.

Peele, S. (1978, September). Addiction: The analgesic experience. *Human Nature,* 61–83.

Peele, S. & Brodsky, A. (1973). *Love and addiction.* New York: Taplinger.

Perloff, E. (1991). *Health and psychosocial instruments (HAPI).* Pittsburgh: Behavioral Measurement Database Services.

Petitti, D. B., Klein, R., Kipp, H., Kahn, W., Siegelaub, A. B., & Friedman, G. D. (1982). A survey of personal habits, symptoms of illness, and histories of disease in men with and without vasectomies. *American Journal of Public Health, 72.*

Petitti, D. B., Wingerd, J., Pellegrin, F., & Ramcharan, S. (1979). Risk of vascular disease in women: Smoking, oral contraceptives, noncontraceptive estrogens, and other factors. *Journal of the American Medical Association, 242.*

Petrie, L. M., Bowdoin, C. D., & McLaughlin, C. V. (1952). Voluntary multiple health costs. *Journal of the American Medical Association, 48.*

Pigott, H. E. (1996, January/February). Market shifts and emerging information technologies: Changing the equation for healthcare entrepreneurial innovations and opportunities. *Behavioral Health Management,* 32–38.

Pittman, D. J. & Tate, R. L. (1972). A comparison of two treatment programs for alcoholics. *International Journal of the Addictions, 18,* 183–193.

Powell, B. J., Penick, E. C., Read, M. R., & Ludwig, A. M. (1985). Comparison of three outpatient treatment interventions: A twelve-month follow-up of men alcoholics. *Journal of Studies on Alcohol, 46,* 309–312.

Practice Directorate. (1992, March). Office helps members on managed care. *APA Monitor, 23*(3), 16–17.

Pro and con: A look at Harvard's new mental health and chemical dependency benefit plan. (1993, June). *Open Minds, 7,* 3.

'Psychological health plan nips insurance premium increases.' (1981). *Employee Health and Fitness, 3*(1), 1-2.

Quill, T. E. (1985). Somatization disorder: One of medicine's blind spots. *Journal of the American Medical Association, 254,* 3075-3079.

Ramcharan, S. (1973). Multiphasic checkup evaluation study: Disability and chronic disease after 7 years of multiphasic checkups. *Preventive Medicine, 2.*

RAND Corporation. (1987, July). A report on the changing practice patterns of primary care physicians in geographical areas with too many physicians. Santa Monica, CA: Author.

Reinhardt, U. E. (1987). Resource allocation in health care: The allocation of lifestyles to providers. *Milbank Quarterly, 65,* 153-176.

Robson, R. A. H., Paulus, I., & Clarke, G. G. (1965). An evaluation of the effect of a clinic treatment program on the rehabilitation of alcoholic patients. *Quarterly Journal of Studies on Alcohol, 26,* 264-278.

Rogers, A. H., Robinson, R. M., & Rossiter, L. F. (Eds.). (1987). *Advances in health services research, Vol. 8.* Greenwich, CT: JAI Press.

Rosen, J. C. & Wiens, A. N. (1979). Changes in medical problems and use of medical services following psychological intervention. *American Psychologist, 34,* 420-431.

Rosofsky, I. (1993). Psychologists should opt out of health care, says Kovacs. *Practice Management Monthly, 1,* 4-6.

Rutan, J. S. & Stone, W. N. (1984). *Psychodynamic group psychotherapy.* Lexington, MA: Callamore Press.

Ryder, C. F. & Getting, V. A. (1950). Preliminary report on the health protection clinic. *New England Journal of Medicine, 243.*

Saeman, H. (1996, January/February). Psychologists frustrated with managed care, economic issues, but plan to "hang tough," survey reveals. *National Psychologist, 5*(1), 1-2.

Saunders, R. & Ludwigsen, K. R. (1992). Mental health in New Jack City. *Independent Practitioner, 12*(3), 97-99.

Saxe, L., Dougherty, D., Esty, K., & Fine, M. (1983). *The effectiveness and costs of alcoholism treatment.* (Health Technology Case Study 22.) Washington, DC: Office of Technology Assessment.

Saxe, L. & Goodman, L. (1988). *The effectiveness of outpatient vs. inpatient treatment: Updating the OTA Report.* (Health Technology

Case Study 22 Update.) Washington, DC: Office of Technology Assessment.

Schlesinger, H. J., Mumford, E., & Glass, G. V. (1980). Mental health services and medical utilization. In G. R VandenBos (Ed.), *Psychotherapy: Practice, research, policy*. Beverly Hills, CA: Sage.

Schlesinger, H. J., Mumford, E., Glass, G., Patrick, C., & Sharfstein, S. (1983). Mental health treatment and medical care utilization in a fee-for-service system: Outpatient mental health treatment following the onset of a chronic disease. *American Journal of Public Health*, 73, 422–429.

Schwartz, W. B. (1987, January 9). Medical cost trend after 1990 disputed. *Wall Street Journal*, B1, B8.

Seligman, M. E. P. (1975). *Helplessness: On depression, development, and death*. San Francisco: Freeman.

Seligman, M. E. P. (1994). *What you can change and what you can't change*. New York: Knopf.

Shapiro, A. K. (1971). Placebo effects in medicine, psychotherapy and psycho-analysis. In S. L. Garfield & A. E. Bergin (Eds.), *Handbook of psychotherapy and behavior change: An empirical analysis*. New York: Wiley.

Shapiro, A. K. & Morris, L. A. (1978). The placebo effect in medical and psychological therapies. In S. L. Garfield & A. E. Bergin (Eds.), *Handbook of psychotherapy and behavior change* (2nd ed.). New York: Wiley.

Sheehan, J. J., Wieman, R. J., & Bechtel, J. E. (1981). Follow-up of twelve-month treatment program for chronic alcoholics. *International Journal of the Addictions, 16,* 233–241.

Shellenberger, R., Turner, J., Green, J., & Cooney, J. (1986). Health changes in a biofeedback and stress management program. *Clinical Biofeedback and Health, 9,* 23–24.

Shueman, S. A., Troy, W. G., & Mayhugh, S. L. (1994). Managed behavioral healthcare. *Register Report, 20*(1), 5–9.

Sifneos, P. E. (1987). *Short-term dynamic psychotherapy: Evaluation and technique* (2nd ed.). New York: Plenum.

Smart, R. G. (1978). Do some alcoholics do better in some types of treatment than others? *Drug and Alcohol Abuse, 3,* 65–76.

Smart, R. G. & Gray, G. (1978). Minimal, moderate and long-term treatment for alcoholism. *British Journal of Addiction, 73,* 35–38.

Smith, M., Glass, G. V., & Miller, T. (1980). *The benefits of psychotherapy*. Baltimore: The Johns Hopkins University Press.

Smith, R. G. (1991). *Somaticization disorder in the medical setting*. Washington, DC: American Psychiatric Press.

Soghikian, K. (1978). The role of nurse practitioners in hypertension care. *Clinical Science and Molecular Medicine, 55*.

Steig, R. & Williams, P. (1983). Cost effectiveness study of multidisciplinary pain treatment of industrial-injured workers. *Seminars in Neurology, 3*, 375.

Stevens, R. (1989). *In sickness and in wealth: American hospitals in the twentieth century*. New York: Basic Books.

Stinson, D. J., Smith, W. G., Amidjaya, I., & Kaplan, J. M. (1979). Systems of care and treatment outcomes for alcoholic patients. *Archives of General Psychiatry, 36*, 535–539.

Stone, W. N. & Rutan, J. S. (1984). Duration of group psychotherapy. *International Journal of Group Psychotherapy, 32*, 29–47.

Strumwasser, I., Paranjpe, N. V., Udow, M., Share, D., Wisgerhof, M., Ronis, D. L., Bartzack, C., & Saad, A. N. (1991). Appropriateness of psychiatric and substance abuse hospitalization: Implications for payment and utilization management. *Medical Care, 29* (August suppl.), AS77–AS90.

Strupp, H. H. (1992). The future of psychodynamic psychotherapy. *Psychotherapy, 29*, 21–27.

Supreme Court to review psychology's arguments in *CAPP v. Rank* case. (1988, December 1). *California Psychologist,* Special Edition: *CAPP v. Rank.*

Tomsho, R. (1995, December 29). At medical malls, shoppers are patients. *Wall Street Journal,* B1, B11.

Trotter, S. (1976, November). Insuring psychotherapy: A subsidy to the rich? *APA Monitor,* 1, 16.

U.S. Civil Service Commission. (1976). Unpublished statistics on the Federal Employees Health Benefits Program, Aetna and Blue Cross-Blue Shield. Washington, DC: U.S. Civil Service Commission, Office of the Actuary.

VandenBos, G. R., Cummings, N. A., & DeLeon, P. H. (1992). Economic and environmental influences in the history of psychotherapy. In D. K. Freedheim (Ed.), *The history of psychotherapy* (pp. 11–31). Washington, DC: American Psychological Association.

VandenBos, G. R. & DeLeon, P. H. (1988). The use of psychotherapy to improve physical health. *Psychotherapy, 25*(3), 335–342.

Walker, R. D., Donovan, D. M., Kivlahan, D. R., & O'Leary, M. R. (1983). Length of stay, neuropsychological performance, and aftercare influences on alcohol treatment outcome. *Journal of Consulting and Clinical Psychology, 51,* 900–911.

Ware, J. D. (1991). Measuring patient function and well-being: Some lessons from the medical outcomes study. In K. Heithoff & K. Lohr (Eds.), *Effectiveness and outcomes in health care.* Washington, DC: National Academy Press.

Ware, J. E. & Sherbourne, C. D. (1991). *The SF-36 Short Form Health Status Survey: I. Conceptual framework and item selection.* Boston: New England Medical Centers Hospital, International Resource Center for Health Care Assessment.

Weiss, J. R. & English, O. S. (1948). *Psychosomatic medicine.* New York: Plenum Press.

Welch, B. L. (1992, Spring). Managed care offset is marketing plan aid. *APA Advance Plan,* 1, 14–16.

Whitaker, C. (1979, August 3–4). The present imperfect. Paper presented at the Fourth Don D. Jackson Memorial Workshop, San Francisco (sponsored by the Mental Research Institute, Palo, Alto, Calif.).

Wilensky, G. R. & Rossiter, L. F. (1991). Coordinated care and public programs. *Health Affairs, 10*(45), 62–67.

Willems, P. J. A., Letemendia, F. J. J., & Arroyave, F. (1973). A two-year follow-up study comparing short with long stay in-patient treatment of alcoholics. *British Journal of Psychiatry, 122,* 637–648.

Wolpe, J. & Lazarus A. A. (1966). *Behavior therapy techniques.* London: Pergamon.

Wright, R. H. (1991, Spring). Toward a national health plan. *Advance Plan,* 1, 14–16.

Wright, R. H. (1992). Toward a political solution to psychology's dilemmas: Managing managed care. *Independent Practitioner, 12*(3), 111–113.

Yates, B. T. (1984). How psychology can improve effectiveness and reduce costs of health services. *Psychotherapy, 21*(3), 439–451.

Youngstrom, N. (1992, March). Model law's intent is protecting public and practitioners. *APA Monitor, 23*(3), 18–19.

Zimet, C. N. (1994). Psychology's role in a national health program. *Journal of Clinical Psychology, 50,* 122–124.